Statistics for Biology and Health

Series Editors
K. Dietz, M. Gail, K. Krickeberg, J. Samet, A. Tsiatis

Springer
New York
Berlin
Heidelberg
Hong Kong
London
Milan
Paris
Tokyo

Statistics for Biology and Health

Lemuel A. Moyé

Multiple Analyses in Clinical Trials
Fundamentals for Investigators

With 33 Illustrations

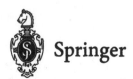
Springer

Lemuel A. Moyé
Department of Biostatistics
University of Texas School of Public Health
Houston, TX 77030
USA
moyelaptop@msn.com

Series Editors
K. Dietz
Institut für Medizinische Biometrie
Universität Tübingen
Westbahnhofstrasse 55
D-72070 Tübingen
Germany

M. Gail
National Cancer Institute
Rockville, MD 20892
USA

K. Krickeberg
Le Chatelet
F-63270 Manglieu
France

J. Samet
Department of Epidemiology
School of Public Health
Johns Hopkins University
615 Wolfe Street
Baltimore, MD 21205-2103
USA

A. Tsiatis
Department of Statistics
North Carolina State University
Raleigh, NC 27695
USA

Library of Congress Cataloging-in-Publication Data
Moyé, Lemuel A.
     Multiple analyses in clinical trials: fundamentals for investigators/Lemuel A. Moyé.
          p. cm. — (Statistics for biology and health)
     Includes bibliographical references and index.

          1. Clinical trials.   2. Multivariate analysis.   3. Clinical trials—Statistical methods.   I. Title.
     II. Series.
     R853.C55M69 2003
     610′.7′27—dc21   2003044598

ISBN 978-1-4419-1836-9   e-ISBN 978-0-387-21813-7

Printed in the United States of America.

9 8 7 6 5 4 3 2 1

www.springer-ny.com

Springer-Verlag   New York Berlin Heidelberg
A member of BertelsmannSpringer Science+Business Media GmbH

To Dixie and the DELTs

Preface

Prefaces are not for those who are in a rush. If you can find a moment for a casual conversation, then I will share with you my reasons for writing this book.

The multiple analysis (or multiple hypothesis testing, or simultaneous testing) issue is the problem of interpreting several (and, often times, many) statistical tests within a single research effort. Many of you who are interested in clinical trials do not know why the concept of multiple analyses is an issue. Alternatively, you may already recognize the difficulty that it presents, but you may view the problem as just one more on a growing list of statistical burdens that you as an investigator must bear in order to have your research results accepted. I know that you also do not have the time or the patience to sit still for a complicated mathematical discussion of this topic. While I may not have met you, you have been foremost in my mind while I was writing this book.

This is a book written for clinical investigators at all levels and research groups within the pharmaceutical industry, as well as medical students, public health students, healthcare researchers, physician-scientists, and regulators at the local, state, and federal levels who must grapple with the multiple analysis issue in clinical trials. Multiple testing has become a serious matter in clinical trial interpretation. Journal readers, editors, peer–reviewers, pharmaceutical companies, federal Food and Drug Administration advisory committee panels, and sometimes even juries struggle with the multiple analysis dilemma. These considerations can appear in several different guises. Two common examples are (1) the interpretation of secondary endpoint analyses, and (2) the evaluation of subgroup results in a clinical trial. Each of us may have a personal philosophy that governs our view of this issue—however, we must carefully measure and recalibrate that view with a well-reasoned and defendable yardstick. This text can serve as a useful metric.

As I have lectured and attended lectures on the principles of statistical analysis in clinical trials, the non-statistical audience has consistently and persistently asked questions concerning the "correct use" of multiple analyses. The questions that are frequently raised are "How should multiple analyses be carried out?" or "How should a reader interpret the multiple analyses executed by others?" Not only have I found that these questions are ubiquitous—they are inescapable! And I have also discovered that, just like discussions involving p-value interpretation, the questions from these audiences are typically sharper and more directed than the answers that they receive from the speakers.

That is not to say that the statistical literature has been mute on the topic. By my count, there are over 300 manuscripts that have appeared in the peer-reviewed literature on multiple analyses. Many of these are elegant mathematical treatises. In addition, there are several books on multiple analyses. One was written in 1981 by R. Miller.[1] Peter Westfall has also been prolific in the area of multiple analyses in general, and has advocated re-sampling procedures to resolve this dilemma in particular.[2] Fine textbooks that they are, it must be admitted that they can be difficult for healthcare researchers with weaker statistical backgrounds to understand. Nevertheless, these physicians and healthcare scientists are often burdened with the task of evaluating research results produced from a multiple analysis setting.

This text was written in order to engage the worker in a discussion of the multiple analysis issue in clinical trials at his or her level. Only a short prior exposure to statistical hypothesis testing is required to follow the discussions in this text. If you do not know much about statistics but must grapple with this multiple analysis issue, then I am willing to play in your ballpark.

A large number of footnotes and several appendices have been included in this text. This additional material (with an occasional anecdote or two mixed in) is intended to be supplemental and not required information. I have included this material in recognition of the fact that readers will have heterogeneous backgrounds with consequent different needs from this book. The unsophisticated reader will have elementary definitions and explanations close at hand in the footnotes. At the other extreme, the appendices provide in-depth discussion and mathematical treatment of the assertions in the body of the text from which a more advanced audience may derive benefit. Both the footnotes and the appendices are available to all, but not all need partake of them. Use them as you like.

I have to confess that there is some unavoidable overlap between this textbook and a prior text of mine, *Statistical Reasoning in Medicine: The Intuitive P-Value Primer*. While the prior book discussed *p*-values in general (describing how audiences should respond to them in clinical research), there are two chapters in that earlier text that deal with the multiple endpoint topic that is a subset of the multiple analysis problem. These same issues are discussed in this book, primarily in Chapter 4. However, the development in the textbook that you now hold is more leisurely, is less technical, and has many more examples.

I have also tried to keep in mind that a little levity every now and then is not such a bad thing. Therefore, you will find an occasional anecdote or aphorism to remind us that, the more serious our undertaking is, the more important is the need for a sense of humor.

Lemuel A. Moyé, M.D., Ph.D.
University of Texas School of Public Health
Houston, Texas, USA
June 2003

---

[1] Miller, R.G. (1981). *Simultaneous statistical inference*, 2nd ed. New York, Springer.
[2] Dr. Westfall's latest text is *Multiple Comparisons and Multiple Tests*, published by SAS Publishing, December 2000.

Acknowledgments

Like the farmer who is thankful for every drop of rain that finally falls on his parched fields, I am grateful for each contribution from my colleagues and friends in this effort. Dr. Anita Deswal helped me to organize the background clinical trial material so necessary for the discussion in Chapter 2 on inference from non-prospectively planned analyses. She also provided many references, insightful observations, and clarifications of the content of Chapter 11. The evaluations of Chapter 5 by Silvia Maberti and Beverly Shirkey were instrumental in the development of my own ideas concerning the complicated topic of dependent analyses in clinical trials. Dr. James Powell is a very good friend who has, time and again, provided important insight for me; in this book, his assistance with the discussion of subgroup analyses was invaluable. Luis Ruedas provided both encouragement and helpful advice.

John Kimmel, the reviewing editor, and many chapter reviewers have provided good questions, challenges, suggestions, and additional references. Their help has improved this book's structure.

There were many others who agreed to review this manuscript during its preparation. Chantal Caverness, Alan Tita, Lise Labishe, Laura Porter, and Jasmin Tito produced very valuable suggestions that strengthened this text's message. If the text is instructive and serves you well, then these hard-working young scientists should get a full measure of the credit. Any problems with the content of the text are mine and mine alone.

Finally, my dearest thanks go to Dixie, my wife, on whose personality, character, love, and common sense I have come to rely, and to Flora and Bella Ardon, whose continued emotional and spiritual growth reveals anew to me each day that, through God, all things are possible.

Lemuel A. Moyé, M.D., Ph.D.
University of Texas School of Public Health
Houston, Texas, USA
June 2003

Contents

Introduction

Multiple analyses in clinical trials comprise the execution and interpretation of numerous statistical hypotheses within a single clinical experiment. These analyses appear in many forms. More prevalent among them are the evaluation of the effect of therapy on multiple endpoints, the assessment of a subgroup analysis, and the evaluation of a dose–response relationship. Both the research and medical communities are frequently exposed to the results of these analyses. Common forums for their dissemination are the presentation of clinical trial results at meetings; the appearance of these results in the peer-reviewed, scientific literature; and discussions before regulatory agencies that are considering the approval of a new intervention. Unfortunately, the result of these analyses is commonly confusion and not illumination.

It is not surprising that the motivation for producing this panoply of analyses is benevolent. By carrying out these multiple hypothesis tests, the physician-scientist may only be indulging her own curiosity or that of her inquisitive co-investigators. On the other hand, she may be dutifully satisfying the demands for additional analyses from her research team leader or from her department chairperson. Peremptory demands for more analyses are generated from journal reviewers and editors, and of course, additional queries often originate from the analysts who work for regulatory agencies.[1] Whatever the driving force for these analyses is, the use of a single clinical trial to address multiple scientific questions proceeds at an accelerating pace. Yet the physician-scientist, while well versed in clinical science and highly motivated to carry out clinical research, is often unprepared for the interpretive complexities presented by the multiple analysis problem.

The multiple analysis issue in clinical trials can appear in many forms. For example, the investigators of a clinical trial can carry out one hypothesis test for each of several endpoints in the study, with little regard to whether the endpoint was created in the design phase of the study or much later during the study's execution or final analysis phase. Another example is the evaluation of each therapy's effect in a clinical trial that has a control group and several different therapy groups. Finally, the examination of a randomly allocated intervention's effect in not just the entire research cohort but in selected subgroups of that cohort constitutes a common illustration of the multiple analysis issue.

Actually, the circumstances of multiple analyses in clinical trials are more complicated than the previous examples suggest because, in reality, these analyses occur not in isolation but in complex mixtures. For example, a clinical trial may report the effect of therapy on several different endpoints and then proceed to report

---

[1] Since regulatory agencies frequently get the dataset of a clinical trial, they are free to carry out their own analyses and to confront the investigator with the results.

subgroup findings for the effect of therapy on a completely different endpoint. Some of these hypothesis tests were designed before the study was executed, while others were merely "targets of opportunity" that the investigators noticed as the clinical trial evaluation proceeded to the end; some of these analyses have small p-values, while others do not.

The development of complex and rapid statistical evaluation systems drive the multiple analysis issue deeper into the heart of the clinical trial, sometimes to the study's detriment. Findings from contemporary clinical trials, based on immature multiple endpoint analyses, have produced confusion in the medical community.[2] In addition, other clinical trial results that focused on the evaluation of subgroup results have led to findings that are difficult to integrate into the current body of scientific knowledge. Multiple statistical analyses create a complex and confusing research environment in which to draw appropriate conclusions.

This complex and germane issue has not been ignored in the statistical literature. There are many fine statistical textbooks and technical articles that address the multiple analysis issue in clinical experiments. However, they are often written of at a level of mathematical complexity that the physician-scientist does not understand. Thus, the investigator, with both expertise and insight into his clinical trial's scientific question, may not find the body of available mathematical material very helpful to him. Without understanding the derivation of the multiple analyses principles, the principles themselves are reduced merely to additional, arbitrary, and perhaps capricious rules that the investigator must follow in the analysis of his data. Produced in a vacuum of understanding, the link between these principles and the investigator is incompletely forged. Remaining weak, this link is easily broken in the tempestuous environment in which clinical research is conducted.

The thesis of this book is that the philosophy and methodology of multiple analyses in clinical trials are within the grasp of all clinical investigators, and that these scientists will understand and absorb these principles without a heavy investment in mathematics. *Multiple Analyses in Clinical Trials: Fundamentals for Investigators* introduces solutions to the multiple analysis issue (including multiple endpoints, combined endpoints, and subgroup evaluations) that are embedded in the bedrock of sound biostatistical and epidemiologic principles. While the issue of multiple testing has often been addressed in arcane, detached, technical language, this text will help clinical investigators surmount the learning curve of multiple analysis procedures and understand the key issues when designing their own work or reviewing the research of others.

The book is aimed at healthcare researchers interested in designing and analyzing clinical research. Basic backgrounds in health care and in statistics (e.g., an introduction to probability and hypothesis testing) are required. *Multiple Analyses in Clinical Trials: Fundamentals for Investigators* is written for advanced medical students, clinical investigators at all levels, research groups within the pharmaceutical industry, regulators at the local, state, and federal levels, and junior biostatisticians. While occasional mathematical developments will be required, they will by and large be relegated to a collection of appendices so as to not interrupt the

---

[2] Specific examples are provided in Chapter 2.

flow of the chapter's discussion. Current examples from the medical literature will be used to demonstrate both good and bad implementation of design principles.

One of the most useful devices to gain a perspective for choosing the best methodological philosophy for clinical trial analyses is to look back for a moment to see how we have arrived at our current "state of the science." The Prologue is a discussion of the roles of biostatistics and epidemiology in clinical research. Since epidemiology and biostatistics have the same common goal when applied to health-care (i.e., to elucidate the true nature of the risk factor–disease relationship), some of their joint history (with both their strengths and their weaknesses) are reviewed as a preamble to consideration of their individual contributions to clinical trial principles. The investigator is reminded that she is in the position to choose the best of both of these disciplines as she develops her own methodological philosophy.

In order to understand multiple analyses, the reader must understand the paradigm of the clinical trial; Chapter 1 provides a quick review of the important principles in clinical trial design and execution. This review will help to ensure that we are all using the same terminology to address clinical trial analysis issues.

Chapter 2 discusses in great detail the need for the prospective planning of statistical analyses in clinical trials. Through a series of examples, this chapter demonstrates the difficulties with drawing conclusions from data-driven analyses (i.e., analyses that are not planned before the experiment, but are motivated by the observed trends that are contained in the incoming data stream); it then develops the critical reasoning that underlies the essential need to have the analysis plan provided in detail before the experiment is carried out. With Chapter 1's review and Chapter 2's principles absorbed, Chapter 3 examines the reasons why multiple analyses in clinical trials are so popular and the difficulties with their interpretation.

Chapters 4 to 6 each discuss a separate dilemma in the application of multiple analyses to clinical trials and provide solutions. Chapter 4 covers the issue of multiple analyses and multiple endpoints. Chapters 5 and 6 focus on multiple endpoints in clinical trials when the statistical hypothesis tests are dependent.[3]

Chapters 7 to 13 apply the principles and theories developed in the first six chapters to current multiple analysis issues in clinical trials. Chapters 7 and 8 concentrate on multiple analyses when the endpoints of the clinical endpoints are put together into a single composite endpoint (e.g., fatal coronary artery disease + non-fatal myocardial infarction). Chapters 9 to 11 focus on the issue of subgroup analyses in clinical trials, and Chapter 12 examines the analysis of clinical trials when there are several treatment groups in addition to the control group. This text culminates with Chapter 13 where combinations of different tools for multiple analyses are forged into constructive combinations that provide clear result interpretations in complicated clinical trial settings. At this point it is my hope that the reader will be able to assemble useful and interpretable analyses for very complex clinical trials.

Multiple Analyses in Clinical Trials: Fundamentals for Investigators is an essentially nonmathematical discussion of the problems posed by the execution of multiple analyses in clinical trials, concentrating on the rationale for the analyses,

---

[3] Two statistical hypothesis tests are dependent when knowledge of a type I error occurring on one of the tests provides information about the occurrence of a type I error on the other.

the difficulties posed by their interpretation, and useful solutions. With its problem sets, it would make a useful textbook for a one-semester course that covers the analysis principles of clinical trials. This course would cover the content of Chapters 1, 2, 3, 4, 5, 7, 9, 10, and 12. A course that requires a more extensive background in clinical trials for its students would cover Chapters 2 to 13.

Prologue
Blossoms on a Healthy Plant

In this prologue, the role of biostatistics and epidemiology in clinical trial design and interpretation will be presented. Although each of these fields has provided an important core component of the foundation of experimental methodology, the philosophies of these disciplines have been criticized. Several arguments against these disciplines' approaches are summarized here in order to provide a balanced perspective on their influence in clinical experiments. Advice is offered to the clinical investigator who attempts to integrate the principles of epidemiology and biostatistics into the design and interpretation of clinical experiments. Finally, a brief review is provided of the important fundamentals of clinical trial design and analysis that will be required for our subsequent discussions of the multiple analysis issue.

Although it is easy to understand why a physician who reviews a detailed report of a clinical trial's results might consider that research effort as primarily a biostatistical exercise, the embedded mathematics are really the culmination of diverse, concentrated nonmathematical efforts. Like the flower that blossoms upon a healthy plant, interpretable biostatistical analyses in clinical trials require a robust supporting structure. The rigorous design and execution of the clinical trial is that framework.

Once the investigators choose the scientific question they wish to answer, many other decisions must be made that have a direct bearing on the interpretation of the experiment. The choices about the number and characteristics of patients to be included, the use of a randomization tool to allocate the therapy of interest, the duration of time over which patients are to be followed, the dosage or duration of the intervention, options for multiple analyses, and many more decisions all are required in order for the final mathematical evaluations to be both interpretable and informative. Since the thinking process used to guide these choices is firmly rooted in the tenets of epidemiology and biostatistics, one cannot understand the important aspects of clinical trials without a working knowledge of the principles that guide each of these areas. We therefore begin with a brief review of the core values of each field and the complicated interactions that these disciplines have had.

Epidemiology and Biostatistics

Epidemiology and biostatistics have a complex history and interrelationship. Unfortunately, these two disciplines are often presented as taking adversarial perspectives on important scientific questions. In fact, each of these fields of study attempts to answer the same question in health care—what caused the event of interest? If the event is the appearance of a disease, both disciplines are interested in identifying

1

the cause of that disease. If the event is a cure or remission of the disease, then these two fields focus on what may have produced the favorable outcome. However, historical controversies involving both biostatistics and epidemiology can make it appear that they are in conflict, acting much like two people riding in the same car, going to the same destination, but fighting each other for control of the steering wheel. These controversies are based on the tools each of them chooses to use.

Association and Causation

Does a risk factor cause a disease? Sometimes the relationship between the risk factor and the disease is merely coincidental. Other times, the risk factor is present in many patients with the disease, but the supposed risk factor does not cause the disease. The question of causality can be a complicated one, and the distinction between a relationship based on association and one based on causation is critical. Associative exposure–disease relationships are linked by the joint occurrence of the risk factor and the disease. The risk factor in the "association" circumstance does not cause the disease; the risk factor and the disease just happen to occur together, appearing jointly.

However, a causal relationship is much different. A risk factor causes a disease if that risk factor *excites the production* of the disease. There is a clear directionality in the risk factor–disease causal connection that is absent in a serendipitous risk factor–disease relationship. The time sequence embedded in the causal relationship is that (1) the disease is absent, (2) the risk factor is introduced, and (3) the risk factor working in ways known and unknown produces the disease.

We are surrounded by relationships that are associative, but not causative. For example, it is common knowledge that the risk of drowning is greatest in the summer months, but we do not say that the summer season itself causes drowning. Smoking is more prevalent in teenagers than in younger children, but we do not say that being a teenager causes smoking. However, we do say that cigarette smoking causes lung cancer. A heart attack can occur in a patient who has hypertension, diabetes mellitus, elevated lipid levels, and who has recently stop smoking. Was it the cessation of smoking that caused the heart attack? A young woman who smoked cigarettes and took birth control pills suffered a stroke after exposure to a cold medicine. What actually caused the stroke? In 1981 there was great concern that coffee drinking caused pancreatic cancer. While an initial report discovered that coffee drinkers had a greater risk of cancer [1], a subsequent reviewing body of scientists ascertained that there was insufficient evidence to determine that coffee drinking actually excited the production of cancer [2], [3].

This problem is complicated by the fact that in research we do not have the opportunity to examine the entire universe of patients who have the risk factor or the entire population of patients who get the disease. Instead, the researcher studies only a sample of these patients. Since the findings of one sample can differ from the findings of another,[1] how is the researcher to determine whether the findings in her sample are due to this sample-to-sample variability that reflects only the play of chance and not a real relationship?

---

[1] The variability from one sample to another in research results is called *sampling error*.

This issue complicates the research effort that seeks to identify the true nature of a risk factor–disease relationship, making the effort a two-step process. First, the investigator must determine whether the findings from the sample are due to the random aggregation of events on the one hand or reflect a true relationship between the risk factor and the disease in the population on the other. Second, the researcher must then deduce whether the relationship identified in the research sample is causal or merely associative.

The classification of a relationship as associative or causal can be a public health urgency. However, this classification can also be a complex, time consuming task, since multiple risk factors and diseases can congregate. This complex coexistence can make it difficult to separate the causal risk factors from the associative ones. Both epidemiologists and biostatisticians are called upon to help disentangle the risk factor–disease connection, and have historically emphasized the use of different research tools (Figure 1).

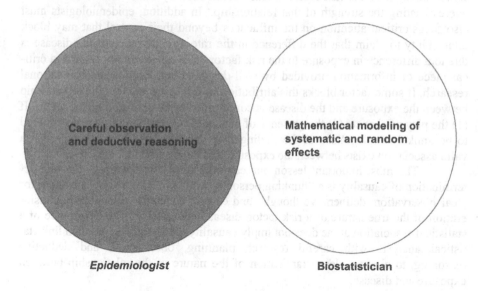

Figure 1. The tools of epidemiology versus the tools of biostatistics.

The Central Core of Epidemiology

The classic epidemiologist is an expert observer. He relies on careful observation and deductive reasoning in the investigation of a risk factor–disease relationship, using research tools to choose the optimal vantage point to view this relationship unfolding before him in the population. Often limited by logistics and ethics, the research effort to identify a cause for a particular disease many times precludes the execution of an experimental study (in which the researcher has control of the risk factor assignment). Instead, the research must be observational, a circumstance in which the epidemiologist has no control of who is exposed to the risk factor. However, if the epidemiologist gives careful consideration to the execution of the observational study, this research tool can illuminate a risk factor–disease relationships with powerful explanatory light.

If the disease is new, a host of risk factors must be excluded. The identification of the bacteria *Legionella pneumophilia* as a cause of an outbreak of a new and unrecognized pneumonia at a veterans' meeting in Philadelphia is a fine example [4]. Yet another example is the identification of the mosquito-borne West Nile Virus as responsible in 1999 for an outbreak of serious morbidity (and, rarely, mortality) in New York City. The tools commonly used by epidemiologists are described elsewhere [5], but include case control studies, cross-sectional studies, historical cohorts, and prospective cohorts.

Recognizing the limitations of these studies, epidemiologists pay particular attention to the types of systematic influences that can inappropriately shift the observed strength of the risk factor–disease connection by either underestimating or overestimating the strength of that relationship.[2] In addition, epidemiologists must also focus critical attention on the influences beyond their control that may block their ability to claim that the difference in the rate of occurrence of the disease is due to a difference in exposure to the risk factor. This *attribution of effect* is a critical piece of information provided by well-designed and conducted observational research. If some factor blocks this attribution of effect we say that the relationship between the exposure and the disease is confounded by or confused by the factor. If (1) the play of chance, (2) the presence of bias, and (3) confounding are determined to be unlikely explanations of the findings, we can then carefully conclude that a valid association exists between the exposure and the disease that may be causal.

The most important lesson one can take from this process is that the determination of causality is a "thinking person's business." There is no substitute for clear observation, deliberative thought, and careful deductive reasoning in consideration of the true nature of a risk factor–disease relationship. The occurrence of a statistical association alone does not imply causality. Epidemiologists often link statistical analysis with careful research planning, observation, and deductive reasoning, to allow a clear examination of the nature of the relationship between exposure and disease.

Scurvy

The impact of clear-thinking epidemiologists on society has been felt for over four hundred years. The beginning of modern epidemiology is traced often to the work of John Graunt and William Petty on developing a rudimentary life table analysis [6].

The powerful combination of deductive reasoning and experimental design was further demonstrated by James Lind. In the eighteenth century, one of the single greatest impediments to the discovery and exploration of new lands in the Western Hemisphere was the ravage of scurvy. The impact of this disease was commonly felt on long sailing voyages to the New World from Europe during

---

[2] These systematic influences are known as *biases*.

which time passengers and crew became vitamin C deprived. The illness, often beginning with bleeding gums, developed into a dreaded and irreversible constellation of symptoms. The worst cases lead to severe pain produced by any physical movement as the body began to swell. The skin would split, producing deep, bleeding gashes. Finally the neck would swell to the point that eating and drinking were impossible. Most of these patients slipped into irreversible coma and subsequently died. Over 75% of passengers and crew aboard these sailing ships were afflicted to some degree with scurvy,[3] a disease that at the time had neither an identifiable cause nor cure.

James Lind, on the *HMS Salisbury* in 1747, observed the ravages of this disease from close range. He decided to conduct an experiment to test the possible effect of several proposed treatments for the illness, in the hope of identifying its cure. Lind chose ten seamen who had nothing in common except that they served on the same ship at the same time and all were debilitated by scurvy. He divided them into five groups of two,[4] and gave each of the groups of sailors a different treatment. The first two sailors were provided rations of sea water. The second two were given oil of vitriol (sulfuric acid) to drink. Patients five and six were administered vinegar. The fourth group was provided "bigness of nutmeg," and the last two were given rations of lemons and oranges. The two sailors who improved were the two who received the citrus fruit. Upon their recovery, they were ordered to care for the remaining eight seamen in the experiment until these others died from the scurvy (or the ineffective therapy). The treatment effect size was dramatic—so dramatic that the use of mathematics was not required to demonstrate it.[5] However, it took the British Admiralty 50 years to finally permit ships to sail with fresh fruits and vegetables, a policy which marked the beginning of the end of scurvy as a serious disease on long sea voyages.

Cholera

Another classic example of epidemiologic deductive reasoning was demonstrated by John Snow in his investigation of cholera from 1830 to 1850. In nineteenth century London, severe gastroenteritis rose to dangerous levels among the local population. Although there were several suspected causes for the episodic outbreaks, one possible cause was believed to be in the water. However, it seemed impossible to demonstrate due to the haphazard organization of London communities that water was a likely source for the disease. Every household required it, but not every household harbored ill family members.

Homes were provided with water service by competing water companies. These companies had different sources for the water they pumped. John Snow made

---

[3] This situation was exacerbated by the fact that sailing ships, having no reliable way to compute the longitude and therefore their own position, were often lost at sea, drifting aimlessly for weeks.

[4] Note that Lind decided to have more than one patient per group. He apparently recognized that a positive finding in a single patient may not be enough evidence to demonstrate the effect of therapy because of sailor-to-sailor variability.

[5] This story is somewhat complicated by the fact that James Lind concluded at first that it was not citrus fruit, but exposure to sea air that produced these two sailors' improvement.

two striking observations about a particular community containing pockets of people with severe acute gastroenteritis. His first observation was that, in this single neighborhood, there were two competing water companies. The Southwark and Vauxhall water company pumped water from the contaminated Thames river—the Lambeth company originally pumped water from the Thames, but later changed its water source to the uncontaminated Thames Ditton. Snow's second observation was that home owners in this neighborhood selected, seemingly at random, one of the two competing water supply companies. This random selection meant that characteristics of households would be equally distributed between the two companies. Thus, the two features of (1) two companies pumping water, one from a contaminated water source, the second from a relatively clean source, and (2) the selection of these companies at random by a neighborhood's dwellings created a near-perfect "natural experiment" within which Snow could observe the relationship between exposure to contaminated water and cholera rates. Again, careful observation and deductive reasoning, in concert with a strong relationship between the exposure and the disease obviated any requirement for complex mathematical analysis.

Causality and Common Sense

The efforts to understand and articulate the arguments that should be used to identify or debunk a risk factor–disease relationship have continuously evolved over the past four hundred years. In 1965, Hill [7] described the nine criteria used to construct a causality argument in health care. These nine rules or tenets are remarkably and refreshingly devoid of complex mathematical arguments. They rely instead on a natural, honest intuition and common sense for the inquiry into the true nature of a risk factor–disease relationship. The nine criteria of Bradford Hill are: (1) strength of association, (2) consistency, (3) specificity, (4) temporality, (5) biologic gradient, (6) biologic plausibility, (7) biologic coherence, (8) experimental evidence, and (9) analogy.[6]

The method for investigating a risk factor–disease relationship that Hill proposed makes good sense to this day. Some of these questions can be characterized as evaluating the direct strength of the evidence for a causal relationship between the risk factor and the disease. For example, we would expect that if the risk factor causes the disease, then the disease occurs more frequently when the risk factor is present then when it is not. We would also expect that a greater exposure to the risk factor produce a greater extent of disease.

Other questions asked by Hill explore the "believability" of the relationship. Some of these are: Is there a discernible mechanism by which the risk factor produces the disease? Have other investigations also shown this relationship? Are there other such relationships whose demonstration helps to understand the current risk factor–disease relationship? The best research efforts are designed to address many of the Hill causality tenets, thereby helping to build (or demolish) a causality argument.

---

[6] These are each defined in Appendix A.

Biostatisticians and Sampling Error

The biostatistician, in general, has a different emphasis from that of the epidemiologist. Since research in healthcare often begins with the selection of a sample from a large population or universe of patients, statisticians have emphasized the effect this sampling process can have on the results of the research effort. The idea that different samples, selected from the same population, can produce different conclusions has motivated biostatisticians to focus on first identifying sources of variability and then measuring and comparing the magnitude of variability from each source. Biostatisticians concentrate on quantifying the likelihood that the research results were produced merely as a product of sample-to-sample variability as opposed to the results being a reflection of the risk factor–disease relationship in the population. Thus, while epidemiologists focus on systematic influences that can affect the study results, biostatisticians concentrate on the possible random influences. This has led to great reliance on the use of sophisticated mathematical modeling by biostatisticians in their attempts to separate the random influences from the systematic influences which are embedded in the risk factor–disease relationship. Logistic regression analysis, Cox proportional hazard modeling, and adaptic Bayes procedures are all tools that help to separate sampling error variability or "noise" produced by the sample from the true population "signal" of an effect that may be embedded in the sample.

Statistics evolved from demography, as the early European tax collectors of four hundred years ago concocted imaginative ways to estimate the population size. These counting tools evolved into surveys of increasing complexity. Concerns about sampling variability, coincident with the development of strategies to win very popular games of chance, accelerated the development of probability laws. The mathematicians, Gauss, DeMoivre, Bayes, and Laplace (among others) developed mathematical tools to compute probabilities based on the nature of the design of the experiment itself. These probabilists carefully considered the experiment (e.g., rolling a fair sided die) and then computed the probabilities of the different possible experimental results. By this process, they developed a new branch of mathematics—probability. Unlike the experiments of James Lind and John Snow, games of chance needed mathematics to help predict results.

Cooperation Between the Disciplines

This difference in emphasis between these two fields can appear to be profound. However, two forces bring epidemiology and biostatistics together. The first is that they each must use the data. Thus, they both have a major interest in collecting data of the highest quality under clearly delineated rules. Second, experienced scientists in each of these fields recognize that in order to provide the clearest answer to the scientific question "Does exposure A cause disease B?" they must borrow from the perspective and tools from the others discipline (Figure 2).

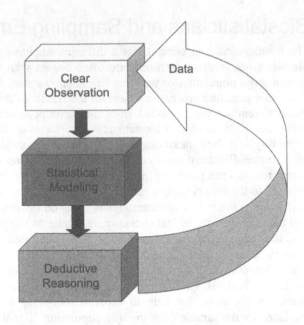

Figure 2. The use of epidemiology and biostatistics in reality.

This means that the skilled epidemiologist recognizes the important information that mathematical modeling can provide in helping to resolve the degree to which sampling error might explain the data. Also, the wise biostatistician realizes that, unless there is considerable attention provided to the research design and execution, the data from that effort will have no scientific value, and her mathematics will be devoid of useful information. These scientists therefore have much in common.

In addition, epidemiology and biostatistics have a common acceptance of experimental design principles. Several of these principles were identified by Young [8] and Johnson [9], early eighteenth-century experimental agrarians. Without the benefit of advanced mathematical tools, these workers enunciated important principles of research upon which epidemiologists and biostatisticians agreed. One principle was that the active research effort must be preceded by careful study and review of the state of the science that had been developed thus far. The second was to acknowledge that poorly designed and poorly executed research leads to incorrect conclusions that may not be recognized at the time as being incorrect. These false conclusions, Young suggested, when accepted by the community would produce a succession of misguided research efforts with unproductive results. This would continue until the false summaries could be correctly identified and extirpated from the knowledge base. These researchers also pointed out the importance of measuring the study endpoint with great attention to detail, since its accurate identification increases the research result's precision. Both epidemiology and biostatistics have accepted and absorbed these principles into their core philosophies.

Finally, both epidemiologists and biostatisticians have faced historically tight, cultural circumscription of their abilities to generalize their own work. Statisticians in general were not allowed to draw conclusions from the results of their early survey data because of the political volatility of these evaluations. While all agreed that the complete collection and correct tabulation of data were well within the statistician's purview, the idea of drawing conclusions from that data was left to the nineteenth-century religious and cultural leaders. Statisticians were called practitioners of "political arithmetic."

Despite this limitation, these epidemiologists and biostatisticians have worked well together in the past. A fine illustration of this cooperative effort was the study of smallpox. Smallpox was one of the great scourges of the sixteenth and seventeenth centuries. Initially identified in China, this disease spread westward over the trade routes, through the Middle East and Turkey, into Europe (and finally, by ship, across to the New World).[7] The disease easily spread from one individual to another by inhalation. Death occurred after the second week of exposure due to pneumonia and subsequent cardiovascular collapse [10]. Those who survived often were hideously scarred for life, a result that was particularly unfortunate in children.

However, from the east there came a persistent rumor of a strange procedure that could offer protection from smallpox. Individuals, it was said, could be protected from smallpox if they would inhale the flaked scales of an infected individual's scabbed skin. The Chinese were known to try to protect themselves in this fashion. The Greeks and Turks attempted protection by first sticking a needle that had previously been pushed into a smallpox pustule of an infected individual, and then pricking their own skin in three different places. This early process was termed *variolation*.

The protective process was refined by taking the pus not of an individual infected by smallpox or variola but from a cow who was afflicted with cowpox, or vaccinia. This inoculation procedure was now renamed *vaccination*. But how could vaccination be demonstrated to work? The joint work of the cleric Cotton Mather, the probabilist Daniel Bernoulli, and the investigator Edward Jenner demonstrated the effectiveness of this vaccine to skeptical officials in a tempestuous environment. In this effort, the probabilists and biostatisticians computed the expected number of deaths, while the epidemiologists counted the observed number of deaths. The comparison of these two estimates provided information about whether vaccination produced fewer "observed cases" than the "expected number of cases," this latter computation being based on the probabilists' theories.

Bernoulli presented his results to the French Royal Academy of Sciences in Paris during a meeting in 1760. At this meeting, he displayed results that he believed demonstrated that variolation would reduce the death rate and increase the population of France. The demonstration of the effectiveness of vaccination to reduce smallpox mortality rates was among the first known collaborations between men of mathematics and men with epidemiologic skills for the scientific demonstration of treatment effectiveness.

---

[7] This is taken from Ed Gehan's and Noreen Lemak's fine depiction in *Statistics in Medical Research. Developments in Clinical Trials*, published in 1994 by Plenum Publishing Company.

Thus, epidemiology and biostatistics, with their common aims, common principles, and joint efforts against common adversaries grew in importance and interdependence in the nineteenth century. However, the joint efforts were soon to be overturned by a controversy that for much of the twentieth century drove a wedge between them.

The Eye of the Beholder

Many workers ascribe the schism between biostatistics and epidemiology to the rise of significance testing, attributed to Ronald Fisher, the agrarian statistician [11], [12]. Certainly, there were important eruptions in the literature over the issue of significance testing, controversies that extend to the present day [13], [14], [15], [16], [17]. Statisticians came to embrace the notion of the null hypothesis, type I and type II errors, and test statistics—many epidemiologists came to abhor them. However, the problem between these two fields is deeper, older, and broader than suggested by a 1930s dispute over the use of test statistics and p-values.

Controversy 1: Biased by Nature?

Recall that carefully crafted research design followed by detailed observation and deductive, disciplined conclusions are the central pillars of epidemiology. As we saw in the case of John Snow's assessment of gastroenteritis, it was actually possible for a discerning epidemiologist to observe an "experiment in nature." However, these skills were indirectly assaulted by the findings of early twentieth twentieth-century physics. Out of this seething cauldron of theoretical and physical investigation spilled new ideas that were to change not just the human appreciation of physics, but also scientific understanding of how we view our surroundings.

At the end of the nineteenth century, physics experiments that delved into the property of matter and light were making observations that were correct but inexplicable by the clockwork accuracy and precision of Newtonian physics. As physicists struggled to understand them, a far-reaching explanation was suggested by the physicists George Fitzgerald and Hendrik Lorentz.[8] These scientists postulated that our measure of physical dimension was not absolute, but asserted that as an object moved its length decreased.[9] This explanation led to the additional conclusions that if the length of an object becomes smaller as its speed accelerates, so that object's volume must also decrease.

Thus, the physical world appeared as it did only because of the position and movement of its observer, a finding that ran against the grain of common sense. August Föppl, in his *Introduction of Maxwell's Theory of Electricity,* stated that "there is a deep-going revision of that conception of a space that has been impressed upon human thinking in its previous period of development."

---

[8] This discussion of physics is from Ronald Clark, *Einstein: The Life and Times.* 1984, New York. Avon Books, Inc.

[9] The Lorentz–Fitzgerald transformation suggested that the length of an object that is moving in one dimension will have its length in that direction decreased by the amount $\sqrt{1 - v^2/c^2}$, where v is the velocity of the object and c the speed of light.

Albert Einstein, in 1905, described what came to be known as the Special Law of Relativity, wherein he determined the changes in physical reality at rates of movement close to that of the speed of light. At these high speeds, termed relativistic speeds, not only are length, area, and volume smaller, but mass is greater and time moves more slowly. In Einstein's General Law of Relativity, published during World War I, the current understanding of the fabric of space itself was demolished. Space could no longer be seen as an empty stage on which objects moved and performed. Instead, space had its own properties, properties that changed when mass was present. In the absence of mass, space can appear alien. Geometry is no longer Euclidean. Parallel lines do not exist. The angles of a triangle no longer have a sum of 180 degrees and perpendiculars to the same line converge.

Certainly, these findings had a major effect on the developing field of physics, itself newly armed with instrumentation that allowed it to probe atoms and look further into the heavens. However, the veracity of these new laws also had a profound impact on all observation-based science. According to physics, physical findings and measurements could no longer be trusted. Concepts easily understood and taken for granted for centuries were found to be inconstant—merely a function of the observation point of the viewer. Two observers could watch an event and have different perceptions, both of which were correct. The stationary person could see two lights flash at once—a second observer moving rapidly would observe that one light appeared before the other. Both are entirely accurate and neither is wrong. The difference in these observations resides in the characteristics of the observation point.

Of course, it had been long appreciated that human senses were "relative." The phrase "one man's meat is another man's poison" spoke to the variability of taste. The fact that animals (like bats) respond to auditory signals to which humans are insensitive is an example of the "relativity" of hearing. However, the mass-, time-, and space-altering findings of physics were an entirely different affair. The absolute immutability of space and time had been accepted and confirmed by centuries of observational evidence. Now it was shown that the conventional belief, deduced from careful observation—observations that had been confirmed and reconfirmed over the centuries—was misleading.

The ability of science to measure the real world had not changed, but the scientific community's absolute confidence in that ability was shaken. The new laws declared that all the systems of measurement used in science were parochial, unsuited to describe nature as a whole. Scientists awakened to the sad reality that they did not see the results of their experiments clearly, but through spectacles fitted over their eyes by their physical viewpoint. This was a major setback to any field that placed its full trust in the power of observation. Epidemiologists had developed principles that would allow the most objective view of a risk factor–disease relationship. They had developed and catalogued an entire system of biases to be recognized, and hopefully prevented. If competing researchers had different research designs and drew disparate conclusions, the best view was accepted to be the one whose point of view was influenced by the least bias. However, this new law from physics suggested that not only did both views contain bias, but that each view, from the position of the observer, could be perceived as correct. It seemed that the platform epidemiologists had been painstakingly and carefully constructing, and from which they would gain an objective view of an exposure–disease relationship that could never be completed. Objective observation was proven to be impossible, and the proof of this counterintuitive finding resided in impenetrable mathematics.

The Supremacy of Mathematics?

The General Law of Relativity dictated that laws are the same for all observers, irrespective of their relative positions, undoing some of the philosophical damage done by the previous Special Law. However, this general law introduced its own set of complexities in some astronomical observations.

Astronomers had lived with the unexplained observation that Mercury's perihelion (or point at which its elliptical orbit came closest to the sun) was not constant as Newtonian mechanics predicted, but steadily advanced and withdrew.[10] The General Law of Relativity (Einstein's second law) suggested that it was not the orbit of Mercury that was perturbed, but rather its position was mistakenly observed; a mistake that occurred because the mass of the sun was bending light. The proof of this second law provided additional difficulties for the observational scientist's approach to scientific questions.

Astronomers had been observing solar eclipses for generations. Now Einstein suggested that specific observations made during these eclipses would reveal what had been hiding in plain view from astronomical observers—that light was being bent when passing through the gravitational field of the sun. In 1919, a scientific exhibition found what Einstein had predicted would be identified. Essentially, based only on his equations, Einstein told astronomers (who had been taking their own observations for years) what to look for, where to find it, and how much of it they would find. These observational scientists found what Einstein said they would find, when they looked where his equations said to look.

While Einstein's general law was being digested by the public, scientists were considering this remarkable demonstration of the power of mathematics. In this circumstance, observation of nature did not lead to a general rule. It was mathematics that dictated where the observers should look. Apparently, mathematical law could predict what would happen (in fact, could find what had been hiding in plain view) that the observers never knew to look for. The directionality of the observation-to-deductive conclusion process was reversed. It was now possible for astute, sensitive mathematicians to teach us about the real world. Observations, having been revealed as flawed, biased, and limited, should perhaps be relegated to a smaller role in a scientific world in which mathematics would reign supreme.

Not only epidemiologists, but the traditional probabilists were threatened by this inexorably progressing ratiocination. The findings of the Russian mathematician Kolmogorov demonstrated that all of probability, with its rich history of observations based on natural phenomena, stock market predictions, and games of chance, was only a subarea of the larger mathematical field of real analysis. Kol-

---

[10] This is a very slow process. Mercury completes one cycle, approaching and then withdrawing from the sun once every three million years.

mogorov, without the benefit of games of chance or other observational devices the early probabilists of the sixteenth-century had used, derived all of the laws of probability from mathematical and functional analysis. In addition, these prodigious mathematical efforts produced new laws of probability that were not available to the observational scientist.[11] Advanced mathematical analysis, functional analysis, and the complicated area of measure theory now jointly subsumed probability, reducing the latter to a mere application. Once again mathematics seemed to be driving out, pushing aside, and supplanting observation-based research.

Hammer Blows

These findings in the first three decades of the twentieth century, stating that (1) all observations are inherently biased; and (2) events in nature can be predicted from cloistered mathematical work, struck the foundations of epidemiology like hammer blows. Epidemiology, already bruised by this philosophical assault, now had to deal with the reverse logic of significance testing proposed by the statistician Ronald Fisher. This new, upside-down paradigm of statistical significance denied the scientist the ability to prove the hypothesis he believed was correct. Fisher substituted, the tepid alternative of disproving a hypothesis the scientist did not believe. Fisher's significance testing appeared to be just the type of indecipherable, mathematical, reverse logic that had already shaken the foundations of early twentieth-century epidemiology. The reaction to Fisher by epidemiologists and other scientists was understandably vehement and severe as in

> What used to be called judgment is now called prejudice, and what used to be called prejudice is now called a null hypothesis ... it is dangerous nonsense ... [18]

Over time, epidemiologists have successfully defended their time-tested methodologic perspective. Of course, the flaw in all of these criticisms of the use of observation as a foundation method of epidemiology, lies in the difficulty in translating findings useful in one field (physics) to that of another (life sciences). While the findings of the relativity laws are in general true, they are most useful in physics. The theoretical physicist may be correct in asserting that every observer is biased and that there is no absolute truth about the nature and magnitude of the risk factor–disease relationship. However, this does not imply that all platforms are equally biased. Epidemiologists never stopped striving to find the most objective position possible. Certainly, if bias cannot be removed it should be minimized. The fact that bias may not be excluded completely does not excuse its unnecessary inclusion.

Second, while mathematicians are capable of predicting results in physics, they have not been able to predict disease in any important or useful fashion. No mathematical models warned obstetricians or their pregnant patients of the impend-

---

[11] An example of this is the strengthening of the law of large numbers, first identified in the seventeenth century and usefully applied for over 300 years. We now know that this familiar law is merely a *weak law* and describe it as the weak law of large numbers. The strong law of large numbers has been deduced from advanced mathematical analysis.

ing thalidomide–birth defect link [19]. Similarly, mathematical models did not predict the birth defects that mercury poisoning produced in Japan [20]. While physics often studies processes that are regular, in which mathematics can reign supreme, real life and its disease processes, on the other hand, have proven to be painful, messy, and chaotic affairs.[12] The substantial role of epidemiology is incontrovertible in the development of the most important new healthcare research tool of the twentieth century—the clinical trial. The time-tested tools of epidemiology continue to prove their utility in the present day.

The Rise and Decline of Significance Testing

The previous section pointed out some of the problems epidemiology faced during the early twenthieth-century and how this discipline has surmounted those problems. Later in the twentieth century, biostatistics faced its own set of difficulties. At the current time, the outcome is less than certain.

Biostatistics fulfills two roles as it guides the investigator's examination of the relationship between the presence of the risk factor and the occurrence of the disease. The first is *estimation*. In order to learn what the odds ratio[13] of an exposure to a disease is in the population, the investigators must follow the proper procedures to obtain an estimate of the odds ratio based on the data in their sample. Estimation theory provides the correct formulas these investigators should implement so that they might obtain an accurate and precise measure of these parameters. The second role of biostatistics is to help the investigators infer what may be observed in the population based on the estimate he or she obtained from the sample. This step of inference, i.e., of extending sample estimates to a larger population, can be difficult, primarily due to the presence of sampling error.

The *p*-value is the accepted measure of the statistical significance of a research finding. It is the probability of a particular type of sampling error. Consider the statistical hypothesis test that is carried out in a clinical trial to assess the effect of therapy on a prospectively defined endpoint. Then, specifically, the *p*-value is the probability that the test statistic in the research sample was produced from a population of patients in which there is no real effect of the therapy at all.

For example, a researcher, studying the effect of an intervention she suspects will postpone mortality in a large population of patients with heart failure, will use statistical principles to compute the difference in the cumulative mortality rates between the control group and the group of patients who received the experimental therapy. She will then compute the test statistic and the *p*-value for that test statistic. When used correctly, this *p*-value will assess the probability that there is no beneficial effect of therapy on the cumulative mortality rate in the large population of patients, but that this population has produced, through chance alone, a

---

[12] It is possible that inclusion of some global climate phenomena can quite possibly reveal patterns in the development of outbreaks of bubonic plague and hanta virus infections.
[13] An odds ratio is a measure of association between the exposure and the clinical event of interest.

sample that falsely suggested that this beneficial effect may be present.[14] The smaller the p-value, the more confident the investigator can be that the effect she has seen in her sample is due not to sampling error, but is instead a true reflection of a population effect. If the experiment was designed and executed well with (1) no systematic bias that distorts the measure of the effectiveness of therapy and (2) no confounding factors that make it difficult to attribute the effect on mortality to the experimental therapy, then the research finding may reflect a population truth.

The development of significance testing is due to the work of Fisher. As he worked through the design and analyses of agricultural experiments in the 1920s, he concluded that one had to consider the likelihood that findings from the research sample were just due to the random play of chance. However, he also stated that if the probability was greater than 0.05 that a population that had no positive findings would produce a sample with positive findings, the research findings should be considered to be due to the random, meaningless aggregation of events.

It was this latter concept that was completely absorbed by the medical research community. No one could have anticipated that "significance testing" would become so firmly rooted among healthcare researchers. Its preeminence is all the more astonishing since the 0.05 threshold set by Fisher was completely arbitrary, with no theory identifying this level as an appropriate threshold for non-agrarian, scientific disciplines. *It cannot be overemphasized that there is no deep, mathematical theory that points to 0.05 as the optimum type I error level—only tradition.*

The underlying motivations for the wholesale embrace of hypothesis testing and the p-value have been discussed by Goodman [21]. His work reveals that, shortly after the development of the p-value, complicated sociologic and scientific groups consisting of government regulators, journal editors, medical researchers, and medical academicians discovered that they shared the common desire for an objective measure of a research effort's results. Their interactions led to the identification of the p-value as an easily computed mathematical entity that seemed devoid of investigator subjectivity. A more thorough discussion of this complex process is available [22].

The technique of significance testing itself was to undergo a refinement into its present form. At its inception, reporting the results of statistical hypothesis testing was somewhat less exact. For example, if it was decided during the design phase of the experiment that the maximum value of the type I error rate was 0.05, the final results were reported as only $p < 0.05$—the exact value was not computed. However, as the use of significance testing grew, the belief that this estimate of the level of significance should be sharpened was encouraged. Also, the availability of more extensive tabulations of probabilities eased the computation for the exact value of this quantity. Thus, it became the custom to report the exact p-value ($p = 0.021$) and not just the inequality ($p < 0.05$). This is how p-values are currently reported.

---

[14] A type I error is when a universe of patients in whom there is no treatment effect produces a sample which contains (just through the play of chance) a treatment effect. A type II error is when a population in which there is a treatment effect produces a sample which contains no treatment effect, again just by chance alone.

The threshold significance level (type I error probability level) was utilized by Neyman and Pearson as a flexible criterion that should be determined in connection with the type II error level. It is interesting to note that Fisher was opposed to the interpretation of the type I error rate as a rejection rate. Instead, he emphasized the significance reflected by the actual p-value, i.e., the smaller the p-value, the greater the strength of evidence that the relationship identified in the sample is not due to chance alone [23].

It is not tragic that the use of p-values accelerated; however, it is unfortunate that they began to take on a new, inappropriate meaning in the medical research community. Medical research journals, that first were willing to merely accept p-values, soon began to require them. Designed to be a measure only of sampling error, the p-value became the ultimate research product distillate, the condensate that remained after the compression of the entire research effort into a single number. This situation degenerated when p-values stampeded over the well-established epidemiologic Hill tenets of causality as reflected in the following statement:

> Since the study found a statistically significant relative risk ... the causal relationship was considered established. [24]

Many workers have substituted the 0.05 judgment for their own thoughtful, critical review of a research effort. In some studies, highly statistically significant effects (i.e., small p-values) are produced from small, inconsequential effect sizes. In others, p-values themselves were meaningless regardless of their size since the assumptions on which they had been computed were violated.[15] Finally, there is the paradox that statistical significance may not indicate true biologic significance.

Many scientists resist the rigidity of the 0.05 p-value threshold, and it was perhaps inevitable that there would be a backlash to the wholesale reliance on them. The common abuse of significance testing has driven some of its critics to conclude that significance testing is synonymous with thoughtless decisions, and some scientific journals have reacted with increasing vehemence against their use. In 1987, for example, a dispute in the literature broke out when the prestigious and well-respected *American Journal of Public Health* solicited an editorial wherein it was suggested point blank that significance testing be purged from articles submitted for review and publication. The ensuing debate was intense [25], [26], [27], [28], [29]. Poole [30] pointed out that the mechanical, reflexive acceptance of p-values at the 0.05 level (or any other arbitrary decision rule) is the nonscientific, easy way out of critical discussion in science.

This distillation effort to reduce a complex research endeavor down to one number is perhaps at the root of the inappropriate role of significance testing. The super-condensation of the results of a research effort down to the p-value may be due to the fact that the p-value is itself constructed from several components. Sample size, effect size, and effect size variability are important pieces of the p-value and are included directly into the p-value's formulation. However, in reality, what

---

[15] This is discussed in greater detail in Chapter 2.

is produced is not a balanced measure of these important contributory components, but only a measure of the role of sampling error as a possible explanation for the results observed in the research sample. Thus, p-values are deficient by themselves in reflecting the results of a research effort, and must be supplemented with additional information (sample size, effect size, and effect size precision) in order for the study to receive a fair and balanced interpretation. These three measures (sample size, effect size, and effect size precision) are all important perspectives that the investigator must jointly consider with the p-value when interpreting research efforts.

Of course, if we are interested only in the size, accuracy, and precision[16] of an effect with no need to make a single decision about the likelihood of that effect occurring in the population, then we do not require a p-value. Other tools, such as confidence intervals, can be employed for this work, and it is to these types of tools some workers (particularly in epidemiology) have turned. However if we are faced with a dichotomous decision—"Does the therapy work or not?"—p-values serve very well when produced from a well-designed, well-executed research effort. This proper implementation precludes their use as tools for thought evasion but, more importantly, protects their function as an appropriate reflection of the community and regulatory standard for type I error rate consideration [31].

Advice to the Physician–Scientist

In the twentieth century, both epidemiology and biostatistics struggled with the correct role of mathematics in their respective fields. Against epidemiology, the criticism was leveled that the tried and true approach of direct observation would eventually be overshadowed by the use of complicated mathematical structures. On the other hand, the unjustified, blanket use of (and blind trust placed in) p-values, elevating their interpretation above other reliable evaluators of research results has troubled many scientists. The researcher may feel trapped between the pressures of epidemiology, with its emphasis on observation and deductive reasoning on the one hand, and biostatistics, with its emphasis on sampling error and mathematical modeling, on the other. The fact that some research journals refuse to accept manuscripts without p-values, while other prestigious journals refuse to accept research results accompanied by p-values deepens the conundrum.

Choosing one philosophy over the other is clearly inferior—both perspectives considered jointly will lead to the most correct interpretation of a study. This suggests that we need not choose only one philosophy, but instead that we synthesize the best elements from both.

How can this be achieved? Consider first that in sample-based research, sampling error is an important issue and must be discerned—we can rely on biostatistics for this. However, the interpretability of the experiment is enhanced and extended if the Hill tenets are embedded in the experiment's design (such as the examination of a dose–response relationship). In addition, the experiment must be well-designed, and executed according to its design (concordantly executed). Fi-

---

[16] Accuracy is a measure of how close the estimate is to the true population value. Precision is how close the estimates are to each other.

nally, the concordant clinical trial's evaluation must be based on the joint consideration of the effect size estimate and that estimate's precision, magnitude of the confidence interval width, the p-value (and, when appropriate, the power). Once we are sure that the findings of a research effort (designed with epidemiologic principles in mind) are not due to random chance, we can then use the tools of epidemiology to determine whether the findings from the study reflect merely an association, or may in fact be causative (Figure 3).

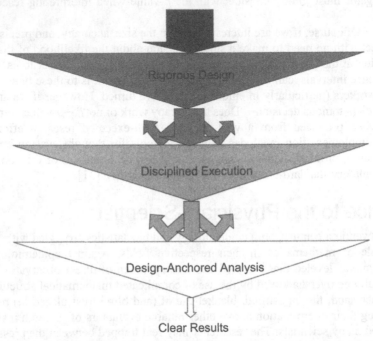

Figure 3. A well reasoned, well conducted clinical trial has the greatest chance of avoiding spurious results and producing a useful product.

References

1. MacMahon, B., Yen, S., Trichopoulos, D., Warren, K., Nardi, G. (1981). Coffee and cancer of the pancreas. *New England Journal of Medicine* **304**:630–633.
2. Kuper, H.E., Mucci, L.A., Trichopoulos, D. (2000). Coffee, pancreatic cancer and the question of causation. *Journal of Epidemiology and Community Health* **54**:650–651.
3. Brown, J., Kreiger, N., Darlington, G.A., Sloan, M. (2001). Misclassification of exposure: coffee as a surrogate for caffeine intake. *American Journal of Epidemiology* **153**:815–820.

4. Fiore, A.E., Nuorti, J.P., Levine, O.S. et al. (1998). Epidemic Legionnaires' disease two decades later: old sources, new diagnostic methods. *Clinical Infectectious Disease* **26**:426–33.
5. Kleinbaum, D.G., Kupper, L.L., Morgenstern, H. (1982). *Epidemiologic Research. Principles and Quantitative Methods*. New York, Van Nostrand Reinhold.
6. Stigler, S.M. (1986). *The History of Statistics—The Measurement of Uncertainty Before 1900*. Cambridge, MA, and London. The Belknap Press of Harvard University Press, p. 4.
7. Hill, A.B. (1965). The environment and disease: Association or causation? *Proceedings of the Royal Society of Medicine* **58**:295–300.
8. Young, A. (1771). *A Course of Experimental Agriculture*. Dublin, Exshaw et al.
9. Owen D.B. (1976) *On the History of Probability and Statistics*. New York and Basal. Marcel Dekker.
10. Beeson, P.B., McDermott, W., Wyngarrden, J.B. (1979). *Cecil Textbook of Medicine* Philadelphia, PA. W.B. Saunders Company. pp. 256–257.
11. Fisher, R.A. (1925). *Statistical Methods for Research Workers* Oliver and Boyd, Edinburg.
12. Fisher, R.A. (1933). The arrangement of field experiments. *Journal of the Ministry of Agriculture* 503–513.
13. Todhunder, L.A. (1949). *History of the Mathematical Theory of Probability,* New York. Else.
14. Berkson, J. (1942). Experiences with tests of significance. A reply to R.A. Fisher. *Journal of the American Statistical Association* **37**: 242–246.
15. Berkson, J. (1942). Tests of significance considered as evidence. *Journal of the American Statistical Association.***37**:335–345.
16. Fisher, R.A. (1942). Response to Berkson. *Journal of the American Statistical Association.***37**:103–104.
17. Birnbaum, A. (1962). On the foundations of statistical inference. *Journal of the American Statistical Association.***57**: 269–306.
18. Edwards, A. (1972). *Likelihood.* Cambridge, UK: Cambridge University Press.
19. Lenz, W. (1962). Thalidomide and congenital abnormalities. *Lancet* 1:45.
20. Pepall, J. (1997). *Methyl Mercury Poisoning: the Minamata Bay disaster*. International Development Research Centre, Ottawa, Canada.
21. Goodman, S.N. (1999). Toward Evidence–Based Medical Statistics. 1: The p-value fallacy. *Annals of Internal Medicine* **130**:995–1004.
22. Gigerenzer, G., Swijtink, Z., Porter, T., Dasxton, L., Beatty, J., Kruger, L. (1989). *The Empire of Chance*. Cambridge, Cambridge University Press.
23. Pocock, R.J., Farewell, V.T. (1996). Multiplicity consideration in the design and analysis of clinical trials. *Journal of the Royal Statistical Society A* **159**: 93–110.
24. Anonymous (1988). Evidence of cause and effect relationship in major epidemiologic study disputed by a judge. *Epidemiology Monitor* **9**:1.

25. Walker, A.M. (1986). Significance tests [sic] represent consensus and standard practice (Letter). *American Journal of Public Health* **76**:1033. (See also journal erratum **76**:1087.

26. Fleiss, J.L. (1986). Significance tests have a role in epidemiologic research; reactions to A.M. Walker. (different views) *American Journal of Public Health.***76**:559–560.

27. Fleiss, J.L. (1986). Dr. Fleiss response (Letter) *American Journal of Public Health.* **76**:1033–1034.

28. Walker, A.M. (1986). Reporting the results of epidemiologic studies. *American Journal of Public Health.***76**:556–558.

29. Thompson, W.D. (1987). Statistical criteria in the interpretation of epidemiologic data (different views) *American Journal of Public Health* **77**:191–194.

30. Poole, C. (1987). Beyond the confidence interval. *American Journal of Public Health* **77**:195–199.

31. Moyé, L.A. (2000). *Statistical Reasoning in Medicine: The Intuitive P-Value Primer*. New York, Springer.

Chapter 1

Fundamentals of Clinical Trial Design

In this chapter, a brief review is provided of the important fundamentals of clinical trial design and analysis that will be required for our subsequent discussions of the multiple analysis issue. The random selection of subjects from the population and the random allocation of therapy is covered. A discussion of the need to blind both patients and investigators to a patient's therapy assignment and the need for a Data and Safety Monitoring Committee is followed by a brief review of interim monitoring procedures that have become so popular in clinical trials. Finally, the effect of sampling errors in clinical trials is developed. Type I and type II errors are defined and the purpose of the sample size computation is reviewed.

1.1 The Definition of a Clinical Trial

The concept of clinical experimentation is not new; experiments have been carried out on humans for hundreds of years.[1] However, this tool was invigorated in the twentieth century through the persistent, patient work of a single epidemiologist— Sir Austin Bradford Hill. Early in the twentieth century, clinical research was restricted, by and large, to case reports and case series (Appendix A). However, in the 1940s, randomization procedures directly applicable to the conduct of healthcare research became available [1]. It was at this time that Hill combined an indispensable feature of laboratory experiments, the control group, with a tool that had been largely exploited in non-medical and agricultural research—the random assignment of the intervention. The joint incorporation of these features into a clinical experiment, produced the first randomized clinical trial [2]. The implementation of this randomization device has both improved the interpretability and increased the controversy of modern clinical experimentation.

The modern clinical trial is an investigational tool that creates a unique research environment. Within it, the simple demonstration of a clinically and statistically significant strength of association between the randomly allocated intervention and the prospectively defined primary endpoint implies that there is a causal relationship between the two. This is a very special situation, and can only be successfully constructed with, (1) a clear statement of the clinical question, (2) a simultaneous focus on epidemiologic and biostatistical principles, and (3) disciplined research execution. Commonly, a clinical trial is an experiment in health care in which an intervention believed to be of benefit to a population is administered in a well-defined fashion so that patients in one group (designated the active

---

[1] The work of James Lind on the *HMS Salisbury* described in the Prologue is an example of a clinical experiment.

group) will receive the intervention while patients in a second group (called the control group) do not. In some circumstances the control group receives only placebo therapy. In situations when it is unethical to withhold therapy, the patients in the control group will receive a competing active therapy.

The advantages of clinical trials have been well established, and information about their goals and interpretations have entered the lay press [3]. Clinical trials can be of all sizes. In the early phases of a drug development program, a clinical trial may contain no more than 50 patients. Sometimes, however, clinical trials are immense, recruiting tens of thousands of subjects. Often these patients are followed for many years, during which time information concerning the benefits and adverse effects of the intervention is collected.

There are several comprehensive references that discuss in detail the methodology of clinical trials, most notably [4], [5], and [6]. This chapter provides a brief overview of the salient issues in clinical trials, serving as a preamble for the discussion of multiple analyses that is the main subject of this text.

1.2 Principles of Randomization

Randomization is a hallmark of modern experimental design. It received considerable attention from Fisher's early research work in agriculture. However, its use in clinical trials did not start until Hill's developmental work. Although its propriety in clinical experiments is still debated, randomization has had a major impact on the development of clinical trials.

In clinical trials, there are typically two levels of randomization that may be used. The first is the random selection of subjects from the population. The second is the random allocation of the experimental intervention. Each of these two levels of randomization has a different goal.

1.2.1 Random Selection of Subjects from the Population

The random selection of subjects from the larger population is not a chaotic or haphazard process. Despite the use of the word "random" the incorporation of this procedure within a clinical trial is well planned and organized. In the idealized clinical trial setting, the goal of the simple random sampling plan is to ensure that every subject in the population has the same, constant probability of being selected for the research sample. However, this worthy goal is seldom if ever achieved.

The simple random sampling mechanism is the best way to ensure that the research sample represents the population at large, and that some findings in the sample can be generalized to the population from which the sample was obtained.[2] There have been several adaptations of the simple random sampling plan that deal with unique and special circumstances (e.g., when there is a concern on the part of the investigators that patients with a certain characteristic of interest will be underrepresented). However, these alterations must be considered very carefully, because

---

[2] We will have much more to say about this generalization process in Chapter 2.

deviations from the simple random sampling schema run the risk of generating a research sample that is not representative of the population.

In addition, the random selection of subjects from the population creates in the sample the property of statistical independence. Statistical independence is the characteristic that permits the multiplication of probabilities that is so useful in the construction of both parameter estimators and test statistics.

1.2.2 Random Allocation of Therapy

In addition, a second level of randomization is critical in clinical trials. This is the random allocation of therapy. As opposed to the random selection of subjects from the population (a process that produced the research sample), the random allocation of therapy occurs within the research sample itself. The simplist application of this device requires that each subject in the sample has the same probability of receiving the intervention. This procedure is intended to effectively decouple the use of the intervention from any patient characteristics. This decoupling in turn allows the effect seen between the active and control groups at the end of the clinical trial to be attributed to the use of the intervention.

This point requires further elaboration. Two important features that lead to the successful interpretation of a positive clinical trial are (1) the identification of an effect at the conclusion of the study, and (2) the attribution of that effect to the therapy that the trial was designed to evaluate. For example, consider a clinical trial that is designed to determine the effect of a therapy to reduce the total mortality rate among patients who have suffered a stroke. All patients who are recruited into the study receive state of the art therapy for their stroke. In addition, some patients received the active therapy while other patients receive an inactive placebo. The investigators follow these patients to the end of the study, carefully counting deaths, and, at the study's conclusion, identify a clinically and statistically different reduction in the total mortality rate observed in the active group. These researchers have completed one part of their mission—they have identified an effect. They now must persuasively argue that the effect is due to the therapy the study was designed to assess.

How can the investigators be sure that the effect observed in their trial is due to the therapy? The only way we have to ensure this is that the two groups must resemble each other in every way and facet except the therapy (control therapy versus intervention therapy). This is what the random allocation of therapy accomplishes. By creating the environment in which the only difference between patients who receive the intervention and those who did not is the intervention itself, the attribution of the reduction in the total mortality to the intervention is clear.

However, the random allocation of therapy also strengthens the interpretation of a clinical trial when the difference in event rates between the two groups is small. In the previous example of a clinical trial that has a control and intervention group and is designed to measure the effect of the intervention on the cumulative total mortality rate, assume now that the difference between the mortality rates for the two groups is disappointingly small. However, this finding may not imply that the therapy was ineffective. For example, if in the absence of randomization, patients in the active group had a greater severity of disease and consequent poorer prognosis than did patients in the control group, then the positive effect of therapy could be overshadowed by the harmful effect of the severity of illness.

The random allocation of therapy all but assures us that characteristics that influence mortality have the same distribution in each of the two groups of patients and will have no more influence in one group than in the other. Since the influences of these characteristics are balanced, they would not blur our view of the effect of the randomly allocated therapy.

It is difficult to overestimate the importance of the random allocation of therapy. Use of this tool not only protects the experiment from the influences of factors known to affect the outcome, but also protects against unidentified influences. This is because the random assignment of therapy does not depend on any characteristic of the individuals. When randomization fails to correct for a variable (such as age), there are techniques that are available that can adjust the analysis for differences produced by the different distribution of age in each of the arms of the trial. However, in randomized experiments, adjusted results will rarely differ markedly from unadjusted results.[3] The random allocation of therapy is a design feature that, when embedded in an experiment, leads to the clearest attribution of that therapy's effect [7].

Large clinical trials attempt to take advantage of both of these levels of randomization. Undoubtedly, the researchers conducting the experiments have little difficulty incorporating the random allocation of the experimental intervention into their study. Proven randomization algorithms are required to be in place at the beginning of the trial, assuring the investigators that every patient who is accepted into the research sample must have their treatment randomly allocated. In addition, once researchers randomize patients, examinations of baseline characteristics in each of the randomized groups are thoroughly reviewed, ensuring that demographic characteristics, morbidity characteristics, and results of laboratory assays are distributed equally across the two groups. These procedures and safeguards ensure that the treatment groups are the same with respect to all other characteristics, traits, and measures.

Unlike the random allocation of therapy, the random selection of subjects from the population in these randomized clinical trials is generally not achieved. It is true that large clinical experiments randomize patients from many different clinical centers. These centers represent different regions of a country, different countries on a continent, and sometimes different continents. This widespread recruitment effort is an attempt to be as inclusive as possible, and the investigators hope that this recruitment process results in an acceptable approximation of this random selection mechanism. However, it must be admitted that this selection mechanism is not random.

One impediment to the random selection of subjects from the population in these large clinical studies is the use of exclusion criteria. Patients who are intolerant of the intervention cannot be included in the study. A patient who is already in one other study cannot be accepted into another trial. Subjects who have life-

---

[3] See the Glidel example in Chapter 2 for an informative counterexample.

threatening illnesses are often excluded as well.[4] Patients who are unlikely to be able to follow the compliance criteria of the experiment (patients who cannot take the intervention consistently or patients who refuse to adhere to a tight schedule of follow-up visits) are commonly prohibited from the study. These exclusion criteria may be necessary for the successful execution of the trial, but each new exclusion criterion weakens the argument that simple random sampling generated the research sample.[5] Thus, although large clinical trials are successful at randomly allocating therapy, they are not so successful in the random selection of subjects from the population [8].

1.2.3 Stratified Randomization

Although the random allocation of an intervention in a clinical trial should produce the same distribution of patient characteristics in each of the two treatment groups (e.g., the same percentage of males in the active and control groups) the desired equal distribution is not ensured. If an imbalance in the use of the therapy occurs on the characteristic of interest, the investigators may not be able to gain a fair appraisal of the drug's efficacy in patients with that trait since, for example, the drug may have been used in more patients with the characteristic than in those without the characteristic.

In order to guarantee that the use of therapy is balanced on a trait of great interest to the investigators, the trial designers can alter the randomization procedure requiring that it now balance the distribution of the drug within each of the levels (or strata) of the patient trait of interest. As an illustration, consider a clinical trial whose goal is to assess the effect of a calcium channel blocking agent on the cumulative incidence rate of congestive heart failure (CHF). There are two types of heart failure in which the investigators are interested: ischemic CHF and non-ischemic CHF. In this setting, stratified randomization is the process that ensures that there are equal numbers of patients assigned to the calcium channel blocking agent as there are to placebo within the stratum of patients who have ischemic cardiomyopathy, and similarly for those patients with nonischemic cardiomyopathy. The equal distribution of patients in these two strata allows a balanced examination of the effect of the calcium channel blocker within each of the two heart failure strata.

1.3 The Use of Blinding

As we stated in the previous section, the motivation for the use of the random allocation of therapy in a clinical trial is to ensure that the only difference between

---

[4] An unfortunate patient who has terminal pancreatic cancer with less than 1 year to live is unlikely to be randomized to a 5-year trial assessing the role of cholesterol reduction therapy in reducing the number of heart attacks, even if the patient has met all other criteria for the trial.

[5] Nonrandomized, observational studies can sometimes do a better job than their counterpart clinical trials in randomly selecting subjects from the population. However, these observational studies are rarely able to randomly allocate exposure in their attempt to assess the relationship between exposure and disease.

subjects who receive the intervention to be studied and those who do not is the therapy itself. Thus, at the time of therapy assignment (commonly referred to as the baseline), the distribution of all patient characteristics (e.g., demographics, lifestyle, previous medical history, and physical examination findings) are the same between the two groups; the two groups of patients are equivalent except for the therapy exposure.

Unfortunately, beginning a clinical trial with equivalent patient groups does not guarantee that the trial will end with this equivalence property intact. If the investigators are to be assured that any difference that is seen between the active group and the control group at the end of the trial can be ascribed to the randomly allocated therapy, the two groups of patients must not only have equivalent characteristics at the baseline; the patients must also have equivalent experiences during the study.

Ensuring this equivalent post-randomization experience can be difficult to accomplish, especially when the patient and/or the physician know the identity of the medication that the patient is taking. Therefore a sequence of procedures has been developed that increases the likelihood that patients will have equivalent experiences during the course of the clinical trial. These procedures are called masks, or blinds. Clinical trials are most commonly either single-blinded, or double-blinded.

1.3.1 Single-Blinded Trials

If a patient knows that she is on placebo therapy, she may believe that her condition is more likely to deteriorate than to improve. This patient may adjust other medication she is taking based on her belief in the ineffectiveness of the study medication. This idea that her condition is worsening can color her reports to the trial investigators about her health, leading her to provide relatively negative quality of life reports and self-assessments. If this conviction takes root in the majority of patients on inactive therapy, the investigators might conclude that the placebo experience is less satisfactory than it actually is.

On the other hand, patients who know that they were assigned to active therapy may be inclined to believe the therapy is helping them (after all, why would the physicians test this medication if there wasn't some feeling among experts in the medical community that the medication would be beneficial?). These patients believe that they are on a positive therapy, and that they will have a resultant positive experience. This belief has its own invigorating effect; if the compound is indeed beneficial, then the actual benefit can be amplified by the patient's conviction that she is improving. If the compound is actually not effective at all (i.e., just like placebo), then this positive belief system can produce its own salubrious effect; an effect that would be mistakenly attributed to the ineffective product.

The influence of these belief systems is strong; if left unchecked, their presence will blur the investigator's view of the therapy's true effect. In order to counterbalance the influence of these belief systems, investigators instituted single-blind trials in which patients were not informed of their therapy assignment. In these single-blind studies, patients do not know whether they are on active therapy or placebo therapy.

It is important to understand that the institution of the single-blind does not keep the individual patient from guessing the identity of their therapy. The single-blind therefore does not block the ignition of the belief system, nor does it stop the generation of its effects within the patient (positive effects if the patient believes that they are on active therapy, negative effects if the patient believes that they are on placebo therapy)—the single-blind procedure distributes these effects. Without knowing the therapy on which they are placed, the patient's ability to guess the therapy identity is dispersed throughout both treatment groups. The effect of the belief system, rather than being concentrated in one treatment group, is randomly distributed throughout the entire recruited cohort.

1.3.2 Double-Blind Studies

In the previous section, the difficulties produced by the knowledge that a patient has about the identity of their assigned study medication in a clinical trial were described. However, physician knowledge of the medication that the patient is taking can also skew the objective evaluation of the effect of the therapy. Physicians commonly agree to be a participant in these studies because they have feelings (sometimes strong feelings) about the effect of the compound that is being studied. These strong feelings can influence the way a physician treats a patient during the course of the study. Such motivations may govern the efforts of physicians to (1) insist that the patient be compliant with their medication, and (2) express to the patient the importance of returning for all of the scheduled follow-up visits that the clinical trial requires.

In addition, doctors may choose to use other concomitant medications much more aggressively in patients who do not receive active therapy. At the end of the follow-up period, these physicians may seek out adverse outcomes more thoroughly from patients who are randomized to the treatment group of the trial that they believe is ineffective and/or produces more side-effects. Each of these maneuvers can adversely affect the assessment of the therapy's influence. In order to distribute these effects randomly among the physicians who treat patients in the study, these physicians are blocked from knowing the medication that their patient is taking. Studies in which neither the physician nor the patient know the effect of the therapy are known as double-blind trials.

Double-blind studies can be difficult to sustain because of the known effects of the medication that are not mimicked by placebo therapy. In a study designed to assess the effect of the angiotensin converting enzyme inhibitor (ACE-i) captopril on reducing the total mortality rate in patients who have CHF [9], patients were randomized to receive either captopril therapy or placebo therapy. After randomization, patients were to be followed for approximately 3 years. However, during the follow-up period physicians involved in treating these patients noted that many of them developed a dry cough unrelated to smoking, seasonal allergic rhinitis, or any other obvious etiology. This so-called "captopril cough" not only threatened to unbind the identity of the study medication to the physician, but threatened to undermine study compliance with the medication since patients were starting to resist taking the drug. This issue was addressed by permitting physicians to decrease the administered dose of study medication in patients who were complaining of cough, temporarily alleviating the troublesome cough, with the hope that they could reinstitute the higher dose at a later time.

If the blinding is to work, the investigators must sometimes go to great lengths to ensure that the identity of the therapy cannot be deduced by its physical appearance. As an illustration of this experience, consider the Treatment of Lead in Children (TLC) trial [10]. This clinical trial recruited children who had been identified as having moderately elevated blood lead levels. The TLC trial instituted the following interventions. First, the houses of each of these children was subjected to a complete lead abatement action[6]. In addition, half of the children were given placebo therapy, and the second half were provided succimer, a lead chelating agent. The clinical hypothesis was that the combination of reduced environmental lead exposure and succimer would have a more beneficial effect on a child's cognitive development than just environmental changes alone.

TLC was designed to blind the identity of the therapy. Thus, the appearances of the placebo and active therapy pills were identical, as were the bottles in which the pills were delivered. However, the nauseating sulfur-enriched odor emanating from some of the bottles permitted an immediate and correct identification of the identity of the active drug, effectively unbinding the therapy assignment. The investigators labored over what to do about this problem since the odor-induced unbinding would block an objective assessment of the effect of therapy. They solved this problem by asking the workers that bottled the study drug to place in the bottom of each bottle a tiny fabric strip that had been exposed to the odiferous sulfur compound. Now, when the bottles were opened in clinic, they would each emit the same odor. They would all reek together!

1.3.3 Arthroscopy and the Art of the Double-Blind

A fine example of (1) the need to maintain that a double-blind in a clinical trial and (2) the lengths to which investigators must go to preserve the double-blind property of a clinical trial is the evaluation of the use of arthroscopic surgery as a tool for relieving the pain and disability associated with osteoarthritis of the knee.

Osteoarthritis of the knee is the result of the chronic strain, weight and stresses placed on this joint from its continual use into and through middle age. Early in life, the knee joint is an example of mechanical efficiency. The distal femoral and proximal tibial surfaces approach each other but do not actually touch, separated by a synovial cavity, itself lined by smooth cartilage and filled with clear synovial fluid. The anterior surface of the joint is protected by the knee cap, the underside of which is lined with cartilage as well. In this environment, the articular surfaces continually glide past each other as the joint flexes and extends. Bone to bone contact is prevented by the presence of the synovial cavity, which acts as a separating buffer zone. The tibial surface therefore sweeps smoothly and easily under the femur.

---

[6] This program consisted of home repainting, replacing old carpets with new carpets, complete home cleaning, and any other environmental changes known to reduce lead exposure in the home's interior.

These mechanics are disrupted by injury and continued use of the joint. Over the course of time, the cartilage, which is consistently and continually worn down by daily joint use, is no longer able to generate new and fully functional cartilage in smooth sheets, but instead produces poorly formed, rough and irregular cartilage. Pieces of cartilage can separate from the synovial membrane. This separated wedge of cartilage can leave sensitive bone uncovered while the cartilage fragment itself floats freely within the synovial cavity. Exposed bone can produce an inflammatory response that, rather than protecting the joint, causes more damage as additional cartilage is dissolved by the release of caustic and lytic enzymes onto the articular surface. Irregularities can develop in the bone underlying the cartilage as well, and new bone growths (called spurs or osteophytes) can push their way into the joint space, squeezing the synovial cavity and reducing the volume of space through which the end of the bone moves. The cumulative result of this process is to convert what was an efficient, functional, buffered joint cavity into an irregular, sharply contoured, debris-filled pseudo-space in which bone movement is restricted, jerky, and irregular. The result is painful swelling and immobility.

To relieve this discomfort, patients commonly resorted to surgery. Under arthroscopic examination, surgeons will perform lavage, which is the removal of unattached macroscopic fragments of cartilage and visualized crystals. In addition, the articular surface will be smoothed, inflamed cartilage is removed, and bone spurs are filed down. This is known as dèbridement. The goal of lavage and dèbridement is to attempt to reproduce a healthier joint, and thereby provide greater use of the knee without the limiting pain and discomfort.

Historical and anecdotal evidence suggested that lavage and dèbridement produced a favorable outcome for the osteoarthritic knee. In order to accurately measure this benefit, several randomized clinical trials were carried out. In these studies, patients randomized to the active group received the arthroscopic surgery, while those in the control group did not. In these studies, patients who received the dèbridement/lavage procedure reported a greater improvement in pain than patients who were in the control group. However, in these studies, it was impossible to separate the effect of the lavage and dèbridement from the influence of the belief that surgery (regardless of what was done during the surgery) would produce an improvement.

In order to address this issue, Moseley et al. [11] carried out a randomized, double-blind, controlled clinical trial on 180 patients who suffer from osteoarthritis of the knee. In order to be recruited into the study, patients had to have at least moderate knee pain despite maximal medical management for at least 6 months, and could not have undergone knee arthroscopy during the previous 2 years. Patients who met all of the entry criteria of this clinical trial were randomly assigned to undergo either arthroscopic lavage and dèbridement, arthroscopic lavage alone, or a placebo procedure. This placebo procedure included a short active intravenous tranquilizer, an opioid, and spontaneous respiration of oxygen-enriched air. Then a standard arthroscopic dèbridement procedure was simulated. Three 1-cm incisions were made in the skin. The surgeon requested instruments and manipulated the knee as though actual arthroscopic surgery was being executed, to the point were saline was harmlessly splashed in a container to simulate the sound of lavage. The patient was kept in the operating room for the standard time and remained in the hospital for the night of the procedure. Post operative care was provided by personnel who were blinded to the therapy assignment.

To assess the effectiveness of this sham surgery in maintaining the blind of the trial, patients were asked if they had experienced the actual surgery or the sham surgery. Patients in the placebo group were no more likely than patients in the dèbridement/lavage and lavage group to correctly identify the procedure that they had undergone, a finding that demonstrated the impact of the blinding procedure.

The primary endpoint of the study was pain assessment at 24 months post surgery. At the conclusion of the trial, the investigators discovered that pain relief was effectively the same between the three groups. Furthermore, at no point during the follow-up period did either the dèbridement/lavage or the lavage group have significantly greater pain relief than those patients who underwent the sham surgery. While there have been several criticisms of this trial, even the critics say that, despite their current popularity, this study has demonstrated that lavage and dèbridement are not very effective for the treatment of most patients with osteoarthritis of the knee [12].

1.4 Interim Monitoring of Clinical Trials

While the effective use of double-blind clinical trial methodology, in concert with the random allocation of therapy, addresses the important issue of attribution of effect in a clinical trial, the implementation of the double-blind technique produces a new problem for the execution of the study. When the investigators design a clinical trial, they first carry out an evaluation of how long it will take them to execute the study. This plan is based on the rate at which they expect to see endpoint events. For example, the investigators may choose to do the final analysis on the cumulative mortality rate at 5 years, anticipating that it will take that long for the effect of therapy on the total mortality rate to emerge in a convincing way. The investigators also appropriately agree to forego the final analyses until the end of the trial. By waiting until the end of the study, the investigators appropriately choose to ignore the random eddies in the data generated by the play of chance that occur as the trial proceeds. These transient trends, appearing and disappearing as the follow-up time progresses, are best set aside since they portray only the random aggregation of data and are not representative of the population at large.

1.4.1 The Need for Trial Monitoring

This is a well-conceived execution plan, but this procedure is based on the assumption that patients must be followed for 5 years before the beneficial therapy effect is persuasively demonstrated. If the trial produces an unanticipated and overwhelmingly beneficial effect as early as 1 year into the study, then the investigators would not know of this early effect until the study has ended after 5 years of follow-up. In this scenario, the trial will have been continued for 4 unnecessary years because the investigators, being "blind" to therapy, would also be "blind" to the effect of therapy. Thus, their dedication to continuing the trial to the end, in concert with the incorporation of the double-blind property, places the investigators in precisely the wrong position to observe this early beneficial effect.

In order to permit the observation of the effect of therapy that may appear early in the trial, while at the same time ensuring the double-blind property remains intact, the trial investigators often create a Data Safety and Monitoring Board (DSMB). This is a relatively small collection of august scientists who have particular expertise in the clinical question the trial is addressing. This distinguished group of scientists commonly includes clinicians, clinical researchers, methodologists (biostatisticians or epidemiologists), and sometimes, an ethicist. The charge of this group is to review all of the data in an unblinded fashion[7] and to determine if either an early therapeutic triumph or early therapeutic catastrophe has occurred.

The mandate of the DSMB has expanded in recent years to review not just the effect of therapy but to examine other barometers of the trial's status as well. It is not uncommon now for DSMBs to review the progress of patient recruitment, to be notified of protocol violations, and to ensure that the statistical and epidemiologic assumptions that underlie the sample size computation are correct. This group then makes recommendations to the investigators and the sponsors of the study concerning the clinical trial's status. It is the responsibility of this group to ensure that the trial is executed according to its protocol and to be on the alert for early signs of therapeutic benefit or harm.

To aid in this review, methodologists have developed statistical monitoring rules that provide an assessment of the early effect of therapy, while simultaneously incorporating the considerable variability associated with the estimate of this early therapy effect. This monitoring rule is a device which is generally established before the trial begins recruiting patients. This guideline specifies how large the test statistic will be allowed to become before the trial is stopped. For this reason, these rules are commonly referred to as stopping rules. However, there are many other considerations that the DSMB must evaluate before the clinical trial is discontinued prematurely. In addition to the magnitude of the test statistic, the merits of the treatment, the availability of alternative treatments, the seriousness of the condition being treated, the clinical importance of the observed difference, and the consistency of the results with the findings of other researchers must all be assessed. Based on careful review of all these considerations, the DSMB will make a recommendation (either continuation or early termination) regarding the safe conduct of the study. Thus the statistical criteria for the early termination of a study are best referred to as *monitoring guidelines*.

1.4.2 Test Statistic Trajectories

Statisticians have developed monitoring guidelines that assist DSMBs in deciding whether a clinical trial should be continued or prematurely terminated. These guidelines are commonly classified into two groups. The first group falls under the rubric of *group sequential procedures*; the second and newer method is termed *condi-*

---

[7] Sometimes even the DSMB is blinded to the identity of the therapy effects. In this "triple-blind study," the DSMB sees the results categorized not as active versus control group findings but, instead, as "Group A" and "Group B."

tional power. Both are easy to conceptualize but can involve some difficult computations. However, since we are simply concerned with the underlying motivations and basic concepts of these useful tools, we will be sure not to lose ourselves in the mathematics.

Let's begin our examination of the concept of monitoring rules with an elementary consideration of the behavior of the test statistic over the course of a clinical trial. Consider, for example, a clinical trial that is designed to test the effect of a therapy that the investigators believe will reduce the cumulative mortality rate in patients with diabetes mellitus. Patients are recruited into the study and then randomized to receive either the control group therapy or the active agent. An equal number of patients are randomized into each group. Appropriately, the test statistic that is designed to be computed at the end of the trial will compare the total mortality rate of the patients randomized to the active therapy to that of the patients who are randomized to control group therapy. Suppose, however, that you have a unique vantage point; you are in a position to compute the test statistic every single day of the trial, plotting its value as a function of time.

What would this plot look like? At the beginning of the study, when no follow-up time has accrued, and there have been no deaths among the small number of randomized participants, the value of the test statistic is zero. However, as more patients are recruited into the study, they accrue follow-up time, experience the effects and consequences of their disease, suffer inevitable morbidity and, ultimately, death. As they die and these deaths are reported to you, the test statistic immediately begins to register the effect of these events. If the total mortality rate is lower in the active group, the test statistic will be positive. Alternatively, the test statistic becomes negative when there are more deaths in the active group than there are in the control group. Thus the test statistic will begin to move away from zero. However, deaths in this sample are not very predictable; in fact, they occur randomly during the follow-up period, and they will commonly cluster. If there has been a recent sequence of deaths in the placebo group, the test statistic will inch its way upward. If a recent cluster of deaths occurred among patients in the active group, the test statistic will decrease, perhaps becoming negative. Thus, the test statistic will wander, with upward movements followed by downward excursions (Figure 1.1).

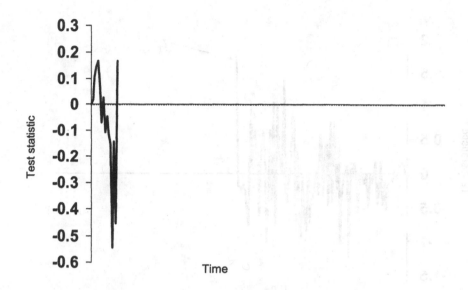

Figure 1.1. Starting to track the random movement of a test statistic over time in a clinical trial.

Imagine the response of the investigators to this preliminary information portrayed in Figure 1.1. These scientists might have difficulty restraining their enthusiasm for the salubrious effect of the active therapy upon the very early evaluation of the test statistic as it crept upward. However, their zeal rapidly evaporates as the test statistic follows its early increase with a prompt reversal and slide to negative values, responding to a spate of deaths that occur in the treatment group. This decline is followed by an upsurge in the test statistic, an increase attributable to more deaths among those patients who were randomized to the control group.

This unpredictable movement of the test statistic is one of the causes of the conundrum a DSMB faces during its deliberations concerning whether a trial should be permitted to continue or be terminated prematurely. Since the excursions of the test statistic are unpredictable, the possibility always exists that its future excursions would reveal that the DSMB drew a wrong and premature conclusion. For example, consider the circumstance of a DSMB asked to make a decision to prematurely halt a clinical trial based on the observed test statistic thus far (Figure 1.2). At the point in time that the DSMB is deliberating (time t_1) the test statistic appears to reach its zenith, with the evidence suggesting that there is not only a beneficial effect of therapy, but an effect that suggests that the trial should end early (Figure 1.2).

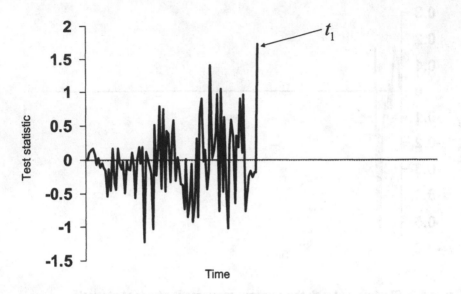

Figure 1.2. The random movement of a test statistic over time in a clinical trial with no treatment effect.

However, when we add the subsequent test statistic excursions (excursions that would not have been observable if the DSMB had decided to terminate the trial at time t_1), the value of the test statistic at time t_1 which appeared to be so suggestive is seen to be merely one random occurrence that was never repeated (Figure 1.3). In fact, if the experiment had been allowed to proceed to its planned end, the conclusion would have been that there is no beneficial effect of therapy on the total mortality rate at all.

If there is no long-term effect of the active therapy, then there will be no long-term reduction (or increase) in the active group event rate. In this situation, the only influence on the test statistic is the random occurrence of deaths which occur unevenly but at equal rates in each of the two groups, excursions that can be all of misleading. Therefore, excursions of the test statistic above zero are matched by movement of the test statistic below zero. Thus, although at any given time the test statistic may appear to be different from zero, if one were to observe the test statistic's excursion over the course of the trial, it would be seen that the excursions above zero are as likely as excursions below zero. It would be easy to identify a time point at which the test statistic is positive, suggesting a beneficial effect of therapy. However, it is equally easy to choose a point in time during which the test statistic is negative, suggesting a harmful effect of therapy.

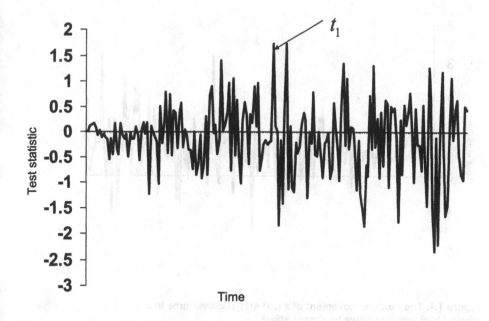

Figure 1.3. The random movement of a test statistic over time in a clinical trial with no treatment effect.

There are other possible scenarios that are worthy of consideration as well. If the therapy has a beneficial effect, it will reduce the number of deaths in the active group, an impact that will drive the test statistic in the positive direction. If we were to plot the trajectory of the test statistic over time in this circumstance, the test statistic will climb to a point above zero. However, the random occurrence of events in the trial will not allow this test statistic's path to be a smooth one. There will also be periods of time during which the test statistic will decrease due to the random aggregation of events, e.g., the unpredictable occurrence of a cluster of deaths of patients randomized to the treatment group. In this case, we say that the test statistic, while still continuing its up-and-down oscillations, will drift upward away from zero. The force and direction of the drift are commensurate with the treatment effect (Figure 1.4).

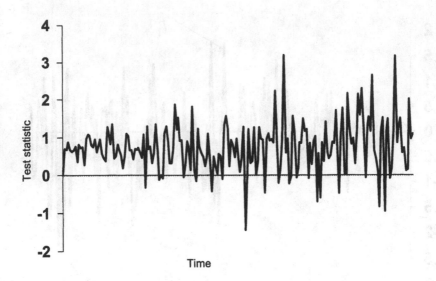

Figure 1.4. The random movement of a test statistic over time in a clinical trial with a positive treatment effect.

If, on the other hand, increased mortality is the result of therapy, the test statistic will move below zero and, for the most part, remain below zero (Figure 1.5).

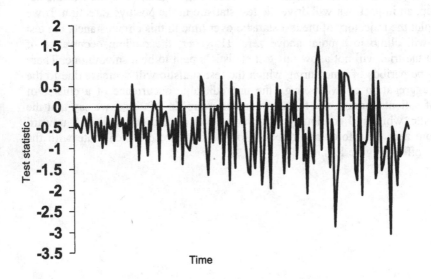

Figure 1.5. The random movement of a test statistic over time in a clinical trial with a harmful treatment effect.

These illustrations suggest that the monitoring process will involve an analysis of the movement that a test statistic undergoes over time. Classical biostatistics are of little use in this sophisticated evaluation, and as clinical trial methodology has expanded to consider this problem, it has borrowed from the deeper regions of probability theory to assemble a discipline that we may call "test statistic trajectory analysis."

1.4.3 Group Sequential Procedures

The first very useful set of stopping rules statisticians have developed are called *group sequential procedures*. Consider a clinical trial that assigns patients to one of two treatments over time. The investigators prospectively agree to monitor the test statistic as the trial progresses. The relevant question for the investigators is how large should the test statistic be in order to justify an early trial termination. The group sequential procedures will tell the investigators, if they choose to stop the trial at some time *t*, before the trial ends, how likely they will be to make a type I error. The specific steps are as follows:

Step 1: Calculate the test statistic at this point in the study
Step 2: If the test statistic is too large, then stop the trial in favor of treatment 1. If the test statistic is too small, then stop the trial in favor of the other treatment.
Step 3: If the test statistic is not in these regions, continue the trial until the next testing period.

Thus, group sequential procedures construct a boundary for the test statistic at each monitoring point in the clinical trial for the investigators. If the test statistic at any of these points is larger than the boundary at that point in time, we say that the monitoring rule suggests the trial should be stopped. Group sequential procedures are a mixture of trajectory analysis (they compute the likelihood that the test statistic would have followed the path it did if there was no treatment effect), and classical statistics (the answer is in terms of type I error rates).

Rules such as those of Lans–DeMets are very popular group sequential procedures [13], [14]. These guidelines are easy to implement and quite intuitive. Consideration of the problem posed by stopping a clinical trial early suggests that if the trial is to be stopped very early the evidence for benefit (or harm) must be overwhelming. We would therefore expect the boundary for the test statistic to be far from zero early in the trial and to get smaller as the trial progresses. Group sequential procedures produce boundary points in such a way that the overall α error rate of the trial is maintained below the maximum level (e.g., 0.05) that the investigators set.

As an example of the implementation of a group sequential procedure, consider a controlled clinical trial which is designed to evaluate the effect of therapy on the total mortality endpoint event rate. The study will have two arms, a control arm and a therapy arm. The experiment will be double-blinded and will have a DSMB in place. This DSMB decides that it will monitor the effect of therapy during the course of the study by evaluating the test statistic at each of five interim points. In order to assist in this effort, and recognizing that these multiple evaluations will have to be disciplined by the presence of prospective guidelines for the test statistic's evaluation, the DSMB chooses to be guided by a group sequential procedure (Table 1.1).

Table 1.1. Type I error at each of five monitoring points during a clinical trial using a group sequential procedure rule.

Monitoring point	Type I error allocation
1	0.0001
2	0.0010
3	0.0060
4	0.0160
5	0.0320

The total type I error expended is 0.05.

Table 1.1 provides the type I error rate threshold that will be used to assess each of the five interim evaluations of the effect of therapy on the total mortality rate. For example, in order to stop the trial early, the results of the first test statistic must produce a p-value of less than 0.0001. For every succeeding analysis, as the quantity of information about the effect of therapy increases, the type I error rate allocation increases. The final evaluation at the conclusion of the trial permits a type I error rate allocation of 0.032. This is less than the traditional level of 0.05 because, rather than allocate a type I error rate of 0.05 level for one and only one evaluation at the end of the clinical trial, the group sequential procedure allocates the error rate over the trial's duration. Thus the total alpha error rate expended over the course of the trial is 0.05.

While the group sequential rule answers an important question, it does not answer other related questions the DSMB commonly asks. Examples of these frequently asked questions are, if the trial is stopped now in favor of the treatment, how likely is it that, if the trial were allowed to continue, the test statistic at the end of the study would lead to the rejection of the null hypothesis? What is the likelihood the trial goes to completion (i.e., the monitoring rule never crosses the boundary) if there is no treatment difference? If the DMSB does not stop the trial now, and there is a treatment effect, how likely is it that the monitoring rule will suggest the trial be stopped at the next monitoring point? We can begin to answer these questions, but in order to do so, we must add to the path analysis component of our methods. This is what stochastic curtailment does.

1.4.4 Stochastic Curtailment

We noted in the previous section that group sequential procedures assess the probability that the path the test statistic has taken is a likely one under the null hypothesis. This is a statement about the past performance of the test statistic. Stochastic curtailment (commonly referred to as conditional power) assesses possible future paths of the test statistic. Stochastic curtailment can be a very illuminating concept [15], [16]. One of the greatest concerns a DSMB has when it considers stopping a clinical trial early is what would have happened if the trial was allowed to continue. Would their decision to end the trial prematurely be confirmed by the test statistic's location at the end of the trial? This path evaluation is of course based on assumptions about the treatment effect. If the investigators assume that no additional treatment effect will be seen for the rest of the trial, then certain test statistic paths become highly probable. This is termed conditional power under the null hypothesis. If, on the other hand, the investigators assume that an additional treatment effect will be seen for the remainder of the study, other test statistic paths become more likely. These procedures have also become valuable in the interim monitoring of clinical trials.

Both group sequential procedures and conditional power procedures take different approaches to assess the current position of the test statistic. To illustrate this perspective, imagine that we are standing at our monitoring point with the test statistic in hand. We can either look backward over the path the test statistic has traversed, or turn and look forward to inspect its possible future paths. The direction we look to for a decision determines the type of monitoring rule that we will use (Figure 1.6). The group sequential procedure would have us look backward over the terrain the test statistic has crossed, and ask How likely is it that we would have taken this path if there is no treatment difference? The conditional power approach is invoked if we instead look forward and ask How likely is it that, if we continue to follow this path, the test statistic will wind up in the critical region at the end of the trial and we will reject the null hypothesis?

1.5 Intention to Treat Analyses

The intention to treat analysis is the generally accepted standard by which clinical trials are evaluated. In an intent to treat analysis, the data for each patient is included in the group to which that patient was randomized regardless of that patient's post-randomization experience. In this context, if a patient was randomized to the control group, and then had a defibrillator implanted, then that patient's data will be included with the control group, even though that patient will have the experience of a patient who has received a defibrillator. Thus, the patient is analyzed as he was intended to be treated. This style of evaluation is very conservative, tending to underestimate effect sizes. However, its value lies in its immunity to post-randomization influences that can influence the effect of the therapy. Alternative approaches to this analysis and their associated problems will be considered in Chapter 9 when we discuss subgroup analysis.

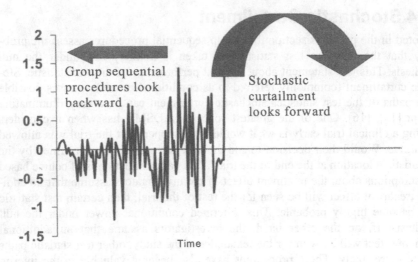

Figure 1.6. The perspective of each of the group sequential procedures and stochastic curtailment procedures in monitoring clinical trial results.

1.6 Measures of Effect

A clinical trial is designed to measure the effect of the intervention it tests. This effect consists of the comparison of the response in the active group to the response in the control group. Outcome variables are typically of two types; continuous or dichotomous. Continuous outcome variables can attain any value in a particular range. Two examples of continuous outcome measures are blood pressure and left ventricular ejection fractions (LVEFs). A dichotomous endpoint variable can be defined as an endpoint that exists in only one of a small number of states. The definitive dichotomous endpoint is of course mortality: the patient is either dead or alive. Another example is the occurrence of a stroke (either the stroke did or did not occur).

How the effect is measured depends on whether the outcome is continuous or discrete. If the outcome is a continuous one, then the effect size can be measured as a change in the continuous variable. Thus, a clinical trial designed to measure the effect of a left ventricular assist device might compare the change in cardiac output from baseline to the end of the study in the active group to the analogous change seen in patients randomized to the placebo group. This is a measure that is fairly easy to compute, understand, and analyze.

The situation is somewhat more complicated for dichotomous endpoints. In these circumstances, the change is not continuous, but abrupt, e.g., an alive patient dies. Instead, epidemiologists commonly use the relative risk to measure the effect of the therapy. The relative risk is the ratio of the cumulative incidence rate of the event in the therapy group to the cumulative incidence rate of the placebo group. This can be approximated by computing the proportion of patients who have an event in each of the treatment and control groups. A fine, in-depth discussion of these principles appears in Piantadosi [6, Chapter 6].

1.7 The Goal of Statistical Hypothesis Testing

Scientific hypothesis testing focuses on the discovery of a relationship in nature. That relationship may be identified by changing factors either one at a time or jointly to amplify the desired effect. In healthcare research, this scenario requires treating some individuals in the standard fashion—these individuals function as the control group. There will be differences among these patients in the control group simply because the individuals differ one from the other. A second set of similar patients (the experimental group) is treated differently from the control group but in a way to produce the desired effect. The clinical hypothesis is that there is a greater difference in results between the experimental and control groups than within these groups.

Another way to say this is that, since the measurement of differences between subjects is the assessment of variability, then the analysis of the experiment's results is simply the comparison of the variability in the results of those patients treated differently to the variability of those who are treated the same. Those individuals who were treated identically will produce not identical but separate results among themselves because of the inherent and natural differences between them. This is random variability. The comparison of those patients treated differently with those treated the same will reveal a second source of variability—that produced by the treatment. The treatment, if effective, generates a new and different separation among the patient results since the findings of those patients receiving treatment are different from those who do not. This new source of variability is called systematic variability because it was deliberately introduced by the investigators (Figure 1.7).

Test statistics are constructed to identify, measure, and compare these two sources of variability. Most test statistics are ratios as portrayed in (1.1). The numerator containing the variability due to both the random changes plus the systematic changes. The denominator contains only the random variability.

$$\text{test statistic} = \frac{\text{systematic changes} + \text{random changes}}{\text{random changes}} \qquad (1.1)$$

If this ratio is large, we conclude that there is more variability produced by the systematic component, then there is random, background variability. Furthermore, if the experiment was well-designed and executed, we then attribute this excess variability to the treatment. By converting the test statistic to a p-value, the sampling error component is added.

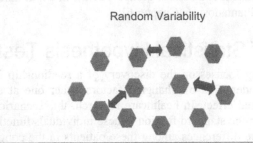

Random Variability

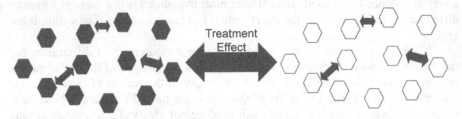

Random + Systematic Variability

Treatment
Effect

Figure 1.7. Comparison of random variability with random + systematic variability.

1.8 Sampling Error and Significance Testing

Sample-based research is the study of a sample obtained from a population. Different samples, obtained from the same population, contain different individuals with different experiences and therefore contain different results. Sampling error is simply this sample-to-sample variability. The symbol α, representing the type I error is the specific sample error that allows a population to generate a sample which contains a spurious relationship that is not seen in the population.

Clinical trial investigators recognize that there are many reasons why the positive findings of clinical experiment may be misleading. For example, they may have selected a population of patients in whom the therapy works but the inclusion and exclusion criteria of the study were too restrictive. The dose of the medication chosen may be effective, but it produces too many side effects. The blinding of the procedure may have been ineffective, leading to a more diligent search for endpoints among the subjects randomized to placebo therapy. These are all problems with the execution of the trial. They can be anticipated and the trial designed to remove them as obstacles to the trial's success. However, there is one problem that, no matter how well the clinical trial is designed, cannot be removed as the generator of false positive results—chance alone. This is an α error.

If an α (or type I) error occurs, then there is no effect of the therapy in the population, but the population produced a sample in which, through just chance alone, the therapy produced an effect. There is no question that the therapy worked in the sample; however, the sample results are not a reflection of the population effect, but instead were generated by the random aggregation of subjects selected for the sample.

The occurrence of a type I error is solely a property of the sampling process. Since sampling is necessary for the research effort, the investigators understand that they cannot remove this possible explanation of these results. They instead decide to measure the possible influence of sampling error. Investigators set the α error level at the beginning of the study, and compute a sample size based on the maximum acceptable type I error rate, as well as on other parameters. At the conclusion of the experiment, the investigators compute the p-value for the result of the study. The p-value is the measure of the type I error rate at the end of the study and is based on the actual research results. If the p-value is less than the α error rate that was prospectively identified, then researchers conclude that it is very unlikely that chance alone produced the findings of the study, and that the results of the study (be they clinically significant or clinically neglible) are truly reflective of what would occur in the larger population from which the sample was obtained.

Therefore, if (1) the systematic explanations for a spurious research finding are removed from the experiment by exceptional planning and good clinical trial execution, (2) the probability of a false finding just by chance alone is reduced to a small level (i.e., the p-value is less than the prospectively set α error rate), and (3) the maginitude of the findings are clinically important, then the medical and regulatory communities are assured that, to a reasonable degree of certainty, the positive results of the trial represent a true population finding.[8]

1.9 Statistical Power

Statistical power, like p-values, is a phenomenon of sampling error. The circumstance in which statistical power is relevant in the interpretation of a clinical trial is when the trial results are not positive, but null; no treatment effect is seen. Of course, there are many systematic explanations for a null finding (the wrong exposure level to the active intervention is but one of many possible circumstance). However, another possible explanation is sampling error. In this circumstance, the therapy is effective in the population. However, the population produced a sample by chance alone in which the therapy was ineffective. This is a type II or beta error. Power is defined as one minus the type II error. High statistical power translates into a low type II error rate.

Since the researcher does not know during the design phase of the study whether the results will be positive or null, she must plan for each possibility. Thus, she should design the study so that the type I error rate will be low (customarily no higher than 0.05) and that the power of the experiment will be high (typically, at least 80%). Each of these considerations are part of the sample size computation.

---

[8] We will have much more to say about the interpretation of p-values in Chapter 2.

1.10 Sample Size Computations

Good clinical trials, regardless of their size, are characterized by careful planning, controlled execution, and disciplined analysis. An important component of the design of a clinical trial is the sample size calculation. The sample size computation is the mathematical calculation that determines how many patients the trial should recruit. It is based on clinical concerns, epidemiologic determinations of event rates, and biostatistical considerations about the role sampling error may play in producing the trial's results.

It can be said that the sample size computation is the forge upon which the clinical trial design is hammered. Since the sample size computation requires a clear set of assumptions about the primary scientific question to be addressed by the study, the expected experience of the control group, the anticipated benefit for the patients randomized to the intervention group, and concerns about type I and type II errors, clearly the investigators and quantitative methodologists (i.e., the epidemiologists and biostatisticians) must be involved and agree on the estimates of these quantities.

However, the sample size computation, although composed only of mathematics, must also reflect the administrative and financial settings in which the trial will be executed. These important logistical considerations, not explicitly included in the arithmetic of the sample size calculation, must nevertheless receive primary attention. The availability of patients may be a question. Alternatively, in the case where a new medication has been developed at great cost, the small number of available doses may preclude recruiting many patients. The financial cost of the trial, and the availability of enough investigators, project managers, and skilled laboratories for executing the protocol also may limit the size of the study.

These latter, nonmathematical considerations must be factored into the final sample size determination in order for the experiment to be executable. They are blended into the plans for the clinical trial in general, and the sample size in particular through several mechanisms during the design phase of the study. Among these mechanisms are (1) re-examination and alteration of the population from which the research sample will be recruited, (2) re-formulation of the primary endpoint of the study, and (3) changing the duration of time over which patients will be followed. Each of these maneuvers is acceptable when considered and finalized during the design phase of the study. For this appropriate mixture of epidemiology, biostatistics, clinical science, and administration to occur, the dialogue between all involved parties should be frank, honest, and collegial. This robust research design with its recomputed sample size will be consistent with epidemiologic, logistical, and financial considerations, making the trial both scientifically rigorous and executable.

1.11 Analysis

The initial description of hypothesis testing by Fisher limited an experiment to a single test of statistical significance on the primary research question of the trial. The application of this rule to a modern clinical trial would require that, at the end of this Herculean effort in which thousands (and, sometimes tens of thousands) of patients are followed for years, the final analysis of the many different outcome varaibles would distill down to a single effect size measurement and p-value.

This ultra-reductionist approach is of course easily criticized as being inefficient. Instead, investigators now execute clinical trials with both multiple treatment arms (e.g., one arm for each dose of therapy and a control arm) and multiple endpoints (e.g., total mortality rate, total hospitalization rate, and quality of life). Also, the effect of therapy can be assessed in the overall cohort or in a subcohort (or subgroup). The creation of these intricate clinical experiments with their complex analyses has created a new host of complications in clinical trial design and interpretation. The focus of this book is on approaches and techniques to address these topics of multiple analyses.

References

1. Yoshioka, A. (1998). Use of randomisation in the Medical Research Council's clinical trial of stroptomycin in pulmonary tuberculosis in the 1940s. *British Medical Journal* **317**:1220–1223.
2. Medical Research Council Streptomycin in Tuberculosis Trials Committee (1948). *British Medical Journal* **ii**:769–782.
3. Brody, J.E. (2002). Ferreting for facts in the realm of clinical trials. *The New York Times* Science Section. October 15, p. D7.
4. Friedman, L., Furberg, C., Demets, D. (1996). *Fundamentals of Clinical Trials*. 3rd Edition. New York, Springer.
5. Meinert, C.L. (1986). *Clinical Trials Design, Conduct, and Analysis*, New York, Oxford University Press.
6. Piantadosi, S. (1997). *Clinical Trials: A Methodologic Perspective*. New York, John Wiley.
7. Berger, V.W., Exner, D.V. (1999). Detecting selection bias in randomized clinical trials. *Controlled Clinical Trials* **20**:319–327.
8. Berger, V.W. (2000). Pros and cons of permutation tests in clinical trials. *Statistics in Medicine* **19**:1319–1328.
9. Pfeffer, M.A., Braunwald, E., Moyé, L.A. et al (1992). Effect of Captopril on mortality and morbidity in patients with left ventricular dysfunction after myocardial infarction–results of the Survival and Ventricular Enlargement Trial. *New England Journal of Medicine* **327**:669–677.
10. Treatment of Lead-Exposed Children Trial Group (1998). The treatment of lead–exposed children (TLC) trial: design and recruitment for a study of the effect of oral chelation on growth and development in toddlers. *Paediatric and Perinatal Eepidemiology* **12**:313–333.
11. Moseley, J.B., O'Malley, K., Petersen, N.H., Menke, T.J., Brody, B.A., Kuykendall, K.H., Hollingsworth, J.C., Ashton, C.M., Wray, N.P. (2002). A controlled trial of arthroscopic surgery for osteoarthitis of the knee. *New England Journal of Medicine* **347**:81–8.
12. Felson, D.T., Buckwalter, J. (2002). Dèbridement and lavage for osteoarthritis of the knee. Editorial. *New England Journal of Medicine* **347**:132–133.

13. Lan, K.K.G., DeMets, D.L. (1983). Discrete sequential boundaries for clinical trials. *Biometrika* **70**:659–663.
14. DeMets, D., Lan, G. (1984). An overview of sequential methods and their application in clinical trials. *Communications in Statistics* **13**:2315–38.
15. Lan, K.K.G. Wittes J (1988). The B-value: A tool for monitoring data. *Biometrics* **44**:579–685.
16. Davis, B.R., Hardy, R.T. (1990). Upper Bounds for type I and type II error rates in conditional power calculations. *Communications in Statistics* **19**:3571–3584.

Chapter 2

Multiple Analyses and the Random Experiment[1]

This chapter describes the difficulty of interpreting clinical trial results when the prospective analysis plan of that trial has been altered. After providing four examples of problematic trial results that had their findings reversed, the necessity of a fixed research protocol is derived from key principles. Investigators generally wish to extend the results from their research sample to the larger population; however, this delicate extension is complicated by the presence of sampling error. No computational or statistical tools can remove sampling error—the best that researchers can do is to provide the medical and regulatory communities with a measure of the distorting effect that sampling error produces. Researchers accomplish this by providing an estimate of how likely it is that the population produced a misleading sample for them to study. However, these estimators are easily damaged and, when damaged, provide misleading assessments. The tools and techniques developed in this chapter to avoid untrustworthy estimation will be the basis of our subsequent work on interpretation of multiple analyses in clinical trials.

How would you react if you overheard the following conversation between two close friends:

> ... and as you know I went to see my physician the other day, but you may not know what it is that he told me. Or, rather, it's not what he told me, but how he decided to treat my stomach cramping and burning that I told you about.
>
> His office was easy to find in a well-kept building, with a nice outer foyer. I didn't even have to wait very long to see him! After I filled out a brief form, his nurse ushered me in to meet this physician for the first time. He was distinquished looking, and when he asked me what my problem was, he spoke in a firm, even voice. Even though I typically do not like doctors, I was becoming more comfortable in spite of myself.
>
> Anyway, he listened patiently to me while I described my problem to him. After his examination, he told me that he thought I had gastro ... something. When he started to speak in English again, he described this problem as a kind of chronic indigestion. The physician then excused himself to make a phone call. Five minutes later, he re-

---

[1] Dr. Anita Deswal was instrumental in describing the results of several of the clinical trials that are discussed in this chapter.

turned with a prescription for me. I asked him who he had called, and he said "oh ... just a colleague who I consult with."

I was pleased with this first encounter—in fact I was feeling so good that when I paid my bill, I joked with the receptionist about the fact that I got to receive the advice of two doctors for the price of one; however, she immediately retorted "The doctor doesn't call another doctor—he calls a fortuneteller!"

What! I just couldn't believe this. This doctor appeared to be so genuine. I had to find out what was going on. After some detective work, I found the address of this fortune teller and slipped into her waiting room, after first calling my doctor and telling him that I had gotten worse while taking his medicine. Sure enough, the phone rang and the fortuneteller, while polishing off some ice cream, mentioned my name on the phone. She repeated out loud his request for a therapy suggestion and seemed to consider it very carefully. However, I almost gasped out loud when, to my horror, she whipped out a pair of dice, threw them across the table, counted the result, and made a decision based on the count. My therapy was not just in the hands of a fortuneteller, but a gambling one at that! Can you believe it?

Wait ... wait ... there's more. I returned the next day to see this doctor, and, I don't mind telling you that I had to really work to control my anger. The nerve of this guy! But he was remarkable—he listened to my explanation of the new symptoms I had, did another brief exam, and then provided a treatment recommendation for me that was the same recommendation that I overheard the soothsayer give to him. Yet, what threw me was that he provided this new recommendation with his usual persuasive combination of tact, firmness, and prestige. He actually felt that the medication that he was prescribing was the best that science could offer; he honestly believed that I would feel better upon taking it. There was no way that I could shake his assurance in his ... his information source. I just took the prescription, paid the bill, and left the office, shaken and diminished by the experience. I trust my physician because ... well, because I guess I have to. What else can I do?

No doubt the first advice we would give this patient would be to find a new doctor! This advise is based on the concept that good physicians do not prescribe therapy randomly. Yet, although we don't use soothsayers, we will see that there are other mechanisms that, while more insidious, are just as effective in injecting randomness into treatment protocols. We will also provide some easy ways to identify this misleading variability and determine how to judge research efforts that have been affected by its presence. As a preamble, we will introduce a forum at which controversial research findings and treatment protocols are debated.

2.1 Introduction

> *When opposing statisticians duel, innocent bystanders get hit in the crossfire.*
> Committee member, FDA Oncology Drugs Advisory Committee,
> December 6, 2001.

In the drive to educate patients about the current epidemics of hypertension, diabetes mellitus, CHF, cancer, and stroke (to name just a few), the public has been conditioned to expect (and perhaps demand) solutions to these public health threats. The scourge of AIDS and the recent occurrence of bioterrorist acts have only amplified this demand. These calls are heeded by teams of research scientists who labor to develop medications and other interventions to rid us of these diseases and their consequences. The implications of these workers' research results have been, and will continue to be, enormous.

However, research results must be evaluated carefully before we accept their conclusions and implications. This review process takes place at several levels. The results and implications of healthcare research activities are the main topic of discussion during scientific meetings that are held at local, national, and international levels. In addition, research results are scrutinized by journal reviewers and editors during the peer-review process. Upon publication, these results are available for general discussion by the medical community.

Another collection of useful discussions focused on medical research is regularly held at public meetings[2] sponsored by the federal Food and Drug Administration (FDA). While most discussions at the FDA concerning the results and implications of a healthcare research study are internal and private, public discussion takes place at regularly scheduled and pre-announced advisory committee meetings. FDA advisory committees are composed of scientists who work neither for the drug companies nor the FDA.[3] On some occasions, these meetings review recent experience with a new class of healthcare interventions. At other times, the advisory committee will be convened to discuss a controversial topic. During these discussions, independent scientists, FDA officials, representatives of the pharmaceutical industry, private physicians, and patient advocacy groups each provide an indispensable perspective on the issue.

Advisory committee meetings serve as crossroads where the requirement to satisfy the needs of a waiting medical community, the dicta of good science, and the desirability of favorable economic incentives can collide dramatically and publicly.

---

[2] These meetings, although open to the public, are primarily attended by representatives of the pharmaceutical industry. Their schedule and agenda are often posted on the FDA website.

[3] Although complete conflict of interest disclosures are required of advisory committee members, their ties with the pharmaceutical industry have been the source of attention by outside advocacy groups, e.g., Public Citizen.

2.1.1 Advisory Committee Discussions

Consider one of the discussions that took place at the May 1996 FDA Cardiovascular and Renal Drugs Advisory Committee meeting. Researchers had carried out a randomized, controlled clinical trial that was designed to demonstrate a medication's ability to increase the exercise tolerance of patients who suffer from CHF [1]. At the conclusion of the body of experiments, the researchers did not identify any important change in exercise tolerance that could be attributed to the randomly allocated medication. However, another examination of these results revealed a striking reduction in mortality.

When the FDA reviewed the data, they confirmed these researchers' findings: the intervention did in fact reduce the cumulative death rate in the research sample. However, to the consternation of the clinical trial investigators and the sponsor, the advisory panel decided not to recommend regulatory approval for the intervention as a proven treatment to reduce mortality in patients suffering from CHF. The panel reasoned that since the findings were for an endpoint (total mortality) that was not a prospectively announced goal of the investigators, the findings must be seen as exploratory and not generalizable to the CHF population at large. The arguments leading to this decision were heated [2], and spilled over into the peer-reviewed literature. This resulted in a letter to the editor [3] and its rejoinder [4], and was followed by manuscripts in the peer-reviewed literature. These manuscripts described the general discussions at the FDA advisory committee meetings [5] and specifically the arguments for [6] and against [7] the approval of the compound carvedilol.[4]

To many people, the advisory committee's finding was both counterintuitive and counterproductive. Certainly, all would agree that saving the lives of patients is a worthy (in fact, the *most* worthy) healthcare goal, and any drug that achieves this goal cannot easily be brushed aside by either regulators or healthcare providers. If, in fact, the drug prevents death, then why should it matter whether the decision to evaluate this effect occurred before, during, or after the study was executed? After all, lives saved are lives saved. Nevertheless, there are important reasons why this controversial research result must be discarded. The purpose of this chapter is to explain in nonmathematical language the critical necessity of a prospectively planned analysis, an analysis plan that was missing in this unfortunate example.

2.2 Prevalent Perceptions

A prospective analysis plan is a plan that identifies the important details of the experiment's design execution and analysis before the research commences. There are many guides written for clinical scientists concerning the correct design, execution, and analysis of research programs. In addition to statements and guidelines issued by government and regulatory agencies [8], there are texts that described the complexity of this work in detail [9], [10], [11]. An important principle enunciated by each of these sources is that of the a priori research plan.

---

[4] This compound was approved for another indication 1 year later.

Of course, it is self-evident that some aspects of the research plan (e.g., the nature of the intervention to be evaluated) must be identified prospectively. However, prospective analysis plans require a great deal more detail than this. The inclusion and exclusion criteria that determine the characteristics of the patients to be randomized (and the population to which the study results can be generalized) must be elaborated. The schedule for follow-up visits, and the activities to be carried out during those follow-up visits must be itemized in detail. The duration of follow-up must be clear. The requirements for laboratory assessments (and who will carry out those assessments) should be articulated. Finally, the analysis plan for the dataset that is collected must be completely specified. Both the analysis variables (the endpoints) and the analysis procedure must be elaborated in detail.

The motivation for this last level of prespecification is unfortunately not always clear and, in fact, its requirement can appear to be a contradiction to the reality of clinical trial execution. After all, wise and seasoned investigators recognize that the experience of their clinical trial can be unpredictable, since there are many influences that can perturb its execution. For example, despite the best efforts of its investigators, a clinical trial may not be able to meet its recruitment goal, thereby providing an inadequate number of patients to estimate the effect of therapy with sufficient precision. Technology (e.g., DNA genotyping) that is capable of illuminating new relationships may not be accessible during the trial's design phase, becoming available only during the second half of the study's execution. A companion clinical trial that is studying a related intervention with a similar goal may provide an insight or analysis that the medical or regulatory community would like to see tested in the current study. Certainly these important events cannot be prospectively anticipated and planned.

Occasionally, a clinical trial produces a surprise. In some circumstances, the beneficial effect of the intervention that the investigators anticipated never materializes [12]. In other trials, a modest result that the trial was designed to identify is overshadowed by an unanticipated, stupendous finding from other analyses [13], [14]. Sometimes the analysis that produced the stupendous finding was planned into the trial's rulebook or protocol during the design phase of the trial, other times it was not.

2.3 Calling Your Shot

Oftentimes, the advice from clinical trial methodologists is that these surprise findings do not carry persuasive weight primarily because they were not planned prospectively [15]. However, to many researchers, this requirement of "calling your shot," i.e., of identifying prospectively what analyses will have persuasive influence, seems much ado about nothing. After all, the data are, in the end, the data. To these critics, allowing the data to decide the result of the experiment can appear to be the fairest, least prejudicial evaluation of the message they contain.

This policy of "let the data decide" also relieves the investigator from the responsibility of choosing arbitrary rules during the planning stage of the experiment, rules that subsequently may be demonstrated by the data to be the "wrong choices." In fact, from the investigator's perspective, it can appear to be far better for her to preserve some flexibility in her experiment's interpretation by saying little during the design of the experiment about either the endpoint selection or the analysis procedures. She then could allow the data she collects to choose the best analysis and endpoint as long as these selections are consistent with the goals of the experiment.

This "let the data decide" point of view may appear to be bolstered by the observation that researchers by and large understand and appreciate the importance of choosing the research sample with great care. Intelligent, well developed methodologies are required to choose the optimum sample size [16], [17], [18], [19], [20]. The sampling mechanism—the process by which patients are selected from the population—requires careful attention to detail. Well-tested mechanisms by which patients are randomized to receive the intervention or the control therapy are put into place in order to avoid systematic biases that can produce destabilizing imbalances. In fact, the fundamental motivation for the execution of the simple random sampling mechanism is to produce a sample that is representative of the population [21]. This effort can be an onerous, time consuming, and expensive process, but investigators have learned that it can pay off handsomely by producing a sample that "looks like" the population at large.

It is therefore understandable why many investigators are convinced that, after winning the expensive and hard fought battle to obtain a representative sample, they have earned the right to report many of their sample's findings with impunity. To investigators, withholding belief in a surprise finding's validity can seem like denying credit to Christopher Columbus for discovering the New World, since his discovery was, after all, "not part of his protocol."

However, the "let the data decide" philosophy often leads to false conclusions, and the experiences of several recent clinical trials have provided useful insight into the hazards of this approach. In each of these settings, a clinical trial that produces an unplanned and surprise result was followed by a second trial that attempted to confirm the first finding. We will review four examples that have recently appeared in the peer-reviewed literature, recalling the comment by Minna Antrim,

Experience is a good teacher, but she sends in terrific bills …

2.3.1 Vesnarinone

Patients with CHF are unable to maintain adequate blood flow through their circulatory system because of the weakened and inadequate pumping strength of their heart. Positive inotropic agents increase the pumping ability of the heart, and these compounds held out initial promise for improving the treatment of CHF. One such positive inotropic drug was vesnarinone.

To study the effectiveness of this compound, patients were recruited into a clinical trial that was designed with three treatment arms. The first arm consisted of control therapy, in which patients with CHF were to receive the best therapy known to be effective in improving outcomes of CHF (known as conventional therapy for CHF) plus a placebo [22]. In the second arm of the trial, patients were to receive, in addition to conventional therapy for CHF, a daily 60-mg dose of vesnarinone. The third treatment arm of this trial consisted of conventional therapy for CHF plus a daily 120-mg dose of vesnarinone. The prospectively stated, primary outcome measure for this clinical trial was the combined endpoint of all-cause mortality and major cardiovascular morbidity.[5] In addition to the primary endpoint, a secondary endpoint of all-cause mortality was chosen. Because of the relatively small number of events, the investigators did not anticipate that they would be able to demonstrate a beneficial effect of vesnarinone on the cumulative total mortality rate. The study was originally designed to randomize 150 patients to each of the three treatment arms, and to follow them for 6 months.

During the trial, the 120-mg treatment arm was discontinued because of the observation of an excess number of deaths occurring in patients exposed to this high dose of drug. At the trial's conclusion, the results of the 60 -mg vesnarinone treatment arm that remained in the trial were compared to those of the placebo group. The administration of 60-mg vesnarinone was associated with a 50% risk reduction in all-cause mortality and major cardiovascular morbidity (95% confidence interval (CI) was 20% to 69% reduction; $p = 0.003$). Thus, the finding for the primary endpoint was achieved. The investigators then turned their attention to an evaluation of the effect of vesnarinone on total mortality. There were only 46 deaths that occurred in this trial, 13 deaths in the vesnarinone group and 33 in the placebo group. However, this translated into a 62% reduction in all-cause mortality (95% CI 28 to 80; $p = 0.002$).

The investigators presented the results of this study before the FDA Cardiovascular and Renal Drug Advisory Committee, positing that this study demonstrated the effectiveness of vesnarinone in reducing the total mortality rate of patients with CHF. This meeting, beginning in the morning, lasted through the dinner hour and into the evening. The review of the data from this trial was punctuated by sharp verbal exchanges between the FDA data reviewers and both the investigators and the pharmaceutical sponsor. The investigators and sponsors argued passionately, but ultimately unpersuasively for the approval of vesnarinone. However, the combination of a small sample size, confusion about endpoint definitions, and concerns for the occurrence of neutropenia persuaded the FDA to request a second, confirmatory study of the mortality effect of vesnarinone.

The Vesnarinone Trial provided the second evaluation of vesnarinone [23]. In that study, 3833 patients with CHF New York Heart Association (NYHA) functional class III or IV and LVEF $\leq$ 30 % were randomized to receive either (1) conventional therapy plus placebo, (2) conventional therapy plus 60-mg of vesnarinone, or (3) conventional therapy plus 30-mg of vesnarinone. The primary endpoint of this study was all-cause mortality, and the goal of the study was to compare the experience of patients who received the 30-mg and 60-mg vesnarinone doses to the placebo experience. The maximum follow-up period was 70 weeks, and it was anticipated that 232 deaths would be required to demonstrate the beneficial effect of vesnarinone on all-cause mortality. In this confirmatory study, however, the mortal-

---

[5] A combined endpoint is used to decrease the required sample size of a trial. By examining the occurrence of either a death or cardiovascular morbidity (essentially giving a cardiovascular event, e.g., a heart attack the same weight as a death in the analysis) more endpoint events occur and therefore fewer patients are required to obtain an adequate sample size. This topic is discussed in Chapter 7.

ity rate was observed to be higher in the patients randomized to 30-mg of vesnarinone (21%) and in those randomized to 60-mg of vesnarinone (22%), than in the placebo group (18.9%). The first trial, which demonstrated a mortality benefit for the 60-mg vesnarinone dose, had its findings reversed by the second trial that demonstrated a mortality hazard for this same dose. The investigators stated, "Examination of the patient populations in the two trials reveals no differences that could reasonably account for the opposite response to the daily administration of 60-mg of vesnarinone."

2.3.2 Losartan

The use of ACE-i therapy has increased dramatically since the 1980s. First approved as a treatment for hypertension, their use expanded into the treatment of other cardiovascular diseases, specifically the treatment of CHF. However, these effective medications also were associated with undesirable adverse events. Among the most common of these were cough, angioedema, and hypotension. As a response to this undesirable profile, angiotensin II type I receptor blockers were developed. It was hoped that this newer class of agents would be safer than the original ACE inhibitors while continuing to confer a survival benefit for patients with CHF. In order to compare the relative safety of angiotensin II type I receptor blockers to that of ACE inhibitors, the Evaluation of Losartan in the Elderly Study (ELITE) I [13] was designed. ELITE I's goal was to compare the effectiveness of the angiotensin II type I receptor blocker losartan to the ACE inhibitor captopril in a randomized, double-blind clinical trial. The primary endpoint of this study was a prospectively designed safety measure; the frequency of an increase in serum creatinine by 0.3 mg/dl or more above baseline.

This double-blind study randomized 722 patients and followed them in a double-blind fashion for 48 weeks. Just prior to the end of the study, an additional endpoint was added. This measure was the composite endpoint of death and/or admission for heart failure. At the conclusion of ELITE I, the investigators determined that the increase in serum creatinine was the same in the two treatment arms (10.5% in each group; risk reduction 2%; 95% CI: –51 to 36; $p = 0.63$). However, the findings for the new composite endpoint were tantalizing. Death and/or heart failure admission occurred in 33 of the losartan-treated participants, while 49 events occurred in the captopril group. This translated into a risk reduction of 32% ; 95% CI –0.04 to 0.55; $p = 0.075$) and suggested that there was a benefit attributable to losartan. The investigators, emboldened by these findings, deconstructed the composite endpoint and discovered that 17 deaths occurred in the losartan group and 32 deaths in the captopril group, a result that produced a risk reduction of 46% (95% CI 5 to 69; $p = 0.035$). These finding received the principle emphasis in the discussion section of the manuscript, minimizing the role of the primary safety endpoint of serum creatinine increase. And, although the need to repeat the trial was mentioned in the abstract, the balance of the discussion focused on the reduced mortality rate of losartan. According to the authors, "This study demonstrated that losartan reduced mortality compared with captopril; whether the apparent mortality advantage for losartan over captopril holds true for other ACE inhibitors requires further study." Others even went so far as to attempt to explain the mechanism for the reduction in sudden death observed in ELITE 1 [24], [25].

To the investigators' credit, ELITE II [26] was executed to confirm the superiority of losartan over captopril in improving survival in patients with heart failure. The primary endpoint in ELITE II was total mortality, an endpoint that required 3152 patients. This was almost five times the number of patients recruited for the ELITE I study. These patients were followed for 18 months, almost twice as long as the duration of follow-up in ELITE I. At the conclusion of ELITE II, the cumulative all-cause mortality rate was not significantly different between the losartan and captopril groups (280 deaths in the losartan group versus 250 deaths in the captopril group, 17.7% versus 15.9%; hazard ratio 1.13 (95% CI: 0.95 to 1.35, p = 0.16). In fact, there was a trend to excess mortality in the losartan group. Thus, losartan did not confer a mortality benefit in the elderly with CHF when compared to captopril as suggested by ELITE I. The investigators conceded "More likely, the superiority of losartan to captopril in reducing mortality, mainly due to decreasing sudden cardiac death, seen in ELITE should be taken as a chance finding."

2.3.3 Amlodipine

In the 1980s, the use of calcium channel blocking agents in patients with CHF was problematic. Initial studies suggested that patients with CHF experienced increased morbidity and mortality associated with these agents [27]. However, additional developmental work on this class of medications proceeded. In the early 1990s, new calcium channel blocking agents appeared. The early data for these compounds suggested that their use may produce improvements in patients with CHF. To formally evaluate this possibility, the Prospective Randomized Amlodipine Survival Evaluation (PRAISE) [14] trial was designed. PRAISE's long-term objective was the assessment of the channel blocker amlodipine's effect on morbidity and mortality in patients with advanced heart failure. The primary measurement in PRAISE was the composite endpoint of all-cause mortality and/or hospitalization.[6] The protocol also stipulated that there would be analyses in the following subgroups of patients; sex, ejection fraction, NYHA class, serum sodium concentration, angina pectoris, and hypertension.

PRAISE began recruiting patients in March 1992. Patients with CHF (NYHA functional class IIIb/IV and LVEF < 30%) were randomized to receive either amlodipine or placebo therapy. The investigators suspected that the effect of amlodipine might depend on the cause of the patient's CHF, so they stratified randomization into two groups, patients with ischemic cardiomyopathy and patients who had nonischemic cardiomyopathy.[7] By the end of the recruiting period, the PRAISE investigators randomized 1153 patients and, by the end of the study, these patients had been followed for a maximum of 33 months.

---

[6] Hospitalization was defined as receiving in-hospital care for at least 24 hours for either acute pulmonary edema, severe hypoperfusion, acute myocardial infarction, or sustained hemodynamically destabilizing ventricular tachycardia or fibrillation.

[7] Stratified randomization is an adaptation of the random allocation to therapy process, and was discussed in Chapter 1.

At the conclusion of PRAISE, the investigators determined that in the overall cohort there was no significant difference in the occurrence of the primary endpoint between the amlodipine and placebo groups (39% versus 42%, 9% reduction; [95% CI −24 to 10], $p = 0.31$). The secondary endpoint of all-cause mortality also was not significantly different between the amlodipine and placebo groups for the overall cohort (33% versus 38%, 16% reduction [95% CI: −31 to 2], $p = 0.07$).

The evaluation then turned to the etiology-specific CHF strata. PRAISE recruited 732 patients with an ischemic cause for their CHF and 421 patients with a nonischemic cause. The analysis of the effect of therapy in these strata revealed that treatment with amlodipine reduced the frequency of primary and secondary endpoints in patients with nonischemic dilated cardiomyopathy (58 fatal or nonfatal events in the amlodipine group and 78 in the placebo group, 31% risk reduction [95% CI 2 to 51% reduction], $p = 0.04$). Further evaluation of these events revealed that there were only 45 deaths in the amlodipine group and 74 deaths in the placebo group, representing a 46% reduction in the mortality risk in the amlodipine group (95% CI 21 to 63% reduction, $p < 0.001$). Among the patients with ischemic heart disease, treatment with amlodipine did not affect the combined risk of morbidity and mortality or the risk of mortality from any cause. Again, the findings for a secondary endpoint overshadowed the primary endpoint's results

A second trial PRAISE-2 [28] was then conducted to verify the beneficial effect on mortality seen in the subgroup analysis of patients with heart failure of nonischemic etiology in PRAISE-1. This trial, while focusing only on patients with heart failure of nonischemic origin, was similar in design to PRAISE-1. The PRAISE-2 investigators randomized 1650 patients to either amlodipine or placebo, following them for up to 4 years. However, the results of PRAISE-2 were quite different from PRAISE-1. Unlike the first study, there was no difference in mortality between the two groups (33.7% in the amlodipine arm and 31.7% in the placebo arm; odds ratio 1.09, $p = 0.28$) in PRAISE-2. Thus, the marked mortality benefit seen in the subgroup analysis in PRAISE-1 for amlodipine was not confirmed in PRAISE-2.

2.3.4 Carvedilol

As a fourth and final example of how surprising results from nonprimary endpoints or other measures can plunge an expensive experiment into controversy, consider the findings of the US Carvedilol program [1]. Up until the 1980s, the usefulness of beta adrenergic receptor antagonists (beta-blockers) in CHF had been intensely debated, with published research efforts yielding inconsistent findings. Although initial studies suggested some positive effect [29], results from each of the Metoprolol in Dilated Cardiomyopathy Study [30] and the Cardiac Insufficiency with Bisoprolol Study [31] did not demonstrate a survival benefit.

In this uncertain environment, private industry developed carvedilol as a nonselective beta and α blocker that was believed to be effective in patients with CHF. The US Carvedilol program was designed to test the effect of carvedilol in patients with heart failure. The core of this program consisted of four prospectively designed, double-blind clinical trials in which 1094 patients were selected for one of four protocols, then randomized to a treatment arm or placebo in the selected protocol. There were 398 total patients randomized to placebo and 696 to carvedilol.

Each of these protocols had its own primary endpoint. Three of the four prospectively stipulated that the change in exercise tolerance over time was their primary endpoint. In none of these three clinical trials did carvedilol demonstrate a statistically significant, beneficial effect. The fourth protocol had as its primary endpoint a measure of quality of life, for which carvedilol did produce a benefit that was statistically significant. However, while the studies were ongoing, it was observed that across all four protocols 31 patients died in the placebo group and 22 patients died in the active group, resulting in a relative risk[8] of 0.65 and a p-value less than 0.001. The program was terminated, and the investigators posited that, since total mortality was an objective of the carvedilol program, then the beneficial effect of carvedilol on total mortality should compel the FDA to approve the drug as effective in reducing the incidence of total mortality in patients suffering from CHF.

In May 1996, the results of this research effort were published in the *New England Journal of Medicine* [1], and brought before the Cardiovascular and Renal Drugs Advisory Committee of the FDA. Although the article describing the results of the trial stated that patients were stratified into one of four treatment protocols [1, p. 1350], it did not state the fact that each of these protocols had its own prospectively identified primary endpoint and that total mortality was not a primary or a secondary endpoint for any of the trials.[9] This discovery produced a host of problems for the experiment's interpretation, and the advisory committee voted not to approve the drug for use in the CHF population. The interpretation of this discordant program was both complex and contentious [2]. In February 1997, these same investigators presented the results to the same committee, this time to successfully apply for a claim that carvedilol reduced the incidence of the combined endpoint of morbidity and mortality in patients with CHF. Much discussion and debate have occurred over the quality of the *New England Journal of Medicine* article and the discussions that took place at these meetings [5], [6], [7].

CAPRICORN (Carvedilol Post-Infarct Survival Control in LV Dysfunction) [32] was a subsequent study designed to clarify the relationship between carvedilol and total mortality. This study recruited 1959 patients from 17 countries and 163 centers worldwide. However, just as in the US Carvedilol program, this study was plagued with unfortunate endpoint difficulties. The first primary endpoint of CAPRICORN was all-cause mortality. However, the investigators decided to

---

[8] The relative risk is based on a Cox proportional hazards model, a detail that should not distract from the discussion.

[9] The investigators stated prospectively that p-values less than 0.05 would be considered significant. Direct interrogation at the meeting revealed that the finding for the prospectively defined primary endpoint in three of the four trials was $p > 0.05$. The fourth study had as its primary endpoint hospitalization for heart failure; the statistical analysis for this primary endpoint was $p < 0.05$. Each of these four studies had secondary endpoints that assessed congestive heart failure morbidity, some of which had p-values less than 0.05, others not. As pointed out by Fisher [2], total mortality was not an endpoint of any of the four studies in the program.

make several changes to the analysis plan of this study during the execution and analysis of the trial. The first change was to replace the analysis plan with its single primary endpoint with a new plan that contained multiple primary endpoints. The new, additional endpoint was a composite or combined endpoint of all-cause mortality and cardiovascular hospitalization.[10] In addition, the type I error level was reallocated so that the new composite endpoint had to have a p-value less than 0.045 and the all-cause mortality endpoint must have a p-value of less than 0.005 in order to be considered statistically significant.[11]

Despite these mid-trial changes, the effect of carvedilol failed to reach the threshold of significance for either of these endpoints. For the new primary composite endpoint, carvedilol use was associated with a relative risk of 0.92 [95% CI 0.80 to 1.07], and for total mortality the relative risk was 0.77 [95% CI 0.60 to 0.98], $p = 0.03$. Thus the findings from the US Carvedilol program were (at least from the sponsor's point of view) positive for a mortality benefit, but from CAPRICORN with its tortured analysis, the result was not positive, creating a substantial discrepancy.

COPERNICUS (CarvedilOl ProspEctive RaNdomIzed CUmulative Survival Trial) [33] was an international study designed to look at the effect of carvedilol on total mortality in patients with advanced heart failure. This study was conducted in over 300 medical centers in 21 countries and enrolled over 2,200 patients with advanced heart failure who had symptoms at rest or on minimal exertion, but required neither intensive care nor intravenous treatments to support heart function. Patients were evaluated for up to 29 months. In COPERNICUS, patients treated with carvedilol showed a significantly lower mortality rate compared to those treated with placebo (11.4% versus 18.5%, respectively; 35% reduction in total mortality). The severity of heart failure was worse in the patients randomized in COPERNICUS than those in either the US Carvedilol program or CAPRICORN, so the results were not directly comparable. Even so, the 35% reduction in mortality observed in COPERNICUS was only half the reduction in total mortality seen in the US Carvedilol program, and completely different from the results of CAPRICORN. Which finding is correct?

2.3.5 Experimental Inconsistencies

In each of these four clinical examples, multiple, prospectively designed, randomized, controlled clinical trials were executed. In the last example, six such trials were carried out (four in the US Carvedilol program plus CAPRICORN, and COPERNICUS). For each of these four examples, the initial trials, carefully designed, executed, and analyzed at great expense, identified a finding that the investigators claimed was positive. In each of these studies, the investigators, rec-

---

[10] In the original analysis plan, only patients who died were considered to have met the primary endpoint. In the new plan, surviving patients could also be counted as a primary endpoint occurrence if they were hospitalized.
[11] The CAPRICORN investigators essentially constructed two coprimary endpoints post hoc. This process will be discussed in detail in Chapter 4.

ognizing the fragility of the findings from these initial studies, argued for a second (and in the case of carvedilol, a third) confirmatory study. Fortunately, they were persuasive in these arguments and the follow-up studies were executed. However, the findings from the follow-up studies reversed the findings from the first studies. In each case we are faced with the same question? How can a collection of expensive, well-designed, clinical studies focusing on the same issue lead to such discrepant conclusions?

The answer to this question must be considered carefully because it has potentially explosive consequences. Most clinical trials do not have follow-up studies executed to confirm their findings—clinical trial results are often accepted at face value. If the first major clinical trial findings for each of vesnarinone, losartan, amlodipine, and carvedilol were overturned when a second study became available, then perhaps we should take the result of any clinical trial with great caution, interpreting its results as being only suggestive of the effect of the drug, rather than as confirmation. This would represent a poor return on the millions of dollars and hundreds of thousands of person hours invested in these endeavors.

However, we do not have to let the situation devolve to that unsatisfactory state of affairs. Lets first ask if there were features of the design, execution and/or analysis of the findings of our four examples that could have predicted the possibility of these disparate conclusions.

2.4 Samples as Reflections

The four examples provided in the previous section, and in fact the overwhelming majority of clinical trials in general, rely on the interpretation of results obtained from a sample of patients taken from a much larger population.

It is clearly impossible for us as researchers to do what we would like to do—study every subject in the entire population. Instead, the researcher selects a sample from that population to investigate. Great effort and expense are exerted to build this sample, and the investigator commonly intends to rely on the entire sample findings. The sample is replete with information and, since the sample was carefully selected, all of this information is used to depict the population. However, no matter how random the sample is, it remains, in the end, only a sample. To many investigators, the sample becomes the population; they believe that every result in the sample reflects a true finding about the population from which the sample was obtained. This is a dangerous trap. It is critical for the disciplined investigator to accept that no matter how carefully they were obtained, representative samples are not populations—they are only the imperfect reflections of populations. For some views of the population, the reflection is a useful and reliable one. For others, the reflection is distorted and misleading.

Imagine for a moment that the population is a complicated, intricately detailed landscape. This landscape has near objects and far objects that are worthy of very careful observation. The investigator–observer must view this landscape through a lens. However, it is impossible to grind the lens so that every object can be viewed with the same sharp detail. If the lens is ground to view near objects, it does not allow a sharp view of items in the distance. If it is ground for the visualization of distant objects, than the observer cannot see the near ones clearly. Thus, if the investigator–observer attempts to use the same lens for viewing everything, some objects will be blurred, and the investigator will be misled about their appearance. A research sample recruited for a clinical trial is a lens that is ground during the design phase of the study. Although the research-lens allows the investigator to see much of the population landscape, it does not permit a clear view of everything.

The limitations of random samples are hidden in plain view all around us. As an example, consider the process by which predictions are made based on early election returns for the mayor of a major US city. On the day of the election, while the polling stations are open, a random sample of voters is taken and these voters are then asked a series of questions about their demographics and their voting preference. When the polls close, these "exit poll results" are announced through the media (and most recently, the internet), providing predictions of the election results. This exercise (barring extremely close contests) represents the success of random sampling. The voting patterns of the individuals in this sample can often be generalized to the larger population of voters with great reliability.

However, we would be remiss if we did not notice that, while these same polls have historically been very reliable for predicting election results, they are unreliable when put to additional uses. For example, would it be constructive for exit pollsters, after collecting information about the annual income of these voters, to proclaim that there is a crisis of poverty in the city because a greater proportion of the sample voters made less money than the pollsters anticipated? The attempt to generalize this type of data would be useless[12] because the sample was not constructed to have its results extended beyond the voting population. In this case, the sampling lens was ground for a view of the voting patterns of the electorate, not for a view of income distribution in the city.

In samples, information is collected about a great many items. However, not every finding in the sample is truly representative of a finding in the population. The absence of this one-to-one relationship between the findings in the sample and the findings in the population means that the sample, however random, is still an incomplete rendition of the population. The random samples on which clinical trial reuslts are based commonly contain meaningless factoids that are not generalizable to the greater population of patients. One of our tasks will be to differentiate the useful representative sample information from the empty sample facts that apply only to the sample and not to the population.

2.5 Representative Samples That Mislead?

Why aren't random samples more representative? In order to begin to understand this, recall that (in health care) research samples, although obtained at great expense, are often miniscule when compared in magnitude to populations (Figure 2.1).

---

[12] The appropriate use of these data would be to categorize voting patterns by income category.

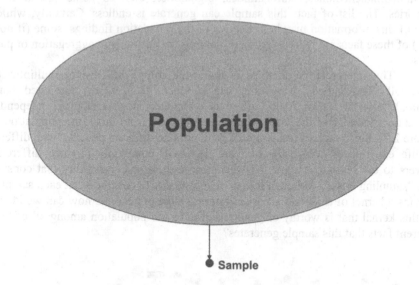

Figure 2.1. One small sample from a large population

Consider, for example, a clinical research program that goes to great effort and expense to identify 300 patients with type II diabetes, randomly allocating these patients to either a new pharmacologic intervention or to control therapy. Despite the great effort that is invested into this enterprise, it must be acknowledged that most of the patients with type II diabetes in the United States will not be included in this sample. Since there are 14.5 million patients with type II diabetes in the United States [34], the research sample contains only 0.00207 % of the total number of diabetics. Put another way, 99.99793% of type II diabetics are specifically not included in the sample. The aggregation of these 300 patients in the sample is merely by chance alone.[13] To what extent can the random selection[14] of these 300 patients be representative of 14.5 million patients? Certainly there will be some nugget of truth about the population of patients with diabetes mellitus contained in this 300 patient sample, but this 300 patient sample will contain many other findings as well. For example, this small sample will certainly generate demographic factoids (e.g., the distribution of age, distribution of gender, ethnicity proportions), findings concerning the presence of risk factors for cardiovascular disease (prevalence of tobacco use, serum lipid levels, obesity, exercise levels, alcohol consumption), facts concerning comorbidity (prevalence of myocardial infarction, hypertension), and

---

[13] This aggregation is by chance alone if every patient in the diabetic population has the same chance of being selected for the research. As discussed in Chapter 1, this would be an ideal set of circumstances.

[14] If the 300 patients were not chosen completely at random from the population of diabetic patients, the findings from that sample are even less likely to represent the population.

facts about the use of therapy for the control of type II diabetes (diet, exercise, insulin, thiazolindienediones, sulfonamides, biguanides, etc.) to name just a few categories. The list of facts this sample can generate is endless. Certainly, while some of this information may be reflective of the population findings, some (if not most) of these facts are representative of nothing but the random aggregation of patients.

This interpretative dilemma is somewhat complicated by the multiplicity of samples the diabetic population can produce. It is easily computed that 14,500,000/300 or almost 50,000 different, completely nonoverlapping, independent, random samples of the same size can be obtained from this same population[15] (Figure 2.2). Since each of these samples will contain different patients, with different life experiences, and different data, they will commonly produce different answers to the same questions. It is this sample-to-sample variability that constitutes "sampling error". Although it may be reasonable to conclude that each sample contains a kernel of truth that accurately portrays the population, how can we identify this kernal that is worthy of generalization to the population among all of the different facts that this sample generates?

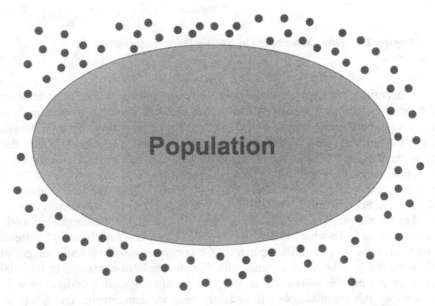

Figure 2.2. There are many possible samples from a large population.

The process whereby the results from a single sample are extended to the much larger population is a fragile process, a process with which sampling error is tightly intertwined. Although sampling error cannot be separated or removed from this process, we can estimate the extent to which it is responsible for the sample's

---

[15] The number of overlapping samples is the combinatoric of a much larger number.

results. We can answer the question "How likely is it that the findings from my sample are due wholly to sampling error?"

Most times, the researcher has the opportunity to collect one and only one sample. In order to increase the accuracy of that sample's ability to answer the scientific question of interest, the research designer crafts and molds the research sample so that it accurately measures the characteristics of the population which are the researcher's primary focus. Experienced research designers focus on a small number of questions so that they can "grind the research sample lens" to focus on the tightly circumscribed areas of interest.

By focusing on this small number of questions, investigators are able to perform important tasks. They can choose the sample so that it contains patients who have the characteristics they wish to study. If the question is "Does patient education about diabetes mellitus improve control of glycosylated hemoglobin levels (HbA1c)?" the sample can be chosen so that the distribution of HbA1c levels in the sample closely mirrors that of the population. The investigators can ensure that there is a broad range of educational backgrounds within their sample of patients. The trial designers can recruit enough patients so that they can address the scientific question with adequate control of the type I and type II statistical error levels.

Focusing at this level of sample construction increases the sample's "population accuracy" for the examination of the relationship between education and HbA1c. However, it does not guarantee that the sample will be able to address other issues involving diabetes mellitus. The sample will be useful for the question it was designed to address, but not much else.

2.6 Estimators

Unfortunately, careful selection of the sample to address the scientific question of interest does not prevent random sampling error from generating the sample's answers. In order to measure the role of sampling error accurately, the investigator turns to the quantitative procedures supplied by the disciplines of epidemiology and biostatistics. These two fields have provided the computations that convert the sample's information (the data) into the best, unbiased estimates of the intervention's effect size (e.g., mean effect, odds ratio, or relative risk) and effect size variability. The researcher relies on the accuracy of these estimators.

It is important to note that these estimators do not remove sampling error. Instead, they channel sampling error into the effect size estimates and the variability of these estimates. For example, if a researcher in a clinical trial estimates the relative risk of therapy attributable to the randomly allocated intervention, the investigator will also have a standard error for this relative risk. The standard error measures the degree to which the relative risk will vary from sample to sample (i.e., sampling variability).

If the researcher also is interested in inference (i.e., statistical hypothesis testing), then statistical procedures will channel sampling error into p-values (the likelihood that there is no effect in the population, but the population has produced a sample in which there is an effect due to chance alone) and power (the likelihood that there is an important effect of therapy in the population, but the population has produced a sample due to chance alone in which no effect of therapy is observed).

Thus, when used correctly, epidemiologic and statistical methodology will appropriately recognize and transmit sampling error into familiar quantities with which research efforts have useful experience in interpreting. Unfortunately, these estimators are commonly corrupted.

2.7 Random Experiments

As pointed out in the previous section, sampling error is appropriately passed through the data collection and research execution to estimators. The measures used to accomplish this are very effective, but rely on a core assumption: only the data can be subject to the random influence of sampling error. This may seem like the only possible state of affairs at first glance. After all, what else could be random in the experiment? In fact, the protocol itself could be random.

2.7.1 What Is a Random Protocol?

The idea of a random protocol may appear to be far fetched. After all, experiments are often planned in great detail. However, protocols don't become random during the clinical trial's design, but instead are transformed to randomness during the experiment's execution. Specifically, the protocol becomes random when researchers examine their data and make protocol changes based on their observations.

A common setting for random research is when the analysis for a prospectively identified primary endpoint is overturned because the randomly allocated therapy did not produce the desired effect on the primary endpoint. In this case, the null findings for the preannounced primary endpoint are replaced by a positive therapy effect for another endpoint. Sometimes that other endpoint is prespecified by the investigators; sometimes it is not.

In fact, overturning the principle analysis of the clinical trial is the thread that links each of the four examples provided earlier in this chapter. For the first vesnarinone study, the null finding for the primary combined endpoint was replaced by the finding for the secondary endpoint of total mortality. In the ELITE-1 trial, the null findings for creatinine levels were supplanted by the findings for total mortality. In PRAISE-1, the finding for the entire cohort (the prospectively designed analysis) was supplanted by the findings for the subgroups based on the etiology of the CHF. Finally, in the situation involving carvedilol, the investigators attempted to replace the null findings for three of the four experiments in the US Carvedilol program with the findings from a post hoc combined analysis of total mortality.

In each of these four cases, the investigators reacted to this unanticipated change by moving the focus away from the principle analysis of the study to the new trend seen in the data. Since the data contain sampling variability, the sampling variability most likely produced the data stream that led to the change in the objective. After all, a different sample from the same population could produce a different data stream that would reveal different trends, and lead to different midtrial endpoint selections by the investigators. This is the hallmark of the random protocol. By letting the data decide the analysis, the analysis, and the experiment, becomes random.

2.7.2 Crippled Estimators in Random Experiments

Unfortunately, our commonly used estimators do not work well in this random environment. The usual estimators whereof we scientists avail ourselves are designed to handle a single source of variability. Specifically, that variability is sampling variability (i.e., that the data in one sample will differ from that in another sample in measuring a predetermined endpoint). These estimators cannot handle the situation in which a different sample with different data would lead to a different endpoint choice. In the environment of random research, our otherwise accurate estimators now function irregularly, returning aberrant estimates of what they were designed to measure.

Of course, in research, the data always contribute to the endpoint. However, in the aberrant examples provided earlier in this chapter, the data did not just contribute to the endpoint—they actually chose the endpoint. Since the data are random, the endpoint selection process has become random, and this new source of variation wrecks the standard computations of relative risks, standard deviations, confidence intervals, and type I and type II error levels. These quantities are still computed to be sure, but their computations can not be interpreted, nor can they be trusted. No longer anchored to its protocol, the research has become discordant and unsystematic.

Drawing conclusions from these estimators is like applying cosmetics using a distorted, blurred mirror. Since the reflection is not a true one, the result is unsatisfactory and, ultimately, the exercise must be repeated.

2.7.3 Untrustworthy

This last point is worthy of elaboration. The difficulty with the estimators' computations in the random experiment is not one of sloppy calculations. To the contrary, great effort is expended on these computations, using modern computing facilities and procedures. However, because the research is no longer protocol-tethered, the computations are uninterpretable, and cannot be corrected.

As an example, consider a medical resident working in an emergency room whose next patient is a young woman who has a tender abdomen. After his evaluation of her, he orders a white blood cell count with differential as part of his clinical workup. The patient's blood is drawn and sent to the laboratory, where the laboratory technician makes a technical mistake with the preparation of the sample. The mistake, which makes it impossible to visualize many of the leukocytes, is subtle but has major implications. Not recognizing his error, the technician proceeds with the white cell count and differential, returning the result to the unsuspecting resident. The resident, assuming the white count that he has been given is accurate, attempts to integrate these results into his information about the patient. Since the blood count is wrong, not only is it unhelpful, but it can direct him away from the correct diagnosis.

Continuing with this analogy, if the resident were to learn that the white blood cell count was inaccurate, what could he do to correct it? In fact, he does not know how to adjust it; there is no known factor that he can add to or multiply the reported white count by in order to obtain the true white blood cell total and differential. He only knows the count is wrong, and that he does not know how to make it right. Therefore, his only alternative is to repeat it.

This is the situation that the medical community is confronted with when it attempts to interpret random research. The estimators of relative risk, standard error, p-values, and confidence intervals have been corrupted by the random protocol that now governs their implementation. Since the estimators are incorrect and uncorrectable, we cannot integrate them into our fund of knowledge, and they must unfortunately be discarded. The experiment must be repeated.

The random research paradigms of the vesnarinone, losartan, amlodipine, and carvedilol examples identified in the previous section require very difficult, obtuse estimators for correct analysis (Appendix B). The correct analysis is difficult to interpret, but this problematic analysis is nevertheless the one that should be used. The fact that the correct estimators are tough to use and interpret is merely an expression that the paradigm of randomness is difficult. The problem is not the estimators—the problem is the paradigm.

The only protection against this dilemma is the prospective specification of the endpoints and the execution of the study in accordance with this protocol. By doing so, the protocol is fixed, and the sampling error contained in the data is isolated from the research procedures and analysis plans. This isolation ensures that the statistical procedures applied to the data provide accurate estimates of effect size, standard errors, confidence intervals, and p-values. The fixed, prospective protocol anchors the researcher, keeping her protocol from drifting with the data. This is the central motivation for the tenet "First say what you will do—then do what you said" in research.

2.8 Collecting the Entire Population

When the sample size equals the population, the situation is quite different, and the concern for random research vanishes. Recall that the root of the difficulty in random research is how to handle sampling error. Therefore, this dilemma is resolved if the researcher can study every subject in the population, and there is no sampling error. In fact, there is no "estimation" since the population parameters are directly measured.

As an example [35], consider a laboratory researcher who is interested in characterizing the measure of abnormal glucose metabolism in diabetic patients admitted to a community hospital during July and August 2002. There are two possible candidates for the research endpoint—HbA1c or fasting blood glucose levels. In this circumstance, there is no requirement for choosing only one prospectively. Here, the sample *is* the population, and the issues of sample extension and generalizing results are not germane. The investigator chooses and studies every member of her population. For her, she does not estimate parameters—she simply measures them. There is no need for standard errors, and no need for inference testing, because sampling error was not involved in the selection of the subjects. There is freedom in choosing (and re-choosing) the endpoint here.

However, this endpoint selection liberty gained by studying the entire population is counterbalanced by the generalizability restriction—the results of this two-month evaluation apply only to this hospital for only the time frame during which the measurements were made. They cannot be applied to other community hospitals, and should not be applied to the same hospital for different time frames.

The distinction between analyzing a sample and analyzing a population is critical. In population research, every result applies to the population (since the entire population was included in the analysis), while only a small number of results from sample-based research can be extended to the population at large. Most medical research is executed on samples derived from much larger populations. However, researchers should not first select their sample, and then treat the analysis as though the sample was the population. They should instead be consistent, recalling that extending results from their small research sample to the large population is a delicate process.

2.9 Regulatory Example

Discussions that occurred at the FDA in 2001 demonstrate the applicability of issues that were developed in this chapter.

Glidel is a medication combining two antitumor compounds (BCNU and carmustine) into a wafer that is placed in the tumor cavity of patients who have just had the brain tumor glioblastoma multiforme (GBM) surgically extracted. It was approved by the FDA in 1996 for use as an adjunct to surgery to prolong survival in patients with recurrent GBM for whom surgical resection is indicated.

The sponsor submitted a supplemental SNDA[16] presenting results from a multi-center, randomized, placebo-controlled trial in a newly diagnosed population of patients with malignant glioma. The endpoint of this trial was survival.

The study was stratified by center and, therefore, indirectly stratified by country. The protocol for this study indicated that an unadjusted log rank test statistic would be used to analyze the survival data. The results of the trial demonstrated that the median survival for patients taking Glidel was 13.9 months (95% CI 12.1 to 15.3) when compared to 11.6 months for the placebo group (95% CI 10.2 to 12.6). The relative risk was 0.77 and the p-value for the log rank test was 0.08, higher than the prospective level of 0.05 that the company had set.

However, upon conclusion of the study, an independent statistician was called in by the sponsor to analyze the data. In the alternative analysis, the therapy effect was stratified by center, producing a p-value of 0.07; an additional analysis, now stratifying by country, revealed a p-value of 0.03. The sponsor argued that since the study was stratified by center (and that this perhaps indicated some stratification at the country level) the appropriate analysis should be the country stratified log rank analysis [36.]. What is the correct conclusion?

---

[16] A new drug application (NDA) is the compendium of material composed of thousands of pages describing the safety and efficacy of the compound that the companies sponsoring the drug submit to the FDA for the regulatory agency's review. A supplemental new drug application (SNDA) is the supporting data for a new indication for the drug that has already been approved.

The advisory committee to whom these data were presented debated their correct interpretation for an afternoon and delivered a split decision to the FDA. The pharmaceutical sponsor argued that since the trial was designed to stratify patients by center (and indirectly by country) the positive country-stratified analysis should be accepted. However, committee members argued that the prospective analysis plan in place at the study's inception required that the unadjusted log rank test should be used. In the end, a 7-6 vote that the trial was not adequate and that the intervention should not be approved was presented to the FDA.

2.10 Additional Comments

Here are some final comments for investigators to consider as they review the published work of others.

2.10.1 Don't Rush to Judgment

There are other explanations for the disparate findings of the four collections of clinical trials that we have reviewed. Factors such as the clinical impression of the benefit of therapy, the needs of the population at risk, changing standards of care for this population over time, the spectrum of adverse effects produced by the therapy, and the cost of the intervention must all be jointly considered as we work to interpret the results of a research effort.

If patient characteristics are substantially different from trial to trial, and the effect of the intervention depends on these characteristics (e.g., comorbidity), then the two trials can come to different conclusions about the effect of the intervention. Another factor to consider in attempting to explain differences between the findings of two clinical trials that examine the effect of therapy for CHF is the time-dependent nature of CHF interventions. Treatment patterns for CHF are not static over time, but dynamic. Since the therapy commonly used in patients changes over time, the effect of the intervention being testing can either be reduced or amplified by the background therapy with which the intervention is concomitantly used. Clinical trials instigated in the twenty-first century are carried out in patients who commonly are taking a combination of digitalis, diuretic, ACE-i therapy as well as beta blockers. This was not the background therapy of ten years ago. Temporal changes in ongoing therapy for heart failure can make an important difference in the identification of a therapy effect.

Carefully considering these factors, both one at a time and then jointly, is an indispensable evaluation process and should not be avoided. However, by even attempting to view these effects in order to draw conclusions about the relationship between the intervention and clinical endpoints of heart failure, we are assuming that sampling error has been controlled enough for us to interpret results in different trials with different population bases. Therefore, we should suspend this clinical judgment until we are satisfied that the underlying methodology of the research is sound. The insistence of the correct research methodology is the bedrock upon which clinical interpretation of the research must rest.

2.10.2 Random Research in Extremis

Data dredging is random research in extremis. This search for a significant finding in the research may be well motivated; the dredgers are driven by the notion that if they work hard enough, long enough, and dig deep enough they will turn up something "significant." However, while it is possible to discover a jewel in this strip-mining operation, it is also more likely that for every rare jewel identified, there will be many false alarms, fakes, and shams [11], [37]. It takes tremendous effort to sort out all of these findings. In his book *Experimental Agriculture* (1849), James Johnson stated that a badly conceived experiment not only wastes time and money, but also leads to (1) the adoption of incorrect results into standard books, (2) the loss of money in practice, and (3) the neglect of further research along more appropriate lines. This is the legacy of random research [38].

It is not enough to design the research well. Believing that well-designed research can overcome subsequent protocol violations is like believing that a well-prepared, well-stocked kitchen will produce a good meal in spite the presence of an inept chef. Both a well-stocked kitchen and a skilled chef are necessary. One alone is not sufficient.

2.10.3 Requirements of Investigators and Readers

Any review of the experience of the vesnarinone, losartan, amlodipine, and carvedilol trials must acknowledge the effort of the investigators in all of these studies. Had they not appreciated the weak methodologic support for the findings from the first study for each drug, no additional confirmatory data would have been collected, and the heart failure community would have been left with the findings of the first vesnarinone study, ELITE-1 and PRAISE-1, and the US Carvedilol program as the final research effort for these interventions. We should be encouraged that the CHF community was willing to invest precious resources into the execution of additional studies in order to obtain the correct results.

Finally, the readers of the medical literature must develop a new skill of discrimination. Keeping in mind that the role of the investigator is not as an "explorer" or "searcher" who stumbles upon an unexpected finding but as a "*re*searcher," who confirms an a priori hypothesis with scientific rigor, readers of the peer-reviewed medical research literature must separate prospectively planned from random analyses. Manuscripts submitted to journals for publication must be rewritten and resubmitted if they do not allow the readers to make these critical distinctions. Confirmatory analyses are those for which there is a prospective specification of an analysis plan in complete detail, including type I error level allocations, leaving nothing in the analysis plan to be determined later by the data. This is the best way to ensure that the estimators the investigators have provided are trustworthy. Data-driven protocol deviations, that are the hallmarks of random research, are alarm bells for type I and type II error level aberrations, and can serve only to produce preliminary, exploratory evaluations.

2.11 Conclusions

Clinical trial interpretation requires judgment; the balancing effort in which we all engage as we weigh a study's strengths against its weaknesses remains a central one. However, just as justice cannot prevail in the absence of the rule of law, causality determinations in clinical trials require the rule of methodology. The first rule that validates the estimators of the effect of the clinical trial's intervention is the presence of a prospective, fixed analysis plan. Allowing data-driven analyses to determine a clinical trial's results, however well intentioned, strikes at the heart of the medical community's ability to generalize results from the research sample to the population at large. Random research, like our physician's gambling fortune teller, misdirects. It misdirects without malice, and misdirects with assurance; however in the end, misdirection is midirection. It holds a great potential for harm, and must be resolutely resisted.

Problems

For each of Problems 1 to 7, answer each of the following three questions:

   A) Is this research result concordant or discordant?
   B) Is this result of the research either hypothesis testing (confirmatory) or hypothesis generating (exploratory)?
   C) Are the effect measures and p-values for these reported results of this experiment all interpretable, or uninterpretable?

1. A multicenter clinical trial is designed to evaluate the effect of exposure to a randomly allocated intervention on the occurrence of sudden cardiac death. The protocol for the study is carefully written, with the prospective primary analysis plan. However, the therapy is determined to have side-effects, and many patients who are randomized to the active group are unable or refuse to continue to take their therapy. When the analysis is carried out with each patient assigned to the randomized treatment group, the effect of the therapy is neither clinically nor statistically significant. However, when the investigators analyze the data by dividing patients into those who have stayed on their medication versus those who do not take active therapy (either by assignment or by choice), the results demonstrate a clinically important reduction in the cumulative incidence of the primary endpoint, $p < 0.025$. The researchers report the "as treated" analysis, and claim that the study is positive.

2. A clinical trial is designed to evaluate the effect of cholesterol-reducing therapy on the occurrence of heart attacks. According to the protocol, the hypothesis test is a one-tailed test for benefit at the 0.025 level. The z-score at the conclusion of the experiment is 1.72 The researchers conclude that since this z-score is greater than 1.645, the experiment is positive.

3. A randomized, double-blind clinical trial is designed to look at the effect of therapy on total mortality in patients who have heart failure. The endpoint for this prospectively designed trial is total mortality and the prospectively declared maximum type I error is 0.05 (two-tailed). However, during the course

of the trial, the investigators believe that the death rate observed in the study will not produce enough deaths to have adequate power for the prospectively identified hypothesis test. They therefore change the endpoint to the combined endpoint of either death or survival and worsening of CHF. At the trial's conclusion, the number of deaths is observed, after all, to be sufficient for a hypothesis test on total mortality. The investigators report the total mortality result, $p = 0.019$.

4. A randomized, double-blind clinical trial is carried out to determine if the administration of a drug known to reduce the occurrence of dangerous heart rhythms will reduce mortality. The prospectively designed hypothesis test is one tailed, and the investigators have a critical region which, if the test statistic is greater than 1.96, the research will conclude that at the 0.025 significance level, the drug is beneficial. At the conclusion of the study, the test statistic is -2.0. The investigators conclude that the drug is dangerous.

5. A clinical trial is executed to determine the effect of diet pills on weight loss. According to the prospectively written protocol, the investigators will declare the study is positive if both the mean reduction in weight for patients in the active group is 5 pounds greater than the mean reduction in the control group and the p-value associated with this difference is less than 0.05. The trial reveals that the active group lost 4.5 pounds more than was lost in the trial with a p-value of 0.045. The investigators declare that the study was positive.

6. A drug company is anxious to demonstrate that their new medication, when given intravenously to patients who are undergoing a cardiac procedure to widen their narrowed coronary arteries, reduces mortality. They execute a clinical trial for which the prospectively determined primary endpoint is a reduction in the 3-month mortality rate, at 0.05 significance level (two sided). The researchers determine that the p-value for the 3-month reduction in mortality is 0.06 (two sided), but the p-value for the 6-month reduction in mortality is 0.04 (two sided). The researches declare that the study is positive.

7. A researcher carries out a clinical trial to assess the effect of inhalation therapy on stress reduction. This prospectively planned study is designed to demonstrate that inhalation therapy reduces a quantitative measure of stress by 30%, with a p-value of < 0.05 (two tailed). At the conclusion of the study, the researcher finds the reduction in stress to be 26% with a p-value 0.06. He notes, however, that the reduction in stress is 55% ($p = 0.039$) for patients greater than 60 years old, a subcohort that made up 40% of the recruited sample. He declares the study is positive.

References

1. Packer, M., Bristow, M.R., Cohn, J.N. et al (1996). The effect of carvedilol on morbidity and mortality in patients with chronic heart failure *New England Journal of Medicine* **334**:1349–55.

2. Transcript for the May 2, 1996, Cardiovascular and Renal Drugs Advisory Committee.

3. Moyé, L.A., Abernethy, D. (1996). Carvedilol in patients with chronic heart failure. (letter). *New England Journal of Medicine* **335**: 1318–1319.
4. Packer, M., Cohn, J.N., Colucci, W.S. (1996). Response to Moyé and Abernethy *New England Journal of Medicine* **335**:1318–1319.
5. Fisher, L.D., Moyé, L.A. (1999). Carvedilol and the Food and Drug Administration Approval Process: An Introduction. *Controlled Clinical Trials* **20**:1–15.
6. Fisher, L.D. (1999). Carvedilol and the fda approval process: the FDA paradigm and reflections upon hypothses testing. *Controlled Clinical Trials* **20**:16–39.
7. Moyé, L.A. (1999). *P*-value interpretation in clinical trials. The case for discipline. *Controlled Clinical Trials* **20**:40–49.
8. FDA Staff (1997). *Statistical Principles for Clinical Trials*. Version 4.
9. Meinert, C.L. (1986). *Clinical Trials Design, Conduct, and Analysis*. New York: Oxford University Press.
10. Friedman, L., Furberg, C., and DeMets, D. (1996). *Fundamentals of Clinical Trials 3rd edition*; New York. Springer.
11. Moyé, L.A. (2000). *Statistical Reasoning in Medicine–The Intuitive P-Value Primer*. New York. Spinger.
12. MRFIT Investigators (1982). Multiple risk factor intervention trial. *Journal of the American Medical Association* **248**:1465–77.
13. Pitt, B, Segal, R., Martinez, F.A. et al. on behalf of the ELITE Study Investigators (1997). Randomized trial of losartan versus captopril in patients over 65 with heart failure. *Lancet* **349**:747–52.
14. Packer, M., O'Connor, C.M., Ghali, J.K., et al for the Prospective Randomized Amlodipine Survival Evaluation Study Group (1996). Effect of amlodipine on morbidity and mortality in severe chronic heart failure. *New England Journal of Medicine*.**335**:1107–14.
15. Moyé, L.A. (1998). *P*-value interpretation and alpha allocation in clinical trials. *Annals of Epidemiology*. **8**:351–357.
16. Lachim J.M. (1981). Introduction to sample size determinations and power analyses for clinical trials. *Controlled Clinical Trials* **2**:93–114.
17. Sahai, H, Khurshid, A. (1996). Formulae and tables for determination of sample size and power in clinical trials for testing differences in proportions for the two sample design. *Statistics in Medicine* **15**:1–21.
18. Donner, A. (1984). Approach to sample size estimation in the design of clinical trials — a review. *Statistics in Medicine* **3**:199–214.
19. George, S.L., Desue, M.M. (1974). Planning the size and duration of a clinical trial studying the time to some critical event. *Journal of Chronic Disease* **27**:15–24.
20. Davy, S.J., Graham, O.T. (1991). Sample size estimation for comparing two or more treatment groups in clinical trials. *Statistics in Medicine* **10**:3–43.
21. Snedecor G.W., and Cochran W.G. (1980). *Statistical Methods, 7th Edition*. Iowa. Iowa State University Press.

22. Feldman A.M., Bristow M.R., Parmley, W.W. et al. (1993). Effects of vesnarinone on morbidity and mortality in patients with heart failure. *New Engand Journal of Medicine* **329**:149–55.

23. Cohn J., Goldstein S.C., Feenheed S. et al. (1998). A dose dependent increase in mortality seen with vesnarinone among patients with severe heart failure. *New England Journal of Medicine* **339**:1810–16.

24. Jensen, B.V., Nielsen, S.L. (1997). Correspondence: Losartan versus captopril in elderly patients with heart failure. *Lancet* **349**:1473

25. Fournier A., Achard J.M., Fernandez L.A. (1997). Correspondence: Losartan versus captopril in elderly patients with heart failure. *Lancet* **349:1473.**

26. Pitt, B., Poole-Wilson P.A., Segal, R., et. al (2000). Effect of losartan compared with captopril on mortality in patients with symptomatic heart failure randomized trial–The losartan heart failure survival study. ELITE II. *Lancet.***355**:1582–87.

27. Multicenter diltizaem post infarction trial research group.(1989). The effect of dilitiazem on mortality and reinfarction after myhocardial infarction. *New England Journal of Medicine* **319**:385–392.

28. Packer, M. (2000). Presentation of the results of the Prospective Randomized Amlodipine Survival Evaluation-2 Trial (PRAISE-2) at the American College of Cardiology Scientific Sessions, Anaheim, CA, March 15, 2000.

29. Waagstein, F., Hjalmarson, A., Varnauskass, E., Wallentin, I. (1975). Effect of chronic beta adrenergergic receptor blockage in congestive cardiomyopathy. *British Heart Journal* **37**:205–11.

30. Waagstein, F, Bristow, M.R., Swedberg, K., et al. (1993). Beneficial effects of metoprolol in idiopathic dilated cardiomyopathy. *Lancet* **342**:144–6.

31. CIBIS Investigators and Committees (1994). A randomized trial of beta-blockade in heart failure: The Cardiac Insufficiency Bisoprolol Study (CIBIS). *Circulation* **90**:1765–73.

32. The CAPRICORN Investigators. (2001). Effect of carvedilol on outcome after myocardial infarction in patients with left-ventricular dysfunction: the CAPRICORN randomised trial. *Lancet* **357**:1385–90.

33. Packer, M., Coats, A.J.S., Fowler, M.B., Katus, H.A., Krum, H, Mohacsi, P., Rouleau, J.L., Tendera, M., Castaigne, A., Roecker, E.B., Schultz, M.K., De-Mets, D.L. for the Carvedolol Prospective Randomized Cumulative Survival Study Group (2001) Effect of carvedilol on survival in severe chronic heart failure *New England Journal of Medicine* **344**:1651–8.

34. Harris, M.I., Flegal, K.M., Cowie, C.C., Eberhardt, M.S., Goldstein, D.E., Little R.R., Wiedmeyer, H.M., Byrd-Holt, D.D. (1998). Prevalence of diabetes, impaired fasting glucose, and impaired glucose tolerance in US adults. The Third National Health and Nutrition Examination Survey, 1988–1994. *Diabetes Care* **21**:518–524.

35. Moyé L.A. (2001). The perils of nonprospectively planned research. Part 1: Drawing conlcusions from sample-based research. *American Clinical Laboratory:* April 2001. 34–36.

36. Questions to the FDA Oncology Drugs Advisory Committee. December 6, 2001.

37. Mills, J.L. (1993). Data torturing. *New England Journal of Medicine.* **329**:1196–1199.

38. Young A. (1771) *A course of experimental agriculture.* J.Exshaw et al. Dublin.

Chapter 3
The Lure and Complexity of Multiple Analyses

This chapter presents the motivations for, and consequences of, executing multiple statistical analyses in clinical trials. Logistical efficiency, the desire to build a causal argument, and the need to explore and develop unanticipated results, are appropriate and powerful factors that motivate the inclusion of multiple analyses in these randomized studies. However, their incorporation may produce results which can be difficult to integrate with the idea of controlling the type I error rate. The need to minimize the type I error rate in a clinical trial is developed, followed by an elementary introduction to one of the most useful tools for controlling type I error rates—the Bonferroni inequality. Alternative methods of controlling the type I error rate are then briefly discussed. The chapter ends by combining (1) the motivation for the prospective plan of an experiment and (2) the need to control the type I error rate into a framework to guide the design of a clinical trial. This final integration (Table 3.3) describes the three ways in which multiple analyses in clinical trials are carried out, and the implications for each of their interpretations. This result will be the basis for the development of the multiple analysis tools to which the rest of the book is devoted.

3.1 Definition of Multiple Analyses

By multiple analyses, we mean the collection of statistical hypothesis tests which are executed at the conclusion of a clinical trial. The term *collection* is deliberately broad, encompassing all of the evaluations that investigators understandably feel compelled to conduct upon the experiment's conclusion. The following are examples of multiple analyses in clinical trials:

> Example 1: A clinical trial is designed to compare the effects of three different doses (D_1, D_2, and D_3) of an intervention to each other and to control therapy on a prospectively chosen endpoint. This setting requires several different pairwise evaluations. Three of them involve the control group (D_1 versus placebo, D_2 versus placebo, and D_3 versus placebo) and three require inter-level comparisons (D_1 versus D_2, D_1 versus D_3, and D_2 versus D_3). Thus, there are six comparisons to be assessed, each leading to a hypothesis test. If there were four doses of the intervention to be evaluated, there would be ten comparisons to assess.

Example 2: A clinical trial is designed to compare the effect of a single dose of an intervention to that of a control group for a prospectively defined endpoint. This comparison is to include not just the entire cohort of research subjects, but also a comparison within males, within females, within different race/ethnicity groups, and within country. Although these additional analyses are traditionally described as subgroup analysis, they fall under our broad rubric of multiple analyses.

Example 3: A clinical trial is designed to compare a single dose intervention against placebo for efficacy. The trial has a primary endpoint of total mortality, but in addition, has included prospectively defined analyses for the secondary endpoints of (1) cardiovascular death, (2) fatal and nonfatal MI, (3) fatal and nonfatal stroke, (4) the cumulative incidence of hospitalization, (5) unstable angina, and (6) revascularization. Each of these secondary endpoints produces a comparison of the effect of the single dose intervention versus placebo.

Example 4: A clinical trial is designed to compare the effect of a medication given immediately after a coronary artery procedure (e.g., coronary artery angioplasty or coronary artery bypass surgery) to placebo. The endpoint for the study is the cumulative mortality rate. The comparison of the mortality rate is to take place at 3 months, 6 months, and 1 year after the procedure. At each of these three time points, the cumulative mortality rate of the intervention group is to be compared to that of the control group.

In reality, these four examples occur not in isolation, but in complicated combinations. For example, a clinical trial may compare the effect of a single dose intervention to a control group on several different endpoints and in several subgroups. Some of the endpoints may have been prespecified in the protocol, while others were not considered until the trial was completed. Likewise, some of the subgroups may have been prespecified, while others were not. This tangle of analyses typically accompanies the execution of a clinical trial as the researchers thoroughly analyze their data. The purpose of this chapter is to (1) review the motivation for multiple analyses, (2) describe the commonly used statistical procedures used to address the multiple analysis issues in clinical trials, and (3) settle on a class of procedures that has the advantage of being easy to understand while simultaneously preserving a comprehensible measure of community protection.

3.2 Why Do Multiple Analyses?

Multiple analyses are a natural byproduct of the complexity of clinical experiments. While investigators describe their motivations to carry out more than one analysis in several ways, there are three primary reasons for the execution of multiple statistical hypothesis tests. They are (1) to provide logistical efficiency, (2) to strengthen the causal argument, and (3) to explore new ideas and establish new relationships between risk (or beneficial) factors and disease. We will briefly discuss each of these in turn.

3.2.1 Logistical Efficiency

One of the motivations that generates multiple analyses is the drive of both the investigator and the sponsor[1] for efficiency. They are each interested in discovering an answer to the scientific question which motivated the trial, but they also require that the experiment should be competently run and analyzed. This translates into ensuring that the clinical trial be as productive as possible, and generate a full return of results to justify the commitment of the logistical and financial resources required for the experiment's execution.

Consider a controlled clinical trial which involves randomizing patients to either the intervention group or the control group, and follows those patients until either the patient dies or the predetermined duration of follow-up has elapsed. The investigators plan only one analysis which assesses the relationship between the use of the therapy and the cumulative incidence of total mortality. For this simple clinical trial with one endpoint and a single analysis, substantial financial, logistical, material, and personnel resources will be consumed. However, once this price has been paid, additional subject measurements can be obtained for a relatively small additional cost.

For example, if the original endpoint was total mortality, what would the additional cost be of collecting the supplementary data that would allow a determination of the cause of death, necessary to create an additional endpoint of cause-specific mortality? The only additional information required for this new endpoint would be the collection of hospital records, death certificates, eyewitness accounts, and a committee to determine and adjudicate the cause of each death. In general, as the investigators add to the number of endpoints, the total cost of the study will increase, but the cost per endpoint or marginal cost will decrease.

There is certainly a supplementary cost for collecting this additional information, but the marginal cost is small compared to the original cost of the trial. Thus, the number of endpoints in the study has doubled but the cost of the experiment has increased by a relatively small amount. The addition of a third endpoint (i.e., total hospitalization) produces yet another increase in the cost of the experiment (a discharge summary will be required for each hospitalized patient), but again the cost of the original experiment is not substantially increased. Thus, one can triple the number of endpoints and increase the number of statistical analyses (and perhaps increase the likelihood of a positive result on at least one),[2] without tripling the cost of the experiment, certainly a cost efficient exercise.

3.2.2 Epidemiologic Strength

An additional motivation for conducting multiple analyses in clinical trials can be found in epidemiology. As discussed in Chapter 1, epidemiologists use a combina-

---

[1] The sponsor of the trial is the organization which funds the study. It could be a government funded study, underwritten by institutes, e.g., the National Eye Institute, or the National Institute of Environmental Health Services. Alternatively, the clinical trial could be funded by a private pharmaceutical company.
[2] We will have much more to say about this concept later.

tion of careful observation and deductive reasoning to determine whether a relationship between an exposure and a disease is causal, an evaluation that is guided by the use of the Hill tenets.[3] Clinical trial designers can implement these investigative tools to cement the causal link between the intervention and patient improvement, but this requires multiple analyses.

For example, one of the causality criteria that is useful in proving that a medication produces a reduction in mortality is the demonstration of a dose–response relationship. If the clinical trial revealed that an increase in the dose of the randomly allocated intervention produced a further benefit, then the causal nature of the intervention–mortality rate relationship is more secure. This investigation could be prospectively embedded into the design of the trial. Elucidating that there is a dose–response relationship requires that (1) the trial have a control group and at least two intervention groups (one receiving intervention dose D_1, and the second requiring intervention dose D_2, where D_1 is less than D_2,) and (2) that the beneficial effect of D_2 exceeds the beneficial effect of D_1. Thus, there are potentially three separate analyses to complete this dose–response evaluation (D_1 versus control, D_2 versus control, and D_2 versus D_1). This approach has been formally addressed in the literature [1].

Another example of an epidemiologic motivation for the execution of multiple analyses is the elucidation of a biologic mechanism. Identifying the physiologic path by which the clinical trial's intervention produces the reduction in morbidity and mortality adds strength to the treatment–benefit causality argument. For example, when HMG-CoA reductase inhibitors (i.e., the "statins") and their effects on cardiovascular disease were first being studied, it was proposed that their effect on the occurrence of atherosclerotic cardiovascular morbidity was mediated by reductions in low-density lipoprotein (LDL) cholesterol levels. Thus, when these compounds were evaluated for their ability to reduce clinical endpoints of interest (e.g., fatal and nonfatal myocardial infarction), the investigators often first demonstrated that this reduction in long-term morbid and mortal events was preceded by a sustained reduction in the LDL cholesterol levels. Although the endpoint of each of these trials was not the change in LDL cholesterol levels, the investigators correctly deduced that they should demonstrate that there was a reduction in LDL cholesterol levels before the reduction in clinical morbidity and mortality produced by the intervention was accepted and understood. This was a tack followed by major clinical trials investigating cholesterol-lowering therapy for patients without a history of atherosclerotic disease [2], or patients with a history of this disease (secondary prevention) in the United States [3], Europe [4], and Australia [5].

Additionally, a causality argument can also be strengthened by the demonstration that several related endpoints, whose occurrence is generated by the same underlying pathophysiology, are simultaneously affected by the intervention. Thus, continuing with the HMG-CoA reductase inhibitor example, the effect of the therapy to reduce not just the cumulative incidence rate of fatal and nonfatal myocardial infarctions, but also the incidence of (1) fatal and nonfatal strokes, (2) unstable angina, and (3) coronary revascularizations provides additional evidence for the causal link between the medication and clinical outcomes of atherosclerotic disease.

---

[3] These nine tenets are listed in Appendix A.

Each additional endpoint requires its own evaluation of the effect of therapy and an additional statistical hypothesis test (to provide some assurance that the finding in the sample is not likely to be due to the play of chance).

Finally, subgroup evaluations have also been an important force in producing multiple analyses in clinical trials. Customarily, the motivation for subgroup analyses is the desire to demonstrate that the response to the medication being evaluated in the clinical trial is uniform and homogenous across ages, gender, ethnicity, and classes of patients who are linked by similar comorbidity. Traditionally, heterogeneity of therapy effect across subgroups in clinical trials has caused concern. The presence of an effect in a sizable subgroup of patients when all other subgroups of patients receive no real benefit of therapy permits speculation that there may be an important treatment effect modification that is subgroup related.[4] Alternatively, profound heterogeneity of effect across several subgroups raises the issue that the finding of the different levels of therapy benefit across the subgroups was just due to the play of chance and not really indicative of a benefit that would be expected in the entire population.

Recently, subgroup analysis has been spurred by the demonstration of heterogeneity in populations. The increased interest in the role of genetics in mediating the effect of a medication, and the interest expressed by the FDA in specifically evaluating the potential differential effect of medications across both gender and race [6] have ignited the interest among clinical trial designers to demonstrate not subgroup homogeneity but heterogeneity. These evaluations would require even more analyses.

3.2.3 The Need to Explore

There is a critical difference between confirmatory research and exploratory research. Confirmatory research executes a protocol that was designed to answer a prospectively asked scientific question. Exploratory research is the evaluation of a dataset for new and interesting relationships that were not anticipated. In Chapter 2, we pointed out that these should be segregated. However, there is room in a clinical trial for both.

Investigators want to cover new ground, and enjoy the exploration process. Exploratory analyses can evaluate the effect of the therapy in subgroups, the effect of the therapy on different endpoints, and the effect of different doses of the medication. Although we will have much to say about the correct place for exploratory analyses in clinical trials, that review must begin with the acknowledgment that exploratory analyses are a sustained, driving force behind many of the statistical analyses carried out in clinical trials.

---

[4] This was the circumstance of the findings in PRAISE–1 in which a reduction in the cumulative total mortality rate was seen in patients with nonischemic cardiomyopathy, but not in patients with ischemic cardiomyopathy (Chapter 2).

3.3 Hypothesis Testing in Multiple Analyses

These well-motivated concerns for efficiency, good epidemiologic evidence necessary to solidify the causal relationship between the intervention and the observed
effect, and the need to explore together demand that multiple analyses remain a
common occurrence in clinical trials. The continued incorporation of multiple
analyses in clinical experiments has led to an increased interest in issues surrounding their use. Since each of these analyses involves a statistical hypothesis test, and
each hypothesis test produces a p-value, a relevant question is how should these p-
values be interpreted?

Some have argued in articles [7] and editorials [8] that these additional p-
values should be ignored. Others have argued that they should be interpreted as
though the value of 0.05 is the cutoff point for statistical significance, regardless of
how many p-values have been produced by the study. This is called using "nominal
significance testing" or "marginal significance." Others have debated whether investigators should be able to analyze all of the data, and then choose the results they
want to disseminate [9], [10], [11].

The discussion in Chapter 2 forces us to reject the results of the investigator who, after inspecting the magnitudes of each of the p-values, makes an after the
fact, or post hoc choice, from among them. This "wait and see what analysis is
positive" approach violates the underlying critical assumption of the p-value construction (i.e., that the data with its embedded sampling error should not choose
either the endpoint or the analysis). This violation invalidates the p-value.

3.3.1 Nominal P-Values

The nominal approach to multiple p-value analysis must now be considered. The
tack of interpreting each of several p-values from a single experiment, one at a time,
based on whether they are greater or less than the traditional threshold of 0.05 may
seem like a natural alternative to the post hoc decision structure that we just rejected. In fact, the nominal p-value approach is very alluring at first glance. The
rule to use nominal p-values is easily stated prospectively at the beginning of the
trial, and is easy to apply at that trial's end.

However, the consequences of this approach must be given careful attention. Consider, for example, two analyses from a randomized clinical trial designed
to measure the effect of therapy of an intervention in patients with atherosclerotic
cardiovascular disease. Let us assume in this hypothetical example that the research
was well-designed with two endpoints in mind: (1) the cumulative total mortality
rate and (2) the cumulative incidence of fatal/nonfatal strokes. We will also assume
that the analysis has been carried out concordantly (i.e., according to the experiment's prospectively written protocol). The first analysis reveals that the
intervention reduces the cumulative incidence rate of total mortality by a clinically
meaningful magnitude, producing a p-value of 0.045. The second analysis reveals
that the intervention reduces the cumulative incidence of fatal and nonfatal stroke in
a clinically meaningful way, again with a p-value of 0.045. The investigators have
clearly met the clinical, statistical, and traditional threshold of results with p-values
of less than 0.05. Should each of these be accepted nominally, i.e., should the inves-

tigator conclude that the study produced evidence that the intervention (when used in the population from which the research sample was obtained) will reduce total mortality and will also reduce the fatal and nonfatal stroke rate?[5]

3.3.2 The Error of Interest: Familywise Error[6]

To evaluate this important question, recall that the p-value for the effect of an intervention on an endpoint measures the probability that the population in which the intervention has no effect generated a sample that, just by the play of chance and the random aggregation of events, shows a positive effect of the intervention. The occurrence of this error is a reasonable event to be concerned about when there is only one endpoint. However, with two endpoints, the event of interest is more complicated, and the nominal interpretation of p-values is unsatisfactory.

In this specific example in which there are two analyses, one on the effect of the intervention on the total mortality rate and the second on the intervention's impact of the fatal and nonfatal stroke rate, a type I error means that the population has produced by chance alone a sample that either (1) gives a false and misleading signal that the intervention reduced the cumulative total mortality incidence rate, (2) gives a false and misleading signal that the intervention reduced the fatal and nonfatal stroke rate, or (3) gives a false and misleading signal suggesting that the intervention reduced both the cumulative mortality rate and the fatal and nonfatal stroke rate. There are three errors of which we must now keep track when there are two endpoint analyses, and the misleading events of interest can occur in combination. Therefore, a more complicated measure of type I error rate is required. This complex measure of type I error rate might be described as an overall research α, but has previously been termed the familywise (type I) error probability (or error level),[7] or FWER [12], [13] and will be designated as ξ.

There is a critical difference between the standard type I error level for a single endpoint and ξ. The type I error probability for a single, individual endpoint focuses on the occurrence of a misleading positive result for a single analysis. This is the single test error level, or test-specific error level. The familywise error level focuses on the occurrence of at least one type I error in the entire collection of analyses. Thus, ξ incorporates the test-specific type I error levels for each of the analyses taken one at a time, and in addition, considers the combinations of type I errors when the statistical hypothesis tests are considered jointly. In the preceding example where there were two endpoints, total mortality and fatal/nonfatal stroke, the occurrence of a familywise error is a measure of the likelihood that we have

---

[5] Recall from Chapter 2 that the p-value should not be considered as a stand-alone integrated measure of strength of evidence. The research can only be accurately interpreted if the sample size, relative risk, the standard error of the relative risk, the confidence interval, and the p-value are jointly interpreted. However, since the focus of this chapter is not the evaluation of the magnitude of benefit but the multiplicity of type I error, these other factors will be deemphasized for the sake of clarity in this discussion.

[6] The terms *error probability*, *error rate*, and *error levels* will be used interchangeably.

[7] This is sometimes called the familywise error rate computed under the complete null hypothesis.

drawn the wrong positive conclusion about the benefit of therapy for total mortality alone, fatal/nonfatal stroke alone, or have made an error about both.

3.3.3 Initial Computations for ξ

The familywise error level can be easily computed if we assume that the result of one hypothesis test provides no information about the result of the other hypothesis test.[8] Recall that the probability of a type I error for the hypothesis test examining the effect of therapy on the cumulative incidence of the total mortality rate is 0.045, and that the same rate has been chosen for the stroke endpoint. First, compute the probability that there is no type I error for the total mortality rate effect and no type I error for the fatal/nonfatal stroke rate effect using the α error levels for each as follows:

P[no type I error for the total mortality effect and no type I error for the fatal/nonfatal stroke rate effect]

= P[no type I error for total mortality effect] * P [no type I error for the fatal/nonfatal stroke rate effect]

=(1 − P[a type I error occurred for the total mortality effect]) *(1 − P [no type I error occurred for the fatal/nonfatal stroke rate])

$$= (1 - 0.045)(1 - 0.045) = (0.955)^2 = 0.9120.$$

Thus, 0.9120 is the probability that there is no false signal from the sample about the beneficial effect of the intervention on each of the total mortality rate and the fatal/nonfatal stroke rate. This situation is the best of all possible worlds. The familywise error level in which we are interested is the reverse of this, i.e., that there is at a type I error for either the total mortality finding, the fatal/nonfatal stroke finding, or both. Thus, we easily compute ξ as

$$\xi = 1 - 0.9120 = 0.088. \tag{3.1}$$

This value of 0.088 is greater than 0.045 (the test-specific *p*-value for each of the two analyses) and presents the results of this experiment in a very different light. By accepting a less than one in twenty chance of a type I error for either the effect of the intervention on either (1) the cumulative mortality rate or (2) the cumulative incidence rate for fatal/nonfatal strokes, we accept almost a one in ten chance of falsely concluding that the intervention will be effective in the population when it is not. Recognition of this error level inflation is the heart of the problem with accepting nominal significance for multiple analyses. For any realistic collection of single

---

[8] The performance of this computation when the result of a hypothesis test for one endpoint provides information about the result of another hypothesis test is the specific subject of Chapters 5–6.

test error levels, the greater the number of endpoints, the larger the familywise error level ξ becomes (Table 3.1)

Table 3.1.   Relationship between the test specific alpha and the familywise error rate.

		Test specific alpha		
	0.05	0.025	0.01	0.001
1	0.050	0.025	0.010	0.001
2	0.098	0.049	0.020	0.002
Number of 3	0.143	0.073	0.030	0.003
tests 4	0.185	0.096	0.039	0.004
5	0.226	0.119	0.049	0.005
6	0.265	0.141	0.059	0.006
7	0.302	0.162	0.068	0.007
8	0.337	0.183	0.077	0.008
9	0.370	0.204	0.086	0.009
10	0.401	0.224	0.096	0.010

Table 3.1 provides the familywise error level as a function of the number of hypothesis tests for different values of the test-specific α. For example, if two analyses each have an α level value of 0.05, $\xi = 0.098$. The entries in Table 3.1 demonstrate that the familywise error level increases with the number of statistical hypothesis tests.

However, Table 3.1 can be used in another manner. Note that if a researcher wishes to keep ξ at less than 0.05, the number of analyses whose results can be controlled (i.e., the number of analyses that can be carried out and still keep the familywise error level ≤ 0.05) depends on the significance level at which the individual analyses are to be evaluated. For example, if each of the individual analyses is to be judged at the 0.05 level (i.e., the *p*-value resulting from the analyses must be less than 0.05 in order to claim the result is statistically significant), then only one analysis can be controlled, since the familywise error level for two analyses exceeds the 0.05 threshold. The researcher can control the familywise error level for two analyses if each is judged at the 0.025 level. If each test is evaluated at the 0.01 level, then five independent hypothesis tests can be carried out.

Note the last column of Table 3.1 in which each test is judged at the 0.001 level. In this case, the familywise error rate ξ can be kept below the 0.05 level, when as many as 50 analyses are evaluated. This is the key to an important criticism of a popular approach to the evaluation of multiple hypothesis tests to be discussed later in this chapter.

3.3.4 FDA and Strength of Evidence

The type of computation that we completed in the previous section is not the only interesting calculation involving type I errors that the investigators of clinical trials face. As another example of this style of reasoning, consider the conundrum that the FDA faces as it attempts to judge the type I error rates across different bodies of evidence.

As it considers whether a new compound is to be approved, most of the FDA's effort is its review of the new drug application (NDA). The new drug application is the tremendous volume of scientific information compiled by the sponsor. This corpus represents all of the relevent evidence that the sponsor believes supports its claim that the compound is safe, effective, and should be approved by the FDA. It consists of thousands of pages of data that describe in great detail the compound's mechanism of action, bioavailability, metabolism, excretion, clinical efficacy, and adverse event occurrences.[9] The NDAs have at their epicenter, the findings of randomized controlled clinical trials. Since the strongest and most interpretable evidence for the benefits and hazards or the compound reside in these trials, these studies are commonly referred to as *pivotal clinical trials*.

In this example, the FDA receives an NDA from each of two sponsors. Each sponsor believes their product is safe and effective for the treatment of CHF. We will assume that the quality of data in the two NDAs is equivalent and meets the FDA's standards. However, the number of pivotal trials in the two NDA's is different. In NDA 1, the evidence that the medication is safe and effective is contained in two well-designed, well-executed pivotal clinical trials. In NDA 2, this evidence is expressed in only one pivotal trial. Each of the pivotal trials is well-designed and concordantly executed with a prospectively declared, persuasive, primary endpoint. Is NDA 1 with its two compelling studies more persuasive than NDA 2 that contains only one pivotal trial?

Our intuition tells us that the strength of evidence for benefit in NDA 1 with its two pivotal studies is greater than that presented in the second NDA which included only one pivotal study. This concept has been quantified by the following argument. Recall that the type I error is the probability that the population (in which the compound is not effective) produces a sample that, just through chance alone, demonstrates an effect. While this event can certainly occur, it is less likely to occur in two independent studies; that would require that the population produce not just one, but two aberrant samples.

Suppose that the investigators in each of the two pivotal studies in NDA 1 wrongly conclude that there is a positive effect of the compound in each of the two studies based on sampling error; this is the same as saying that a type I error has occurred for each of these trials. Assume that these two studies are independent of each other,[10] and each is carried out at the prospectively set 0.05 type I error rate. In

---

[9] These NDAs used to be delivered to the FDA's offices in Rockville, Maryland, in trucks. They are now delivered on small sets of compact discs (CDs).

[10] This means that there is nothing about the design or the execution of the two studies that links them in such a way that the results of the first study predict the results of the second study.

this setting, the probability of "two type I errors" is $(0.05)(0.05) = 0.0025$. Some have argued that, if an NDA is to be approved based on the findings of one rather than two pivotal trials, then the strength of evidence presented by the one pivotal study must match that strength that is created by two pivotal studies. Therefore, if a single pivotal study is to have the same strength of evidence as two pivotal clinical trials, than that single trial, to be equally persuasive as two studies, should be carried out with a prospectively set α error level of 0.0025.

This finding is not a standard for the prospectively set type I error level for a single pivotal study. However, this calculation is commonly used to impress upon the sponsor the importance of retaining tight control on the type I error rate for its single pivotal trial.

3.4 Is Tight Control of the FWER Necessary?

The previous section focused on the problems which arise from the application of nominal statistical testing to multiple analyses carried out in clinical trials. However, the simple computations presented there demonstrate that it is too difficult to keep the familywise error level for even a moderate number of statistical hypothesis tests at an acceptably low level unless the test-specific α levels are exceedingly small. This conclusion excludes the nominal significance testing approach as a useful procedure to draw reliable conclusions about the population based on the research sample in a clinical trial.

The rejection of this nominal testing approach will come as a disappointment to many. This is because (1) p-values are so easily generated, one for each hypothesis; (2) the 0.05 level of statistical significance applied to each test is both traditional, standard, and requires no additional computations; and (3) the prospective statement that each of the many hypothesis tests to be carried out in the clinical trial will be judged nominally avoids the random research paradigm that we so heavily criticized in Chapter 2. Thus, the application of nominal testing at the 0.05 level is an easy analysis plan to execute, requiring very little new judgment, while simultaneously avoiding the difficulty of letting the results dictate the decision rule. In fact, the only difficulty with nominal testing in multiple analyses is that the familywise error level becomes very large very fast for test-specific α rates at 0.05. In light of the three advantages of the nominal testing approach mentioned in this paragraph, it is reasonable to explore just how lethal the criticism of uncontrolled type I error growth really is. In fact, why be concerned about accumulating type I error at all?

This has been a question to which several responses have been clearly expressed in the statistical and epidemiologic literature. Nester [7] has argued that hypothesis testing is an innovation which serves no good useful purpose. He suggests that it is (1) their ready availability and (2) the expectation of the statistical and medical community for the widespread use of tests of significance that stampedes modern-day researchers to require that hypothesis testing be the central feature of their clinical trial analysis. This of course is a general criticism of the use of hypothesis tests in any form, suggesting perhaps that hypothesis tests have been incorrectly applied for so many years that their correct use at this late date may serve only to satisfy a moribund tradition.

Others have criticized the tight control of type I error levels on different grounds. Examination of Table 3.1 reveals that the greater the number of analyses carried out, the larger the familywise error level becomes. A corollary to this observation is that in order to control ξ, the researcher should keep the test-specific α level for each individual test low. An immediate consequence of this strategy is that results accompanied by merely intermediate levels of statistical significance will be ignored since their p-values will exceed the very small test-specific α levels required to keep ξ low. This is a major criticism of type I error control argued by Rothman [8]. The core of this contention is that tight control of type I error rates leads the investigator to inappropriately miss potential positive effects.

Pocock and Farewell [14] also described the problems confronting medical researchers who try to control the familywise error rate in a multiple statistical analysis setting. They presented an illustration in which an investigator is confronted with a study in which there are 34 related response variables recorded to characterize the treatment effect of an intervention on peripheral muscular and nerve function in patients with diabetes mellitus. The investigator had no a priori reason to examine this constellation of variables in any single specific manner, but desires to carry out a statistical hypothesis test for the effect of therapy on each one. The application of Table 3.1 to this example leads to the conclusion that, in order to keep the familywise error level at the 0.05 level, the significance level used to judge each of these tests (i.e., the test level significance levels for each test) would need to be very small.[11]

Yet another example provided by the same author considers the evaluation of a therapy that holds promise for the treatment of arthritis. As with the previous illustration, arthritis is a disease for which there are multiple outcome measures and no clear a priori choice as to which endpoint is the best endpoint among multiple measures of disease progression. Thus, in this circumstance where there is genuine interest in the treatment effect but no a priori reason to select one endpoint over the other, Pocock and Farewell suggest that each be interpreted nominally, i.e., their significance is accepted or rejected based on nominal testing at the 0.05 level of significance.

Thus, not only does it appear that the control of type I error rate blocks the use of the nominal testing procedure, but in addition type I error rate control leads to insensitive result interpretation. These are important criticisms which any proponent of α error rate control must address.

3.5 Community Protection

The fundamental reason for controlling type I error rates in clinical trials is that the type I error is the probability of a mistaken research conclusion for the treatment of a disease, a mistake which has both critical and ethical implications for both the population of patients to be treated and for the medical community. While sample-based research cannot remove the possibility of this mistake, the magnitude of this

---

[11] More specifically, the type I error level for each test would be approximately $0.05/34 = 0.0015$. The simple mathematics of this computation will be developed in Section 3.7.

error rate must be accurately measured and discussed, so that the effectiveness of a therapy can be appropriately balanced against that therapy's risks.[12]

It is easy for the lay community to focus on the potential efficacy of new interventions for serious diseases [15]. However, it is a truism in medicine that all medications have risks. In a clinical trial, this truism is the foundation of the observation that all interventions have adverse effects[13] associated with them. These adverse effects range from troublesome symptoms (e.g., occasional dry mouth) to serious problems (e.g., fatigue, blurred vision, palpitations, vomiting, and diarrhea) to life-threatening injuries (e.g., toxic megacolon, primary pulmonary hypertension, acute liver failure, and birth defects). Many times these adverse events occur so frequently that clinical trials can identify them and can, therefore, accurately predict their occurrence in the population at large. It is important to acknowledge that regardless of whether the drug is effective or not, the population will have to bear adverse events.

In addition to the occurrence of specific, anticipated adverse events, there are circumstances in which serious adverse events occur in large populations without warning. This can happen when the clinical studies (completed before regulatory approval of the compound was granted) were not able to discern the occurrence of these adverse events because the studies contained too few patients.

Consider the following illustration: The background rate of acute liver failure leading to liver transplant or death is on the order of 1 case per 1,000,000 patients per year in the United States. Assume that a new drug being evaluated in a pre-FDA approval clinical trial increases this incidence by tenfold, to 1 case per 100,000 patients exposed per year, representing a ten fold increase in risk. The magnitude of this intervention's effect on the annual incidence of acute liver failure is a critical piece of information that both the private physician and the patient require as they jointly consider whether the risk of this drug is worth its benefits.

However, an important consequence of this tenfold increase in acute liver failure is that (on average) 100,000 patients would need to be exposed to this drug in order to be expected to see one case of acute liver failure per year. This is a large number of subjects, far larger than the number of patients required in the clinical trials in which the safety and efficacy of the drug are demonstrated. Thus, the large increase in the rate of acute liver failure produced by the intervention, representing an adverse effect of public health importance, would be invisible in small clinical trials which recruit and follow less than 1000 patients for 6 months. If this drug were approved and released for general dispersal through the population for which the drug is indicated, patients would unknowingly be exposed to a devastating, unpredicted adverse event. The fact that a clinical trial, not designed to detect an adverse effect, does not find the adverse effect is characterized by the saying "ab-

---

[12] We are setting aside the kinds of errors in clinical trial design that would produce a reproducible, nonrandom bias. An example of such a bias would be to choose a dose of medication to test in a clinical trial that is too small to be effective.

[13] According to the FDA, an adverse effect is defined as an undesirable side effect, reasonably believed to be associated with the drug. It is important to note that the FDA does not require that the drug be shown to cause the adverse effect—only the association between the two needs to be demonstrated.

sence of evidence is not evidence of absence" [16]. This summarizes the point that the absence of evidence within the clinical trial that the drug is associated with a serious adverse event is not evidence that the compound has no serious side effect.[14]

Thus, we expect adverse events to appear in the population regardless of whether the intervention demonstrates benefit or not. Some (perhaps the majority) of these adverse events are predictable. Others may not be. In addition, the financial costs of these interventions are not inconsiderable and must be weighed in the global risk–benefit assessment. Therefore, regardless of whether the medication is effective, the compound is assured to impose an adverse event and a finan-cial/administrative burden on the patients who receive it. The occurrences of these events represent the risk side of the risk–benefit equation.

The use of the intervention is justified only by the expectation that its benefits outweigh these health and financial costs. If the clinical trial which bears the burden of demonstrating the effectiveness of the compound is positive, then the research sample has demonstrated that the desired and anticipated benefit of the compound has been observed. But how likely is it that the population will see the same magnitude of benefit demonstrated by the clinical trial? This is the issue that type I error examines. A type I error is defined to mean that, even though a positive finding was seen in the sample, there will be no positive effect seen in the popula-tion.[15] Thus, even though the trial was positive, and the investigators drew the understandable conclusion that the compound was effective, the type I error's oc-currence directs that this observation of benefit is not true therapy effectiveness. It is instead merely the random, unpredictable, and irreproducible aggregation of events. The patient community, when exposed to this medication is guaranteed to experience the adverse event burden and the financial burden of the therapy; the occurrence of a type I error ensures the community will see no beneficial effect.[16]

Recall that the possibility of a type I error cannot be expunged from an ex-periment. It is intrinsic to the process of carrying out research on a sample. The situation is even more complicated when there are multiple analyses carried out in a clinical trial. Consider our first example in which a clinical trial demonstrated that the effect of a therapy was shown to be positive for each of (1) total mortality ($p = 0.045$) and (2) fatal/nonfatal stroke ($p = 0.045$). The p-value for each of these is ac-ceptably low, however the probability that in the population at least one of these beneficial effects will not take place is 0.088. This means that there is an almost 1 in 10 chance that the population will receive either (1) no beneficial effect on the cumulative total mortality rate or (2) no beneficial reduction in the fatal/nonfatal stroke incidence rate or (3) no beneficial reduction in both. It is this familywise er-ror level of 0.088 that must be compared to the risk of the medication because the

---

[14] The statistical power computation for this example appears in Appendix D.

[15] A type I error in this context means that a population in which the intervention has no beneficial effect produced a sample that, due just to the play of chance, demonstrated that the intervention was effective.

[16] A possible argument that a type I error may be helpful (e.g., an investigational agent that is less expensive and safer than the standard of care is mistakenly found to be more effective than the currently used agent) would be evaluated in a noninferiority trial, which is beyond the scope of this text.

familywise error level most accurately measures the likelihood of a type I error for all of the claimed benefits of the intervention. By not keeping track of (and ultimately controlling) ξ, we turn a blind eye to the likelihood that the therapy will not have the beneficial effects that were suggested in the sample-based research effort, thereby exposing patients to only harm.

The consequence of a type I error for efficacy in a clinical trial that is designed to measure the true risk–benefit balance of a randomly allocated intervention is the reverse of the Hippocratic Oath, succinctly summarized as "first do no harm".[17] In clinical trials, type I errors represent ethical issues as much as they do statistical concerns, and, in these studies which are commonly the justification for the use of interventions in large populations, the familywise error level must be controlled within acceptable limits.

3.6 Efficacy and Drug Labels

It may be surprising, but the notion of multiple analyses and type I error control can be embedded in the drug labels that are assembled in the *Physician's Desk Reference (PDR)*. The label or package insert provided for each prescription drug in the United States is the description of the compound that both the FDA and the sponsoring pharmaceutical company have agreed provides for the safe and effective use of the drug in patients. This agreement often occurs after months of negotiations between the FDA and the pharmaceutical company. The final form of the label is based on the understanding between the two parties that (1) it is the sponsor that owns the label, (2) the FDA sets minimal standards for the label to which the sponsor must adhere, and (3) the sponsor can exceed these standards if it desires.

Since the wording of the label is critical, there are strict rules describing its organization and contents. These rules are delineated in the Code of Federal Regulations. The label itself is divided into several components; among the most prominent are the following sections: description, indications, contraindications, warnings, adverse events, and precautions. The portion of the label of interest to us here is the indication section. It is the indication section of the label that describes the benefits of the drug that the FDA and the sponsor reasonably believed would occur in those patients who use the drug as directed (Appendix C). The code of federal regulations devoted to the indications section of the drug label describes the source of the information that substantiates the claim for benefit.

> *(2) All indications shall be supported by substantial evidence of effectiveness based on adequate and well-controlled studies as defined in Sec. 314.126(b) of this chapter unless the requirement is waived under Sec. 201.58 or Sec. 314.126(b) of this chapter.*

---

[17] This problem is exacerbated by the inability to measure type I error accurately. As demonstrated by the vesnarinone, losartan, amlodipine, and carvedilol examples provided in Chapter 2, the inability to measure the type I error rate accurately because of experimental discordance led to conclusions which were not reproduced in subsequent experiments.

Thus, the source of the information about benefits from a drug should be from adequate and well controlled clinical trials. The definition of an adequate and well-controlled clinical trial is provided in another regulation (available in Appendix C). The salient point here is that these adequate and well-controlled clinical trials should provide substantial evidence for the claimed benefit of the drug. It is important to note that no statistical criteria are listed in these regulations for the determination of whether a clinical trial provides efficacy for a compound or not. However, a guidance issued to industry by the FDA provides instruction:

> *4. Multiplicity Adjustments*
> *If the trial contains multiple tests of significance for any reason (e.g., three or more treatment arms, multiple primary endpoints, interim data analysis, model fitting, subgroup analyses) the analysis plan should include an adjustment to avoid inflation of the type I error rate. A particular adjustment approach should be specified in the protocol before examination of the data.*
>
> Source: Draft Guidance. Developing Antimicrobial drugs—general considerations for clinical trials.
> http://www.fda.gov/cder/guidance/2580dft.pdf

Thus, the FDA, although not mandated by law or regulation to require that type I error rate be reduced, is sufficiently concerned about the damaging effects of type I error rate inflation to suggest that it be closely monitored and controlled.

3.7 The Bonferroni Inequality

The previous section's discussion provides important motivation to control the type I error level in clinical trial hypothesis testing. One of the most important, easily used methods to accomplish this prospective control over type I error rate is through the use of the Bonferroni procedure [17]. This procedure is developed here.

Assume in a clinical trial that there are K analyses, each analysis consisting of a hypothesis test. Assume also that each hypothesis test is to be carried out with a prospectively defined type I error probability of α; this is the test-specific type I error level or the test-specific α level. We will also make the simplifying assumption that the result of each of the hypothesis tests is independent of the others. This last assumption allows us to multiply type I error rates for the statistical hypothesis tests when we consider their possible joint results.

Our goal in this evaluation is to compute easily the familywise type I error level, ξ. This is simply the probability that there is a least one type I error among each of the K statistical hypothesis tests. In probability theory, the occurrence of at least one event is defined as the *union* of events.

An exact computation for the familywise type I error rate is readily available. Let α be the test-specific α error probability for each of K tests. Note that the type I error rate is the same for each hypothesis test. We need to find the probability that there is not a single type I error among these K statistical hypothesis tests. Under our assumption of independence, this probability is simply the product of the probabilities that there is no type I error for each of the K statistical tests. Write

$$(1-\alpha)(1-\alpha)(1-\alpha)\dots(1-\alpha) = \prod_{j=1}^{K}(1-\alpha). \tag{3.2}$$

Therefore ξ, the probability of the occurrence of at least one type I error, is one minus the probability of no type I error among any of the K tests, or

$$\xi = 1 - \prod_{j=1}^{K}(1-\alpha) = 1 - (1-\alpha)^{K}. \tag{3.3}$$

Finding the value of ξ exactly requires some computation. Bonferroni simplified this using Boole's inequality which states that the probability of the occurrence of at least one of a collection of events is less than or equal to the sum of the probabilities of these events. This is all that we need to know to write

$$\xi = P[at\ least\ one\ type\ I\ error] \leq \sum_{i=1}^{K}\alpha_{i}. \tag{3.4}$$

If each of the test-specific type I error levels is the same value α, (3.4) reduces to

$$\xi \leq K\alpha. \tag{3.5}$$

The degree to which this approximation is accurate is worthy of a brief examination (Table 3.2). For each of four different test-specific type I error levels, a comparison of the exact computation for the familywise error level and the Bonferroni approximation is provided. For each combination of type I error level and number of multiple analyses, the Bonferroni approximation is always at least as large as the exact computation as provided in (3.3). The correspondence between the Bonferroni and the exact FWER is closest when the type I error for each individual test is low.[18] A greater divergence between the two measures is seen as the type I error rate for each individual test increases to 0.05.
Equation (3.5) of course can be rewritten as

$$\alpha \leq \frac{\xi}{K}, \tag{3.6}$$

expressing the fact that a reasonable approximation for the α level for each of K hypothesis test can be computed by dividing the familywise error level by the number of statistical hypothesis tests to be carried out. This is the most common method of applying the Bonferroni approach.

---

[18] This is because the higher powers of α (α^{2}, α^{3},...,α^{K}) become very small when α itself is small. When these powers of α are negligible, (3.3) more closely resembles (3.5).

Table 3.2. Relationship between the exact familywise error rate and Bonferroni approximation.

Number of multiple analyses	Type I = 0.005*		Type I = 0.01		Type I = 0.03		Type I = 0.05	
	Exact	Bonferroni	Exact	Bonferroni	Exact	Bonferroni	Exact	Bonferroni
2	0.0100	0.0100	0.0199	0.0200	0.0591	0.0600	0.0975	0.1000
3	0.0149	0.0150	0.0297	0.0300	0.0873	0.0900	0.1426	0.1500
4	0.0199	0.0200	0.0394	0.0400	0.1147	0.1200	0.1855	0.2000
5	0.0248	0.0250	0.0490	0.0500	0.1413	0.1500	0.2262	0.2500
6	0.0296	0.0300	0.0585	0.0600	0.1670	0.1800	0.2649	0.3000
7	0.0345	0.0350	0.0679	0.0700	0.1920	0.2100	0.3017	0.3500
8	0.0393	0.0400	0.0773	0.0800	0.2163	0.2400	0.3366	0.4000
9	0.0441	0.0450	0.0865	0.0900	0.2398	0.2700	0.3698	0.4500
10	0.0489	0.0500	0.0956	0.1000	0.2626	0.3000	0.4013	0.5000

As an example, consider an investigator who wishes to carry out a clinical trial to test the effect of a new medication on each of three endpoints. The trial has three different treatment arms: intervention dose 1, intervention dose 2, and placebo. Each of the three treatment comparisons must be made against each of the three endpoints, producing a total of nine analyses to be executed. The Bonferroni adjustment for multiple analysis testing provided in (3.6) demonstrates that if the familywise type I error rate is to be maintained at the 0.05 level, then each hypothesis test will need to be evaluated at the $0.05/9 = 0.0056$ level of significance.

There have been two major criticisms of the application of this Bonferroni correction for multiplicity. The first (as we saw earlier in this chapter) is the small test-specific type I error level required in order to ensure control over the familywise error level for a large number of analyses. This resultant small test-specific type I error level is the genesis of the argument that the application of this procedure leads to the inappropriate disregard of promising, positive findings in the data.

This criticism returns us to the argument made by Pocock and Farewell [14] suggesting that nominal testing should be permitted when there are many different hypothesis tests to be examined. The specific example provided by these workers was a study that had 34 different endpoints to measure neuropathy in diabetic patients, each of which was to be treated as a primary outcome. To keep the familywise type I error rate at 0.05, the Bonferroni correction requires that each test-specific α level should be set at $0.05/34 = 0.0015$. This is a very conservative estimate, demanding that each test provide overwhelming strength of evidence to demonstrate benefit. Pocock and Farewell contend that one should not divide the total 0.05 type I error rate among these endpoints.

However, to let this argument devolve into a debate between no control versus strict control of the familywise error level is to miss the point—the root of the problem here is the large number of these neuromyographic "endpoints" with no justification for the choice of any single one of them. There is no information denoting which of these 34 measures (or small subset of these measures) would provide the most promising and revealing effect of the intervention. As a preamble to any multiple analysis in this example, effort must be exerted to choose the most useful and most informative of these myographic measures. This work may take months or even years to accomplish, but it must be completed. Without it, the researchers run the unacceptable risk of finding a beneficial therapy "effect" for an endpoint that in the long run holds no importance for the medical or regulatory communities. It would be best if investigators did not short-circuit the learning process by reporting results for several endpoint measures that are of unproven clinical importance. Endpoints should be chosen for their value to patients and the medical community, not merely because they can be measured.

A second criticism of the classic Bonferroni approximation is that the Bonferroni computation makes a critical assumption that the statistical hypothesis tests are independent of each other. If among the K multiple analyses, the findings of one hypothesis test provides useful information about the findings for another hypothesis test, then the Bonferroni computation produces a type I error rate threshold for each hypothesis test which is too low, providing an estimate of the test α level which is too conservative. This will be explored and a solution provided in Chapters 5 and 6.

3.8 Who Was Bonferroni?

It seems only fair to stop and say a few words about the Italian mathematician whose recognition of an application of Boole's inequality has risen to prominence in clinical research. His full name was Carlo Emilio Bonferroni, and he was born on January 28, 1892, in Bergamo, Italy.[19] After studying the piano at the Conservatory in Torino, and completing a tour of duty in the Italian army engineers corps during World War I, he studied mathematics and became an assistant professor at the Polytechnic in Torino.

The primary field of applications for Bonferroni's mathematics was finances. He accepted the chair of financial mathematics in 1923 at the Economics Institute in Bari, transferring to Firenze where he remained until his death on August 18, 1960. During his tenure at Firenze, he wrote one article in each of 1935 [18] and 1936 [19] in which he established some inequalities helpful to him as he developed statistical estimates useful in municipal and national financial computations. This work contained the genesis of the idea that led to the inequality that now bears his name.

The use of Bonferroni's inequality comes from two papers by Dunn. The first [20] is a manuscript in which she considers confidence intervals for k means and mentions a Bonferroni inequality. Two years later, she considers a subset of m statistical hypotheses tests among k means, describing the method of comparison as "so simple and so general that I am sure it must have been used before this" [21]. The most common form of the usage of Boole's inequality is termed the Bonferroni method or the Bonferroni adjustment. Bonferroni also worked out a more general

---

[19] The source of this material is a lecture given by Michael E. Dewey from the Trent Institute for Health Services Research, University of Nottingham. The lecture may be found at http://www.nottingham.ac.uk.~mhzmd/bonf.html.

form of testing for simultaneous inference, as well as an adaptation for confidence intervals which has never become popular.[20]

3.9 Alternative Approaches

The area of multiple testing in clinical trials has been one of fervent activity in the statistical research literature. Before we proceed, we should take a moment to explore some alternative strategies in multiple statistical analyses, including the identification of procedures which may serve to improve the Bonferroni adjustment.

3.9.1 Sequentially Rejective Procedures

One of the many criticisms of the Bonferroni approximation is that it is too conservative. This conservatism leads to an unacceptably high possibility of missing a clinically important finding. An important segment of the statistical literature has focused on this weakness and has identified more powerful procedures. Two useful reviews of these procedures are those of Zhang et al. [22] and White [23]. While the statistical tools described in these articles often have the analysis of variance as their developmental base, it has been proposed that they can be useful in clinical trials as well.

One of these well-developed procedures compares successively larger p-values with increasing α threshold levels. These devices have been termed *sequentially rejective procedures*, and, in general, are easy to apply. Assume that there are K statistical null hypotheses to be carried out in a clinical trial and each statistical hypothesis generates a p-value. Let p_1 be the p-value for the first hypothesis test $H_{0,1}$, p_2 be the p-value for the second hypothesis test $H_{0,2}$, concluding with p_k as the p-value for the Kth and last hypothesis test $H_{0,K}$. These p-values must first be ranked from the smallest to largest. We will denote $p_{[1]}$ is the smallest of the K p-values, $p_{[2]}$ is the next largest p-value … out to $p_{[K]}$ which is the maximum p-value of the K p-values from the clinical trial.

Once the p-values have been ranked, several evaluation procedures are available to draw a conclusion based on their values. One device proposed by Simes [24] compares the jth smallest p-value, $p_{[j]}$ to $\xi j/K$. The procedure is as follows:

(1)   Rank order the K p-values such that $p_{[1]} \leq p_{[2]} \leq p_{[3]} \leq \ldots \leq p_{[K]}$

(2)   Compare the smallest p-value, $p_{[1]}$ to the threshold ξ/K. If $p_{[1]} \leq \xi/K$, then reject the null hypothesis for which $p_{[1]}$ is the p-value.

(3)   Compare $p_{[2]}$ to $2\xi/K$. If $p_{[2]} \leq 2\xi/K$, then reject the null hypothesis for which $p_{[2]}$ is the p-value.

---

[20] As an aside, it is interesting to note that Dr. Bonferroni, as a professor was so concerned about the cost of higher education for his impoverished students that he produced by hand a copy of his textbook for each one.

(4)   Compare $p_{[3]}$ to $3\xi/K$. If $p_{[2]} \leq 3\xi/K$, then reject the null hypothesis for which $p_{[3]}$ is the p-value.

(5)   Continue on, finally comparing $p_{[K]}$ to ξ.. If $p_{[K]} \leq \xi$, then reject the null hypothesis for which $p_{[K]}$ is the p-value.

The procedure ceases at the first step for which the null hypothesis is not rejected. Thus, as j increases, p-values that are increasing are compared to significance levels which are themselves increasing. If the tests are independent one from another, then the familywise error level ξ is preserved. This procedure is more powerful than the Bonferroni procedure.

Holm [25] developed a similar procedure. Again, successively larger p-values are compared with increasing α threshold levels. Holm's procedure consists of the following steps:

(1)   Rank order the K p-values such that $p_{[1]} \leq p_{[2]} \leq p_{[3]} \leq \cdots \leq p_{[K]}$

(2)   Compare the smallest p-value, $p_{[1]}$ to the threshold ξ/K. If $p_{[1]} \leq \xi/K$, then reject the null hypothesis for which $p_{[1]}$ is the p-value.

(3)   Compare $p_{[2]}$ to $\xi/(K-1)$. If $p_{[2]} \leq \xi/(K-1)$, then reject the null hypothesis for which $p_{[2]}$ is the p-value.

(4)   Compare $p_{[3]}$ to $\xi/(K-2)$. If $p_{[2]} \leq \xi/(K-2)$, then reject the null hypothesis for which $p_{[3]}$ is the p-value.

(5)   Continue on,

If at any point in the testing procedure the null hypothesis is not rejected, then all hypothesis testing ceases and the subsequent larger p-values are all judged to reflect statistical insignificance. Holm's procedure has been generalized to multiple hypothesis testing situations where each of the α have different weights. In addition, both Hommel [26] and Shaffer [27] have refined these tools. Sequentially rejective devices are in general more powerful than the Bonferroni procedure [23].[21] It has been suggested that because these methods are easy to apply and less conservative then the classic Bonferroni procedure, they are preferable for hypothesis testing in which familywise error rate control is critical [22].

3.9.2 Who Chooses the α Level Threshold?

These sequential rejective procedures are theoretically sound and mathematically reasonable. However, other criteria must be weighed before we choose to adopt them (or any other statistical computation) as useful procedures to carry out in a clinical trial. One of these other criteria is an assessment of whether the evaluation

---

[21] More powerful in this context means that for the same α level, effect size, standard errors, and sample size, these procedures are more likely to reject the null hypothesis and produce a positive result.

process involved in selecting the thresholds of significance is consistent with good clinical trial decisions.

As we review the sequential rejective procedures as outlined above, we see that the first step required by all of them is the rank ordering of the K p-values obtained from the statistical hypothesis tests. In the sequential rejective procedures, the first p-value tested must be the smallest p-value. This means that the investigator does not choose the order of hypothesis testing, nor does she choose the threshold of significance for each of the hypothesis tests. Since the data determine the magnitude of the p-values, and therefore the rank ordering of the p-values, then the data determine the order of hypotheses to be tested. We must also recognize that, as the significance level threshold varies from endpoint to endpoint, the link between the endpoint and the significance threshold is not set by the investigator but, again, is set by the data.

This latter point is of critical concern to us. An advantage of the sequentially rejective procedure is that, when prospectively identified, the analysis plan is fixed. There is no doubt about how the analysis will be carried out at the end of the study, nor is there any doubt about the choice of the type I error probability thresholds when sequentially rejective evaluations are prospectively set in place. However, the type I error level thresholds are set automatically. There is no place for prospective input by the investigators, the medical, or the regulatory community for the selection of α error rate thresholds that are a standard of community and regulatory protection.

Consider, for example, an investigator who is interested in testing the effect of a new therapy on reducing the consequences of diabetes mellitus in a clinical trial. He has chosen to focus on two analyses for which he has adequate statistical power. The first is to measure the effect of therapy on reducing the cumulative incidence of total mortality. His second endpoint is a new measure of evolving kidney disease. Certainly, epidemiologic considerations, effect size magnitudes, and the variability of these effect sizes are important measures to evaluate when considering the study's findings. However, p-values will also play a role in the assessment of this concordantly executed study. What α level thresholds should be prospectively set by the investigators for each of the two endpoint analyses?

The medical and regulatory community must ultimately be persuaded of the endpoint's relevance as a measure of disease if the community is to accept the result of the study. Assume that the investigators wish to control the familywise error level at 0.05. A Bonferroni adjustment would set the level at 0.025 here. Is this appropriate? The second endpoint is new. Since this endpoint's implications are untested and uncertain, it will require a stronger level of evidence for the beneficial effect of this intervention. The newer the endpoint, the less experience the judging scientific community has with its interpretation. Therefore, in order for the finding of a beneficial effect to be persuasive, the magnitude of the benefit must be large. Only in the presence of a strong sign of benefit will a new endpoint form the basis of an argument that the clinical trial's intervention has produced a result worthy of acceptance.

In this example, total mortality is the most persuasive of the two endpoints to the medical and regulatory community. The medical community is willing to accept a higher threshold of type I error rate for total mortality (at least up to the 0.05 level) because it has a greater understanding of the implications for the diabetic community if the cumulative incidence rate of total mortality is reduced. The investigators, therefore, will require a larger p-value and a consequent smaller effect size for the effect of this intervention on the total mortality rate. On the other hand, the investigators will require a larger effect size and a smaller p-value for the efficacy of therapy on the newer endpoint. They may even reject the Bonferroni adjustment and choose a different split for the type I error probability assignment (e.g., evaluate the effect of therapy for the total mortality endpoint at 0.045, and the new endpoint with an α of 0.05).[22]

The point is that the investigators have an important contribution to make in deciding the α error probability threshold for the statistical hypothesis tests. Their input in this matter is both appropriate and necessary in clinical trial planning. However, a sequentially rejective procedure as described above ignores these concerns, leaving the investigator out of the a priori decisions about the significance levels against which each of these two endpoints will be tested. Effectively, using a sequentially rejective procedure removes the determination of community-based protection levels from the investigators and places it in the hands of the data-set.

In a clinical trial, the choice of an α level threshold is not solely a statistical decision, but a clinical decision as well. This clinical decision is based on (1) the persuasive power of the endpoint to the medical and regulatory community, (2) the anticipated effectiveness of the intervention, (3) the medical community's experience with the intervention, and (4) the likelihood of the occurrence of unpleasant if not dangerous adverse effects. If there are to be different α thresholds for each of the multiple endpoints as the sequential rejective procedures demand, then those levels should be set by the investigators and not by the data. At first glance, it is possible to envision that the sequentially rejective procedures might be attractive in the post hoc setting of a clinical trial. In this circumstance, non-prospectively stated analyses have led to a collection of p-values to which no a priori thought has been given for their interpretation. It is possible that this collection of p-values could be subjected to any of the previously mentioned sequentially rejective procedures to produce some adjustment in statistical testing. However, as we have pointed out in Chapter 2, post hoc analyses are generally unreliable in clinical trials—not because of multiple testing issues, but because the data, having driven the analysis, produce untrustworthy estimators. Fine as these sequentially rejective procedures are, they do not repair the damage done by a data-driven analysis.

There is no question that the sequentially rejective procedures generally have more statistical power than the Bonferroni approach. However, while maximum statistical power is a useful and good criterion for developing a statistical test, it is not the only good criterion governing its use in a clinical trial. After all, in a given hypothesis test, a one tailed 0.05 level test is more powerful for testing for benefit than is a two-sided test, ceteris parabus; and there have been advocates of the use of the one-tailed testing in clinical trials [28], [29], most recently by Knott-nerus [30]. Yet, in spite of this well-known fact, the medical and regulatory

---

[22] This α error probability division will be discussed in detail in Chapter 4.

community continue to correctly reject the principle of one tailed testing in clinical trials. This is because the concern for ethics and the possibility of doing harm is more pressing than the need to produce increased statistical power from a statistical hypothesis test [31], [32].

The fact that the sequentially rejective procedures lock the investigator into an analysis procedure is not bad; the problem is that the investigator is locked out of choosing the details of this plan. Therefore, while sequentially rejective procedures might be useful in statistics in general, the fact that they take control of hypothesis testing away from the investigator will severely limit their utility for us here.

3.9.3 Resampling P-Values

One important new alternative to multiple comparisons is the use of the resampling tool. This approach has been developed by Westfall et al. [33], [34], [35] and has figured prominently in the methodologic literature evaluating the multiple analysis issue. These workers focus on the smallest p-value obtained from a collection of hypothesis tests, using the resampling concept as their assessment tool.

Resampling is the process by which smaller samples of data are randomly selected from the research data set—this essentially treats the research data sample as a "population" from which samples are obtained. Resampling is allowed to take place thousands of times, each time generating a new "subsample" and a new p-value from that subsample. Combining all of these p-values from these subsamples produces, in the end, a distibution of p-values. The adjusted p-value measures how extreme a given p-value is, relative to the probability distribution of the most extreme p-value. This is a reasonable perspective,[23] and the use of these adjusted p-values has been suggested as a test statistic [36].

We certainly should bow to the reality of the situation; the "natural" reaction of an investigator who, when faced with a long list of p-values, is to scan the list of p-values for the smallest one, concentrating on the hypothesis test that produced the minimum p-value. The resampling frame captures the degree of surprise one should have when evaluating this smallest p-value. It does so by comparing its magnitude to its average value (i.e., averaged over all of the smaller datasets obtained in the resampling process). As with the sequentially rejective procedures, the investigator does not take part in choosing the order of hypothesis testing. We will therefore not use it as a basis for our further discussion of multiple analyses.

The Bonferroni adjustment for multiple hypothesis testing has been available for more than 50 years. Miller [37] undertook a review of the use of this procedure. At the time of his review, 25 years ago, he identified over 255 manuscripts covering the topics of multiple analysis in general and the use of the Bonferroni procedure in particular. He concluded from this effort that the Bonferroni procedure has held up quite nicely. Others have evaluated the performance

---

[23] In fact, these issues have been discussed in a textbook (Westfall, P.H., and Young, S.S. (1993). *Resampling–Based Multiple Testing: Examples and Methods of P-Value Adjustments*. A procedure in SAS/STAT software PROC MUTLTEST, that performs these analyses has been available now for almost 10 years.

of the Bonferroni procedure; as examples, consider [38], [39], [40]. However, we will follow the advice of Simes [41]. Although several methods have been developed for multiple statistical inference, the Bonferroni procedure is still valuable, being simple to use, requiring no complicated assumptions about the probability distribution of the sample data, and allowing individual alternative hypotheses to be identified. For these reasons, when the hypothesis tests are independent from each other, this simple device will be the tool by which we construct multiple analyses. However, we will insist that the investigator be incorporated into the prospective choices for the test-specific α error levels.

3.10 Conclusions

As complicated as they are now, clinical trials are likely to become more complex in the future. In fact, the drive for logistical efficiency together with the sound desire to satisfy epidemiologic requirements for solid causality arguments all but ensures the increased intricacy of these experimental designs. However, as pointed out in Chapter 2, this complexity must be prospectively embedded into the research design.

After completing Chapters 2 and 3, we may clearly describe the challenges and difficulties of using multiple analyses in clinical trials (Table 3.3). If the analyses are post hoc evaluations, with no prior planning, then the estimators of effect from these assessments are untrustworthy. Any hypothesis testing based on these estimators is also unreliable, and the analyses results are best viewed as exploratory. This was the result of Chapter 2. In these circumstances, the results of hypothesis tests might best be reported as z scores, with no p-values, since the ability to extend the findings of an exploratory analysis to the population from which the sample was derived is impaired.

If the analysis is planned prospectively and the experiment is executed concordantly (i.e., is executed according to the protocol), then the estimators derived from the analysis are trustworthy. However, with the execution of each hypothesis test in a multiple analysis plan, there is further inflation of the type I error rate, and with each inflation there is erosion of the persuasive force of the research effort. Thus, prospective identification of hypothesis testing in clinical trials with subsequent concordant execution is not enough to produce useful positive results—it is necessary, but not sufficient.

The key to producing useful results from multiple analyses in a clinical trial environment is not just prospective planning, but the prospective inoculation of the trial with familywise error level protection. Embedding familywise error level control a priori into a clinical trial program avoids both the random research paradigm and type I error inflation. This strategy provides results in a multiple analysis setting that can be balanced against the risk of the therapy. Procedures for how to implement this will be the topic of Chapter 4.

Table 3.3 Consequences of Alternative Multiple Analyses Strategies

Strategy	Consequences
Analysis plan is based on incoming data (Random research) ⟹	Untrustworthy estimates of effect size, standard errors, confidence intervals and p values
Prospective choice of analyses but no a priori alpha allocation ⟹	Trustworthy estimates are obtained but type I error inflation and degradation of risk-benefit assessment
Prospective choice of analyses with a priori alpha allocation ⟹	Trustworthy estimates are obtained with good familywise error rate control and realistic risk-benefit appraisal

Problems

1. A physician is interested in estimating the prevalence of hypertension in his clinic for a 1 year period. He has his staff count the number of patients who visit his clinic for the year, and also count the number of those patients who are diagnosed with hypertension. He would like to know if the prevalence of hypertension at his clinic is 20%. Why is the computation of a test statistic and a type I error rate irrelevant here?

2. A researcher in gynecology would like to study the effect of a new medication for the treatment of carcinoma in situ. If the medication is successful, it will reduce the spread of cervical cancer within the uterus. Not knowing which measurement is best, the researcher measures twelve different estimates of the ability of the cancer to spread, intending to carry out twelve hypothesis tests. The goal of this research is to generalize its results to the population of patients who have cervical cancer, but no effort is made to control the familywise error rate. If testing for each of the twelve results is to occur at the 0.05 level, show that the probability of drawing at least one wrong conclusion about the population based on these twelve hypothesis tests is 0.46.

3. Compare the probability of making at least one type I error to the Bonferroni approximation when the test-specific type I error rate is 0.10 for seven independent statistical hypothesis tests. Make the same comparison for a test-specific type I error of 0.05 and, finally, for a test-specific type I error of 0.01. What would you conclude about the accuracy of the Bonferroni approximation and the exact computation of the familywise error rate as a function of the test-specific error rate?

4. From an investigator's point of view, what is the fundamental difference between controlling the familywise error rate in a clinical trial using the sequentially rejective procedures/resampled p-values versus a Bonferroni type rule?

5. How does the risk–benefit assessment of a new therapy studied in a clinical
    trial degrade when there is no control of the familywise error level?
6. Explain in words how the sequential rejective procedures conserve the family-
    wise error rate ξ.

References

1. Budde, M., Bauer, P. (1989). Multiple test procedures in clinical dose finding
    studies. *Journal of the American Statistical Association* **84**:792–796.
2. Shepherd, J., Cobbe, S.M., Ford, I., et al. (1995). Prevention of CAD with
    pravastatin in men with hypercholesterolemia. *New England Journal of Medi-
    cine* **333**:1301–7.
3. Sacks, F.M., Pfeffer, M.A., Moyé, L.A., Rouleau, J.L., Rutherford, J.D., Cole,
    T.G., Brown, L., Warnica, J.W., Arnold, J.M.O., Wun, C.C., Davist, B.R.,
    Braunwald. E. (1996). The effect of pravastatin on coronary events after
    myocardial infarction in patients with average cholesterol levels. *New England
    Journal of Medicine* **335**:1001–9.
4. Scandinavian Simvastatin Survival Study Group. (1994). Randomized trial of
    cholesterol lowering in 4444 patients with CAD: the Scandinavian Simvastatin
    Survival Study (4S). *Lancet* **344**:1383–9.
5. Long-Term Intervention with Pravastatin in Ischaemic Disease (LIPID) Study
    Group. (1998). Prevention of cardiovascular events and death with pravastatin
    in patients with CAD and a broad range of initial cholesterol levels *New Eng-
    land Journal of Medicine* **339**:1349–1357.
6. Food and Drug Modernization Act of 1997. (November 21, 1997). Public
    Law.105–115;21USC 355a;111Stat. 2295.
7. Nester, M.R., (1996). An applied statistician's creed. *Applied Statistics* **45**:
    4401–410.
8. Rothman, R.J. No adjustments are needed for multiple comparisons. *Epidemi-
    ology* **1**:43–46.
9. Fisher, L.D., Moyé,L.A. (1999). Carvedilol and the Food and Drug
    Administration Approval Process: An Introduction. *Controlled Clinical Trials*
    20:1–15.
10. Fisher, L.D. (1999). Carvedilol and the FDA approval process: the FDA para-
    digm and reflections upon hypothesis testing. *Controlled Clinical Trials* **20**:16–
    39.
11. Moyé, L.A. (1999). P–Value Interpretation in Clinical Trials. The Case for
    Discipline. *Controlled Clinical Trials* **20**:40–49.
12. Hochberg, Y., Tamhane, A.C. (1987). *Multiple Comparison Procedures*, New
    York , Wiley.
13. Westfall, P.H., Young S.S. (1993). *Resampling Based Multiple Testing: Exam-
    ples and Methods for P-Value Adjustment.* New York. Wiley.
14. Pocock, R.J., Farewell, V.T. (1996). Multiplicity consideration in the design
    and analysis of clinical trials. *Journal of the Royal Statistical Society A*
    159:93–110.

15. Adams, C. (2002). At FDA, approving cancer treatments can be an ordeal. *The Wall Street Journal.* December 11, p 1.

16. Senn, S. (1997). *Statistical Issues in Drug Development.* Chichester, Wiley, Section 15.2.1.

17. Miller, R.G. (1981) *Simultaneous Statistical Inference,* 2nd ed. New York Springer.

18. Bonferroni, C.E. (1935). Il calcolo delle assicurazioni su gruppi di teste. In *Studi in Onore del Professore Salvatore Ortu Carboni.* Rome, 13–60.

19. Bonferroni, C.E. (1936). Teoria statistica delle classi e calcolo delle probabilità. *Pubblicazioni del R Istituto Superiore di Scienze Economiche e Commerciali di Firenze* **8**:3–62.

20. Dunn, O.J. (1959). Confidence intervals for the means of dependent, normally distributed variables. *Journal of the American Statistical Association* **54**:613–621.

21. Dunn, O.J. (1961). Multiple comparisons among means. *Journal of the American Statistical Asssociation* **56**:52–54.

22. Zhang, J., Qwuan, H., Ng, J., Stepanavage, M.E. (1997). Some statistical methods for mulitple endpoints in clinical trials. *Controlled Clinical Trials* **18**: 204–221.

23. Wright, S.P. (1992). Adjusted P–values for simultaneous inference. *Biometrics* **48**:1005–1013.

24. Simes, R.J. (1986). An improved Bonferroni procedure for multiple tests of significance. *Biometrika* **73**:819–827.

25. Holm, S. (1979). A simple sequentially rejective multiple test procedures. *Scandinavian Journal of Statistics* **6**:65–70.

26. Hommel, G. (1988). A stepwise rejective multiple test procedure based on a modified Bonferroni test. *Biometrika* **75**:383–386.

27. Shaffer, J.P. (1986). Modified sequentially rejective multiple test procedures. *Journal of the American Statistical Association* **81**:826–831.

28. Bland, J.M., Altman, D.G. (1994). Statistics notes: One and two-sided tests of significance. *British Medical Journal* **309**: 248.

29. Dunnett, C.W., Gent, M. (1996). An alternative to the use of two-sided tests in clinical trials. *Statistics in Medicine* **15**:1729–1738.

30. Knottnerus J.A., Bouter L.M. (2001). Commentary The ethics of sample size: two-sided testing and one-sided thinking. *Journal of Clinical Epidemiology* **54**:109–110.

31. Moyé, L.A. (2000). *Statistical Reasoning in Medicine: The Intuitive P-Value Primer.* New York, Springer. Chapter 6.

32. Moyé, L.A., Tita, A. (2002). Ethics and Hypothesis Testing Complexity *Circulation* **105**:3062–3065.

33. Westfall P.H., Young S.S., Wright S.P. (1993). Adjusting *p*-values for multiplicity. *Biometrics* **49**:941–945.

34. Westfall, P.H., Young, S. *P*-value adjustments for mulitple tests in multivariate binomial models. *Journal of the American Statistical Association* **84**:780–786.

35. Westfall, P.H., Krishnen, A., Young, S.S. (1998). Using prior information to allocate significance levels for multiple endpoints. *Statistics in Medicine* **17**:2107–2119.
36. Berger, V. (1998). Admissibility of Exact Conditional Tests of Stochastic Order. *Journal of Statistical Planning and Inference* **66**: 39–50.
37. Miller RG. (1977). Developements in multiple comparisons 1966–1976. *Journal of the American Statistical Association* **72**:779–788.
38. Edwards, D., Berry, J.J. (1987). The efficiency of simulation–based multiple comparisons. *Biometrics* **43**:913–928.
39. Einot, I., Gabriel, E.R. (1975). A study of powers of several methods of multiple comparisons. *Journal of the American Statistical Association* **70**:574–583.
40. O'Brien, P.C. (1984). Procedures for comparing samples with multiple endpoints. *Biometrics* **40**:1079–1087.
41. Simes, R.J. (1986). An improved Bonferroni procedure for multiple tests of significance. *Biometrika* **73**:751–754.

Chapter 4

Multiple Analyses and Multiple Endpoints

Multiple analyses in clinical trials comprise the execution and interpretation of numerous statistical hypothesis tests within a single research effort. This definition of multiple hypothesis testing encompasses combinations of analyses involving multiple endpoints, comparisons of endpoint findings among multiple treatment arms, and subgroup analyses. However, our study of multiple analyses will not begin by first considering these complex combinations of analyses, but will instead focus on one of the most commonly occurring multiple analyses circumstances in clinical trials—multiple endpoints. This chapter's goal is to provide a paced development for how one chooses and analyzes multiple endpoints in a two-armed (control and treatment group) clinical trial. The only mathematical tool we will use is an understandable adaptation of the Bonferroni multiple comparison procedure, an adaptation which is both easy to compute and interpret.

4.1 Introduction

In Chapter 3, we acknowledged the inevitability of multiple analyses in clinical trials. Since additional endpoints can be added to the design of a clinical trial relatively cheaply, the inclusion of these additional endpoints can be cost effective. In addition, epidemiologic requirements for building the tightest causal link between the clinical trial's intervention and that trial's endpoints serve as powerful motivators for the inclusion of multiple analyses. These carefully considered, prospectively designed evaluations may provide, for example, information about the relationship between the dose of a medication and its effect on the disease, or evaluate the mechanism by which the clinical trial's intervention produces its impact on disease reduction. The cost of carrying out these analyses is commonly small compared to the overall cost of the clinical trial.

However, we have also observed that increasing the number of hypothesis tests also increases the overall type I error level. In clinical trials, measuring the type I error level is a community obligation of the trial's investigators; the type I error level measures the likelihood that an intervention, known to produce an adverse event and a financial burden, will have no beneficial effect on the population from which the sample was derived. Thus the type I error level is an essential component in the risk–benefit evaluation of the intervention and must be both accurately measured and tightly controlled. While the prospective design and concordant execution of a clinical trial ensures that the estimate of the type I error level at the experiment's conclusion is trustworthy, this research environment does not guarantee that the type I error level will be low.

We must also acknowledge that it is standard for supportive analyses to be executed in clinical trials. Such epidemiologic elaborations, e.g., an examination of the dose–response relationship or the evaluation of subgroup analyses, play an important role in elucidating the nature of the relationship between the intervention and the disease. These analyses must therefore figure prominently in any multiple analysis structure that we provide for the design and evaluation of clinical trials.

In this chapter, we will develop the requisite skills to control and manage type I error rates when there are multiple endpoints in a two-armed clinical trial. In doing so we will adhere to the familywise error level (ξ) as the primary tool to manage type I error level control.

4.2 Important Assumptions

Since effective type I error level management can only occur when the estimates for α error rates are both accurate and trustworthy, we will assume that trials for which these management skills are developed in this chapter are prospectively designed and concordantly executed. This permits us to steer clear of the problems presented by the random research paradigm.[1] In addition, we will assume that, in this chapter, the clinical trial endpoints are independent of each other.

Finally, although the focus of this chapter is type I error levels, this emphasis should not be interpreted as denying the time-tested advice that experimental interpretation is an exercise involving the joint consideration of effect sizes, standard errors, and confidence intervals. *P*-values are necessary components of this evaluation, but they are not the sole component. They do not measure effect size, nor do they convey the extent of study discordance. A small *p*-value does not, in and of itself, mean that the sample size was adequate, that the effect size is clinically meaningful, or that there has been a clear attribution of effect to the clinical trial's intervention. These other factors must themselves be individually considered by a careful, critical review of the research effort. This inclusive effort provides the clearest interpretation of the implications of the research sample findings for the population from which the sample was obtained.

4.3 Clinical Trial Result Descriptors

In order to continue our development we will need some unambiguous terminology to categorize the results of clinical trials. It is customary to classify clinical trials on the basis of their results, e.g., positive trials or negative trials. Here we will elaborate upon and clarify these useful descriptors.

4.3.1 Positive and Negative Trials

Assume that investigators are carrying out a prospectively designed, concordantly executed clinical trial in order to demonstrate the effect of a randomly allocated in-

---

[1] The difficulties of random research are examined in Chapter 2.

tervention on the clinical consequences of a disease or condition. For ease of discussion, we will also assume that the clinical trial has only one prospectively designed endpoint that requires a hypothesis test. Define the hypothesis test result as positive if the hypothesis test rejects the null hypothesis in the favor of benefit. Since the clinical trial had only one hypothesis test, and that hypothesis test result was positive, the clinical trial is described as positive. This definition is consistent with the customary terminology now generally in use, and we will use it in this text.

The commonly used descriptor for a negative statistical hypothesis test can be somewhat confusing, requiring us to make a simple adjustment. Typically, a negative hypothesis test result is defined as a hypothesis test which did not reject the null hypothesis and therefore did not find that the clinical trial's intervention produced the desired benefit for the population being studied. However, this terminology can cause confusion since it is possible for a hypothesis test result to demonstrate a truly harmful finding.[2] The hypothesis test that demonstrated not benefit but harm must also have a descriptor. We will define a negative hypothesis test result as a hypothesis test result that has demonstrated that the intervention produced harm. Thus, a positive trial demonstrates that the intervention produced the desired benefit, and a negative trial demonstrates the trial produced a harmful result. However, some additional comments are required concerning hypothesis test results that do not reject the null hypothesis.

4.3.2 Null Results Versus Uninformative Results

Just as the interpretation of hypothesis tests results that are positive if there is no consideration of the type I error can be confusing, the evaluation of hypothesis test results that do not reject the null hypothesis can be complex as well. In this latter circumstance, there should be adequate consideration given to the occurrence of a type II error. A type II error occurs when the population in which the intervention produces an effect generates a research sample that, through chance alone, displays no intervention effect. Therefore, when the research sample finding does not reject the null hypothesis, it becomes important to consider how likely it is that this finding could have been produced by chance alone. If there is inadequate power (i.e., a high type II error rate), then the result of the trial is uninformative.

The correct interpretation of a statistical hypothesis test that does not reject the null hypothesis depends on the size of the type II error rate. For example, consider a study that is required to recruit 3868 patients in order to demonstrate with 90% power and an α error level of 0.05 that an intervention reduces total mortality by 20% from a cumulative mortality rate of 0.20.[3] Unfortunately, during the execution of their clinical trial, the investigators are only able to recruit 2500 of the required 3868 patients. At the conclusion of the study, the investigators find that the

---

[2] An example of a negative trial is the CAST study (Preliminary Report: Effect of encainide and flecainide on mortality in a randomized trial of arrhythmia suppression after myocardial infarction. 1989. *New England Journal of Medicine* **321**:406–412). CAST demonstrated the harmful effects of arrhythmia treatment in patients who had suffered a heart attack.

[3] An elementary discussion of sample size and power computations is provided in Appendix D.

relative risk of the clinical trial's intervention for the cumulative mortality event rate is 0.85, representing a 15% reduction in the total mortality rate produced by the intervention. However, the investigators cannot reach a definite conclusion about the effect of therapy. This is because their inability to recruit the remaining 1368 patients has dramatically reduced the power of the hypothesis test from 90% to 49%, (or alternatively, increased the type II error rate from 10% to 51%). Stated another way, although it was unlikely that a population in which the intervention was effective for mortality would produce a sample of 3868 patients in which the intervention was ineffective, it is very likely that the same population would produce a sample of 2500 patients in which the intervention was not effective. In this case, although the investigators were unable to reject the null hypothesis of no effect, the low power level requires them to restrict their comments about this finding to only that the study was uninformative on the mortality issue.

The use of the term *uninformative* is consistent with the commonly used admonition at the FDA "Absence of evidence is not evidence of absence" [1]. In the circumstances of the preceding clinical trial, this aphorism may be interpreted as the "absence of evidence (of a beneficial effect of the intervention in the research sample) is not evidence of absence (of a beneficial effect of the intervention in the population)." The absence of evidence of the effect in the sample is only evidence of absence of the effect in the population at large in the high-power environment of a well-designed and concordantly executed clinical trial.

Occasionally, a hypothesis test result will not reject the null hypothesis, but there will be adequate power. This result we will describe as a "null" finding.[4] Thus, we see that clinical trials whose results are based on statistical hypothesis tests can have those results classified as either positive, negative, null, or uninformative (Figure 4.1).

4.4 The Strategy for Multiple Endpoint Analysis

Assume that in a clinical trial with two treatment arms (intervention and control) there are K prospectively declared endpoints. Assume also that the effect of the intervention will be evaluated by a hypothesis test for each of these endpoints. Let each of these hypothesis tests be independent from each other and carried out with the same prospectively defined, test-specific type I error level of α. The investigators require a strategy that allows them to draw useful conclusions about the type I error level from this collection of hypothesis test using ξ, the familywise type I error probability. Recall from Chapter 3 that the familywise error level, which is the probability that there is at least one type I error among the K independent hypothesis tests, is computed as

$$\xi = 1 - (1 - \alpha)^K. \tag{4.1}$$

---

[4] A null finding, since it occurs in the presence of adequate power has been described as a finding that demonstrates that neither therapeutic intervention nor therapeutic calamity has occurred.

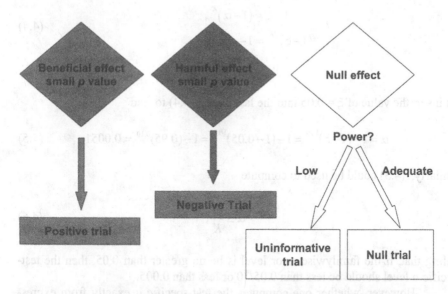

Figure 4.1. The correct interpretation of primary endpoint hypothesis tests from a clinical trial.

For example, in the circumstance where there are ten hypothesis tests to be executed, each at the test-specific α level of 0.05, we may compute

$$\xi = 1 - (1-\alpha)^K = 1 - (1-0.05)^{10} = 1 - (0.95)^{10} = 0.401. \qquad (4.2)$$

Thus, the probability that there is at least one type I error among the 10 independent hypothesis tests is 0.401. Alternatively, one could use the Bonferroni inequality to compute

$$\xi \leq K\alpha \qquad (4.3)$$

and therefore calculate the upper bound for the familywise type I error rate from ten hypothesis tests as $\xi \leq 10(0.05) = 0.50$. Finally, one can fix the familywise error level $\xi = 0.05$ and compute the value of the test-specific α level by solving (4.1) to find

$$\xi = 1 - (1-\alpha)^K,$$
$$1 - \xi = (1-\alpha)^K,$$
$$(1-\xi)^{1/K} = 1 - \alpha, \tag{4.4}$$
$$\alpha = 1 - (1-\xi)^{1/K},$$

and insert the value of $\xi = 0.05$ into the last line of (4.4) to find

$$\alpha = 1 - (1-\xi)^{1/10} = 1 - (1-0.05)^{1/10} = 1 - (0.95)^{0.10} = 0.0051. \tag{4.5}$$

Similarly, (4.3) could be used to compute

$$\alpha \leq \frac{\xi}{K}, \tag{4.6}$$

finding that, if the familywise error level is be no greater than 0.05, then the test-specific α level should be less than 0.05/10 or less than 0.005.

However, whether one computes the test-specific α exactly from expression (4.4) or approximately from (4.6), the α level at which each hypothesis test must be evaluated become prohibitively small as the number of analyses increase. These error rates threaten to make the concept of familywise type I error probability management unworkable and impractical for many clinical trial circumstances in which the endpoints are considered independently of each other. Thus, if the familywise type I error probability computations are to be useful, we must deal directly with the issue of its rapid inflation in response to the increased number of multiple analyses. We will use two helpful tactics in producing constructive control of familywise error levels—triage (discussed in Section 4.5) and uneven error rate allocation (presented in Section 4.9).

4.5 Tactic 1: Triage the Endpoints

An important part of any useful strategy to limit the familywise error level for the investigators of a clinical trial must center on control of the number of endpoints. It is critical to understand that endpoint control does not mean endpoint reduction. Endpoint control means the deliberate, prospective selection of that small number of endpoints on which the benefit of the clinical trial's intervention will be judged from among the many endpoints the investigators will measure. Thus, control here does not mean reducing the number of endpoint evaluations and endpoint hypotheses tests to be executed, but does require that the investigators prospectively decide on the few endpoints that will form the basis of the declarative statement at the trial's end about the worth of the intervention (positive, negative, null, or uninformative).

4.5.1 The Process of Endpoint Triage

This strategy of endpoint control permits the investigators the freedom to completely evaluate and analyze all of their endpoints measures—measurements that have been designed and collected at great expense. As stated in Chapter 3, there are compelling logistical, financial, and epidemiologic reasons for this task to be completed. However, carrying out this understandably large collection of endpoint evaluations must be reconciled with the requirement of familywise type I error level control. Investigators can accomplish the reconciliation; however, that effort requires careful, detailed planning among the investigators as well as a full series of discussions within the research community and, if appropriate, the regulatory agency.

The goal of these early discussions is for the investigators to choose the endpoint measures that they believe will provide a comprehensive view of the effect of the therapy to be tested in the clinical trial. This evaluation will commonly generate a large number of endpoints. In fact, it will produce as many endpoints as the investigators believe are necessary to shed light on the nature of the relationship between the intervention and the disease. During this early stage of the research design, the investigators should also acknowledge that there will be a collection of post hoc endpoint analyses at the end of the trial. They may not be able to identify these evaluations yet, but the investigators can easily anticipate that some will be necessary.[5]

Once this exhaustive process of endpoint identification has concluded, the investigators should then choose the small number of endpoints for which a type I error rate will be allocated. It is over this final subset of endpoints that the familywise error level will be controlled. Therefore, the effect of therapy on this small number of signature endpoints will ultimately determine if the clinical trial is judged as positive, negative, null, or uninformative.

4.5.2 An Example of the Endpoint Triage Process

Consider the following illustration: Investigators are interested in designing a clinical trial in order to assess the effect of a new oral therapy to reduce the clinical complications of type II diabetes mellitus. In this trial, patients will be randomized to receive conventional therapy for diabetes mellitus, or conventional therapy plus the new medication. Since diabetes mellitus is a disease which ultimately affects every organ system in the body, there is a large number of potential endpoints from which the investigators can choose. A series of discussions among the investigators and other endocrinologists produced the following list of endpoints: total mortality, cardiovascular mortality, total hospitalizations, fatal and nonfatal myocardial infarction, fatal and nonfatal stroke, end-stage renal disease, microalbuminuria, nontraumatic amputations, retinopathy, blindness, plasma HbA1c levels, plasma glucose levels, plasma insulin levels, three measures of quality of life, and 34 electromyographic measures of peripheral neuropathy. The investigators are inter-

---

[5] These post hoc endpoints will have to be interpreted very carefully—the appropriate evaluation will be provided later in this chapter.

ested in measuring each of these endpoints in the study. However, they also under-stand that with 50 endpoints, the test-specific α for any of these endpoints will be approximately $\alpha \leq \xi/50 = 0.05/50 = 0.001$. The investigators believe they will not be able to achieve the required minimum sample size for this test-specific α level of 0.001 using the effect sizes they believe the intervention will produce for these pro-spectively identified endpoints.

The trial designers recognize the importance of reducing the familywise error level, and begin the process of choosing from these 50 endpoints a small number of selected endpoints. These signature endpoints are chosen to demonstrate in the clearest manner the effect of therapy on the clinical consequences of diabetes mellitus. The investigators believe that, if the intervention produces a benefit among these signature endpoints, the investigators will be able to make a very per-suasive argument to the medical and regulatory communities that this new medication is an effective treatment for type II diabetes mellitus. They settle on five primary endpoints: total mortality, total hospitalizations, microalbuminuria, reduc-tion in HbA1c, and one measure of quality of life. It is important to note that each of the original 50 endpoints will be measured and reported, but only the 5 primary endpoints will have a prospective allocation of an α error rate. If ξ is to be 0.05, then assuming that there will be an equal test-specific α rate that will be prospec-tively allocated for each of these five endpoints reveals that

$$\alpha = 1 - (1 - \xi)^{1/5} = 1 - (1 - 0.05)^{0.20} = 0.0102.$$

Alternatively the upper bound on the test-specific α could have been computed as $\alpha \leq \xi/5 = 0.05/5 = 0.01$. In any event, this is a level of type I error rate for which the investigators are confident they will be able to recruit sufficient numbers of pa-tients to test each of the five statistical hypotheses.

4.5.3 Other Motivations for Triaging Endpoints

There are, of course, other reasons to reduce the number of endpoints in a clinical trial that are not quite so mathematical. Allocating a collection of type I error rates across each of 50 endpoints is possible. However, this decision requires that each endpoint be obtained and evaluated with the same high quality that is worthy of a primary endpoint and that this standard be consistently maintained throughout the trial. This goal is worthy—after all, any endpoint worth measuring is worth measur-ing correctly—but this may be a practical impossibility in a world of resource constraints. Serum measures should be evaluated by laboratories that have both an excellent tradition of quality and a fine research track record. If total mortality is an endpoint, then death certificates will be required, as well as the verification that every patient for whom there is no death certificate is alive.[6] This can be an expen-sive and time-consuming effort. If, for example, the cumulative incidence of total

---

[6] Since patients who have no death certificate may nevertheless be dead, it is imperative to confirm that patients without death certificates are in fact alive.

hospitalizations is to be an endpoint, then discharge summaries will be required of each patient who was hospitalized (with the coincident verification that the absence of a discharge summary actually means the patient was not hospitalized). Again, this can be a resource-intensive and a financially draining activity.

    The limited resources available to a clinical trial require that these resources be deployed selectively to be effective. The selection of a smaller number of signature endpoints allows the trial to focus its resources on the collection of this manageable number of endpoints with consistent attention to detail.

4.5.4 Endpoint Triaging and Labeling Indications

The notion of choosing carefully from among a collection of possible endpoints is a lesson that the pharmaceutical industry has understood and embedded into their clinical trial programs. In order to gain approval of its product by the FDA, the pharmaceutical company sponsoring the intervention must demonstrate that use of the product produces a favorable risk–benefit balance. This risk–benefit evaluation is a complex calculation that includes many components: however, one essential requirement is that the data must clearly demonstrate the benefits of the compound. Clinical trials that contain the balance of the information about the risk and benefits of the compound (known as pivotal clinical trials) are commonly the main source of these data. If the medication is determined to provide a favorable risk–benefit balance for an endpoint, the drug company may win permission to disseminate information about the compound's ability to favorably affect that endpoint's measure. This is one type of "indication" for the compound.

    As pointed out in Chapter 3, there are federal regulations and guidelines that govern the criteria to be met by the sponsor in gaining a new indication for the therapy in question. Thus, pivotal clinical trials, although permitting the measure of many endpoints are, nevertheless, designed to focus attention on a small number of key endpoints. Each endpoint for which an a priori α error probability has been allocated is a candidate for consideration as a potential indication for the use of the drug. Since the sponsor's resource investment in the compound is considerable, and the financial investment can run into tens of millions of dollars, the selection of these endpoints is made very carefully.

4.6 Endpoint Descriptors

The previous section described a process of dividing all of the endpoints of a clinical trial into two groups of endpoints: (1) prospectively selected endpoints and (2) post hoc, exploratory, or data-driven endpoints (Figure 4.2). The prospectively chosen endpoints are selected during the design phase of the trial, and are themselves divided between endpoints that will accumulate type I error rate and those that will not. The endpoints for which type I error rates will be accrued are termed the *primary endpoints*. The remaining prospectively selected endpoints are *secondary endpoints*. Finally, the *exploratory endpoints* are selected during the execution and analysis of the trial. Each of these endpoint classes (primary, secondary, and exploratory) has an important role to play in the interpretation of the results of a study.

4.6.1 Primary Endpoints

Primary endpoints are the primary focus of the study. Being prospectively chosen, statistical estimates of the effect of the clinical trial's intervention on these primary endpoints (along with that effect's standard error, confidence intervals and p-values) are trustworthy. In addition, since type I error is prospectively allocated to these primary endpoints, these tools permit an evaluation of the likelihood that the effect produced by the clinical trial's intervention would not be seen by the population, an evaluation that can be directly integrated into the risk–benefit assessment of the compound being studied. In a very real sense, the clinical trial's primary endpoints represent the axis around which the trial's logistical machinery revolves. The findings for the primary endpoints of the study will determine whether the study is positive, negative, null, or uninformative, thereby serving as the ruler against which the trial's results will be measured. The analyses of these primary endpoints are often described as confirmatory analyses, because the analyses confirm the answer to the scientific question which generated the clinical trial.

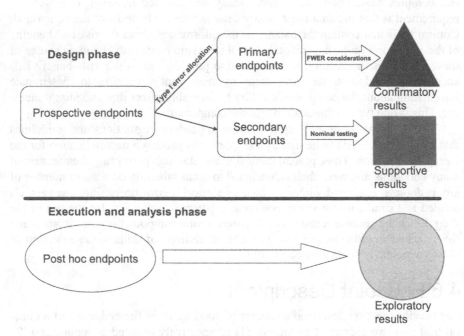

Figure 4.2. Description and purpose of endpoints in a clinical trial.

This definition allows us to consider as a candidate primary endpoint an endpoint for which an α error probability is allocated prospectively, but for which there will be inadequate power as a primary endpoint. A circumstance in which this could occur is when a rare endpoint may have an α error rate allocated prospectively, but the required sample size of the study to examine the effect of the intervention on this endpoint may be prohibitively large. A priori α error probability allocation in this circumstance provides the environment in which the effect of therapy for this endpoint could be considered positive (or negative). However, if the null hypothesis is not rejected for this analysis, the conclusion can only be that the analysis is uninformative. We will provide specific examples of this strategy later in this chapter.

4.6.2 Secondary Endpoints

The endpoints of the clinical trial that were prospectively selected during the trial's design phase, but had no a priori α allocated to them, are termed *secondary endpoints*. These endpoints, being prospectively selected, produce trustworthy estimators of effect size, standard error, confidence intervals, and *p*-values, all of which measure the effect of the clinical trial's intervention. However, drawing confirmatory conclusions about the effectiveness of the intervention being studied by the clinical trial, based on the results of secondary endpoints in general, cannot be permitted, since conclusions based on these secondary endpoints will increase the familywise error level above acceptable levels.

The role of analyses carried out on secondary endpoints is to provide support for the conclusions drawn from the trial's primary endpoints. Secondary endpoints can provide important information about the nature of the biologic mechanism of action of the compound that is being studied in the clinical trial. If they are endpoints that are related to the primary endpoint, they can add additional persuasive force to the argument for the beneficial effect of therapy, a force that is bolstered by the reliability of their effect size estimates. Typically, there are more secondary endpoints than primary endpoints. Again, *p*-values are of limited value with secondary endpoints since their interpretation produces unacceptable increases in ξ.

An example of the useful role that secondary endpoints can play is provided by one of the major trials that evaluated the effect of blood pressure control of the incidence of stroke. While the control of chronic elevations in diastolic blood pressure (DBP) was a significant and well accepted public health activity in the 1980s, the beneficial consequences of isolated elevations in systolic blood pressure (SBP), a finding of greater prevalence in the elderly, had yet to be rigorously evaluated. To investigate the risks and benefits of reducing isolated SBP elevations in this population, the Systolic Hypertension in the Elderly Program (SHEP) was initiated [2]. This was a prospective, randomized, double-blind, placebo controlled clinical trial that was designed to examine the effect of reducing SBP elevations in the elderly. SHEP recruited 4736 subjects who were at least 60 years old to either active antihypertensive control or placebo therapy. The primary endpoint of SHEP was prospectively specified as total (fatal and nonfatal) stroke. The α error level that was allocated to the primary endpoints was 0.05 (two-sided). Prospectively defined secondary outcomes were (1) sudden cardiac death, (2) rapid cardiac death, (3) fatal myocardial infarction, (4) nonfatal myocardial infarction, (5) left ventricular failure, (6) other cardiovascular death, (7) transient ischemic attack, (8) coronary artery therapeutic procedures, and (9) renal dysfunction.

The results of the study were positive (Table 4.1) [2]. The SHEP clinical trial produced a reduction in the primary endpoint of the study (total stroke) as a consequence of antihypertensive therapy. Thus, SHEP is considered to be a positive trial. Its secondary endpoints are, in general, supportive of the finding for the primary endpoint, suggesting that the effect of therapy may be a global effect on the reduction of major atherosclerotic cardiovascular disease.

Table 4.1. Results of the Systolic Hypertension in the Elderly Program.

Endpoints	Active Group (2375 patients events)	Placebo Group (2371 patients events)	Relative risk	95% confidence interval lower bound	upper bound	P Value
Primary endpoint						
Total stroke	103	159	0.64	0.50	0.82	0.0003
Secondary endpoints						
Sudden cardiac death	23	23	1.00	0.56	1.78	
Rapid cardiac death	21	24	0.87	0.48	1.56	
Nonfatal myocardial infarction	50	74	0.67	0.47	0.96	
Left ventricular failure	48	102	0.46	0.33	0.65	
Other cardiovascular disease	21	25	0.87	0.49	1.55	
Transient ischemic attack	62	82	0.75	0.54	1.04	
Coronary artery procedures	30	47	0.63	0.40	1.00	
Renal dysfunction	7	11				

Segregation of primary endpoint from secondary endpoints.

4.6.3 Exploratory Endpoints

By their very nature, nonprospectively defined, exploratory endpoints can simultaneously be the most exciting yet the most problematic analyses in clinical trials. Our examination of the difficulties inherent in random research[7] revealed that the analyses of these endpoints, endpoints that were chosen not during the design phase of the study but that arose from the examination of the data while the research is under way or upon its conclusion, will produce estimates of effect size, standard error, confidence intervals, and p-values that are unreliable and untrustworthy. Thus, upon the conclusion of these exploratory evaluations, the investigators will not know the true measure of the effect of the clinical trial's intervention on these exploratory endpoints in the population.

However, these chronic difficulties with exploratory endpoints should not be construed to mean that they have no useful role to play in clinical trials or that the results of these analyses should not be reported. Quite the contrary—they are an important research tool, and their inclusion in research can serve a very useful function. Much like the first step out onto uncharted terrain, exploratory analyses often provide a preliminary examination of what may become a promising line of re-

---

[7] Chapter 2 explored the difficulties involved in attempting to generalize results from the research sample to the population at large when the results were not prospectively chosen but instead were produced from the research data stream.

search. Thus, these analyses can prove to be the first data-based view of future investigations.

It cannot be denied that sometimes unforeseen, curious, and unanticipated findings will occur during a clinical trial's execution. One example is when the Data Safety and Monitoring Board's[8] review of an ongoing study reveals that the therapy being evaluated in the clinical trial may be having an unforeseen effect.[9] Another example is when investigators in clinical trial A report a relationship between the intervention and an endpoint. Investigators in clinical trial B testing the same intervention as in trial A, had also measured the endpoint reported in trial A, but made no prospective plans for its analysis. However, based on the findings from clinical trial A, they now feel compelled to carry out the evaluation that was conducted in trial B.

Circumstances such as these create an understandable demand from the medical community (and often from regulatory agencies) that the clinical trial report its nonprospectively planned analysis. Certainly, no clinical trial wishes to be accused of withholding, hiding, or refusing to carry out analyses requested by the medical community. In these cases, exploratory endpoints may reveal a surprise finding that, when fully and properly developed in future clinical trials, can lead to important conclusions. On the other hand, it must be admitted that the exploratory result generating the excitement may be due to sampling error. The untrustworthy estimates of effect sizes, confidence intervals, standard errors, and p-values produced by exploratory analyses preclude our ability to distinguish between these two possibilities. Therefore, the result must be repeated. The exploratory analyses represent "search," not "research."

There are other difficulties with these post hoc endpoints. With no prospective plan and prior discussion of the exploratory endpoint, the clinical trial may not have recruited sufficient numbers of patients to reduce the standard error of the estimate of the intervention's effect for this endpoint (i.e., the estimate of the effect may not be precise). In addition, there may be insufficient financial resources available in the trial to permit the best possible measurement of the endpoint. An example would be a decision made during the course of a clinical trial to identify the number of silent, asymptomatic heart attacks which occur annually in the recruited population. This new activity requires that electrocardiograms be obtained, transported, interpreted, and archived on a yearly basis for each randomized patient. Without a budget allocated for this effort, it can be impossible for the clinical trial's administrators to put together the funds for the comprehensive execution of this new, midtrial effort. The result is an incomplete dataset and an unreliable analysis.

We have discussed at length the inability to extend the results of an exploratory endpoint's analysis from the sample to the population. Setting this aside for a moment, sometimes the inclusion of a post hoc endpoint can make it difficult to understand the implications of the exploratory endpoint's analysis within the trial itself. Consider the following illustration:

---

[8] The Data Safety and Monitoring Board (DSMB) was briefly discussed in Chapter 1.

[9] Minoxidil, a preparation used to help attenuate baldness was originally used as an antihypertensive agent.

Example: A clinical trial is designed to evaluate a medication as an effective tool for weight loss. Overweight patients are recruited into the study with the understanding that they will have their weights measured initially and then be placed on either the placebo therapy or the active medication for three months. After three months, all patients will have their weights measured again. The investigators plan to measure the baseline–to–three month weight change in the active group, make the same measurement in the placebo group and then compare the two differences. This comparison of the change in weight between the active and placebo groups is the prospectively designed primary endpoint. The experiment proceeds.

Toward the conclusion of the study, the investigators learn of the possibility that the medication could raise pulmonary blood pressures, and wish to use their study to investigate this occurrence. The investigators therefore add the echocardiographic endpoint of increased pulmonary artery pressure to their study and, even though the trial is almost over, proceed to obtain echocardiograms on the patients in the clinical trial.

It is understandable why the investigators added the echocardiographic endpoint to their study. During the course of the trial, the concern for elevated pulmonary artery pressures raised a new safety issue about the active medication currently being evaluated in the clinical trial. By measuring whether trial participants who were on the active medication had a greater likelihood of experiencing increased pulmonary artery pressures, the investigators hoped to (1) obtain useful information about a potential risk of this drug, thereby providing an essential new insight into the risk–benefit assessment of the study medication, and (2) give important clinical information directly to each individual patient in the study about their health status. At the beginning of the study, these patients signed informed consent statements that mentioned nothing about the possibility of experiencing pulmonary artery pressure elevation. They now need to know whether they have been injured by a drug they volunteered to take.

However, there remain two fundamental difficulties raised by the inclusion of this endpoint which cloud its scientific interpretation. The first is that some patients who were recruited into the study may have had longstanding pulmonary artery pressure elevations. Since these elevations occurred before the trial began, it would be wrong to attribute the elevated pulmonary pressures of these patients to the weight loss medication being studied in the trial. However, obtaining an echocardiogram late in the trial does not enable the investigators to distinguish elevated pressures which first occurred during the course of the trial from elevated pulmonary pressures that occurred before the trial's initiation. The best tool to identify the critical timing of the occurrence of elevated pulmonary pressures would have been a baseline echocardiogram. This early measurement would have permitted the investigators to exclude those patients from the study who had pre-existing elevated pressures, leaving the study free to measure only new occurrences of elevated pulmonary pressures. However, this useful tool could only have been implemented if the decision to obtain echocardiograms had been made before the trial began. Thus, the decision to measure the echocardiographic endpoint post hoc ensured that it would be difficult to correctly attribute any finding of excess pulmonary pressure to the randomized group which received the active medication.

A second difficulty posed by the exploratory echocardiographic endpoint is that, in order to have an accurate depiction of the finding in the sample, patients would need to agree to return at the end of the study for the diagnostic echocardiogram. However, the patients in this trial did not consent to join the study to have echocardiograms carried out—only to get their weights remeasured. In addition, there is the additional, sad consideration that, if the medication is dangerous, patients may be too sick to return for the echocardiogram. Thus, if a sizable fraction of the participants either refuse to return or are unable to return for their evaluation, then the investigators cannot be sure of the actual findings in the research sample.

The desire to measure the medication's effect on pulmonary pressure was laudable and the data was necessary to arrange the appropriate care for the trial participants. However, its scientific contribution is ambiguous. The post hoc decision to incorporate the echocardiographic endpoint into the trial all but ensured that the exploratory endpoint's analysis would not provide an accurate assessment of the effect of the therapy on pulmonary pressure.

Investigators want to explore, perhaps need to explore, and nothing that we have said here will stop them from exploring. However, investigators must discipline themselves in the explorative process. The evaluation of exploratory endpoints in clinical trials can be exciting. However, the practical difficulties with their measurement, and the theoretical obstacles to their clear interpretation, limits exploratory endpoints to hypothesis generation and not hypothesis confirmation.

4.6.4 Choose Wisely

It is important to recognize that the use of this triage system does not prohibit the investigators from measuring multiple endpoints. In fact, investigators should be encouraged to measure as many endpoints as required to build the tightest causal link between the clinical trial intervention being evaluated and the disease process that intervention will affect. These investigators, having made the investment in time to understand the disease process, having committed the intellectual energy in appreciating the direct and indirect effects of the clinical trial's intervention, and having gained important experience with the persuasive power of the candidate endpoints, have earned the right to bring this unique combination of talents to the endpoint selection process. However, these investigators must organize the endpoints in a way that permits overall conservation of the familywise error level.

4.6.5 Planning Well to Learn Well

Prodigious work and effort awaits the clinical trialist as she prepares to design her research. It can take her a long time to clearly articulate the study question that the clinical trial will address. Weeks more will be invested in identifying and absorbing the pertinent medical literature. She must also find the fellow investigators and health workers necessary to share the burden of the trial's execution. There remains the inescapable task of finding funding for the study. Finally, her team must prepare for the arduous task of recruiting and following patients in the study. We have further increased this burden's weight by now forcing her to go through a prolonged examination of all of the potential endpoints of the study, a process requiring the complete immersion in the endpoint triaging system outlined in this chapter.

Many new investigators do not understand how deep (or cold) these waters can be when they first take the plunge into clinical trial research. Investigators whose fundamental interest and drive is in generating new knowledge about the disease (and its treatment) often become impatient with time-consuming planning meetings and costly pilot studies. After all, they just want to do the experiment and gain the knowledge. The realization of the labor involved is often a numbing shock.[10]

However, the product of this planned effort can be remarkable. In 1998, I was asked to participate in the Nobel Laureate Lectureship at McMurry University in Abilene, Texas. This university-sponsored activity featured the 1986 Nobel Laureate for Physiology and Medicine, Dr. Stanley Cohen of the Vanderbilt University School of Medicine. I, along with another invited guest, was asked to give one of two introductory or "warm-up" lectures as a preamble to Dr. Cohen's talk that would itself be the main event of the afternoon. Before these lectures began, we two introductory speakers and Dr. Cohen found ourselves together engaged in idle banter. Now, the question on both my mind and that of the other introductory speaker was just what distinguished Dr. Cohen from his competitive colleagues. What was special about Dr. Cohen's research ideas and philosophy that led to his winning the Nobel Prize? One of us marshaled the courage to ask him.

Dr. Cohen's response was memorable for its honesty, frankness and humility. From the mid-1960s up to the present, he said, research in biochemistry and physiology had undergone revolutionary changes. Technological advances now permitted the automation of physiologic experiments, and the newly developed capacity to computerize research analysis meant that studies, that before would have taken days to carry out, now could be executed in hours.

These new abilities produced an interesting change in the way many physiologists approached their research. In prior years, when experiments required a good deal of time to execute, these research efforts were designed slowly and carefully. With the need for slow execution pushed aside by technical advances, the scientists no longer felt bound by the requirement for time-consuming research design. They could now execute experiments one after the other in rapid fire succession.

Dr. Cohen, however, chose a different strategy. Rather than quickly execute a quickly executable experiment, he would instead invest much of his time and best effort into preexperimental thought, with attention focused on each of the possible outcomes of the experiment. Specifically, he would carefully consider the implication of every possible result of the experiment, mentally working to convert

---

[10] One young investigator, having just completed the monumental task of participating in the design, execution, and analysis of an industry-sponsored clinical trial, when asked about his willingness to help with another exclaimed, "The government hasn't printed enough money to persuade me to do that again!"

each result to a new piece of knowledge gained about the underlying physiology. If he could not in his own mind link each possible experimental result to new, reliable information to be added to the physiology corpus of knowledge, he would redesign the experiment so that this linkage was achievable. Dr. Cohen would go through this mental–experimental design process for days (sometimes for weeks) completing these linkages and matches. Only when he was sure that each possible experimental result would teach him something that was both new and worth knowing would he proceed with the experiment's execution. This was, in Dr. Cohen's view, the only noteworthy distinction between the character of his Nobel Prize–winning work and those of his competitors. After listening to and absorbing his self- effacing answer, it was then time for us to give our talks.

Clinical investigators want to learn; they know they must execute the experiment for the ultimate learning to take place. Methodologists not only endorse the drive of researches to learn—we share it. We only add that the best learning follows the best planning.

4.7 Mapping Out the Manuscript

The use of the system described above defines a hierarchy of clinical trial endpoints that can easily be ranked in terms of their persuasive power: Primary $\rightarrow$ Secondary $\rightarrow$ Exploratory. It is essential that this plan be fully described in the clinical trial's protocol. The protocol is the book of rules which governs the conduct of the trial. In it, the specification of each endpoint's ascertainment, verification, and analysis is laid out in great detail.[11] A well-written protocol serves as an indispensable anchor for the study, keeping the trial analyses from being cast adrift in the eddies of the clinical trial's incoming data stream. In addition, the protocol provides a guide for two important clinical trial publications.

4.7.1 The Design Manuscript

Occasionally, the clinical trial's investigators will choose to publish the protocol of their study. This choice offers several important advantages. The first is that appearance of the protocol in the peer-reviewed medical literature broadcasts to the research and the medical community that a trial is being conducted to answer a scientific question. In addition, important facts concerning the design of the trial that are of interest to other researchers in this field can be addressed in great detail. Assumptions underlying the sample size computation, aspects of the inclusion and exclusion criteria, and endpoint determinations are carefully described. In effect, a design manuscript is a message to the medical community from the investigators

---

[11] Of course, in general, post hoc exploratory endpoints are not defined in the prospectively written protocol. However, in some cases, the protocol may discuss an analysis even though neither the endpoints of the analysis nor the details for the analysis are known during the design phase of the trial. An example is the decision to store blood drawn in a clinical trial from each study participant at baseline for future genetic analyses whose details are not developed sufficiently while the protocol is being written. While these analyses are ultimately exploratory, they must (1) be discussed in the protocol and (2) be disclosed in the patient consent form.

that says "Here is the research question we wish to address. This is how we have decided to address it. Here are the rules of our trial. Be sure to hold us to them."[12] Examples of design manuscripts are [3] and [4] in hypertension, [5] and [6] in the therapy for CHF, [7] in cancer therapy, and [8] in the treatment of hyperlipidemia, just to name a few.

Design manuscripts can be particularly useful for clinical trials evaluating disputed areas of medicine, arenas where strong, vocal, and influential forces have long made known their points of view before the trial was conceived. At its conclusion, an expertly designed, well-conducted, and concordantly executed clinical trial will be criticized by some because that trial's results don't conform with the critics' preconceived ideas. This level of criticism increases in direct proportion to the controversial nature of the scientific question the clinical trial was designed to answer. Much of this criticism, being essentially nonscientific in nature, cannot be avoided. However, one particularly sharp but easily anticipated criticism is that the clinical trial's investigators tuned and adjusted their analyses to the incoming data stream, thereby ensuring that the investigators' own preconceived biases and notions would be validated by the clinical trial's results.

The publication of a design manuscript can blunt these criticisms precisely because the design manuscript will lay out the plan of analysis publicly before the data are collected and any analyses are attempted. In this desirable circumstance, the investigators are only required to execute their prospective analysis plan, thereby demonstrating to the medical community that the analysis plan, published before the study ended, matches the analyses published at the trial's conclusion.

4.7.2 Laying Out the Manuscripts

Delineating the prospective primary and secondary endpoints, while simultaneously acknowledging the need and limitations of exploratory analyses, are processes that will bear much good fruit for the diligent investigator. One example of this planning's satisfying product is that the description of these endpoints actually sets the stage for the layout of the clinical trial's main manuscript.

This main manuscript (often referred to as the "final manuscript"[13] is the focal point toward which the various logistical, statistical, and clinical work in the trial converges. This final manuscript describes the final results of the study; specifically, it details the findings of the primary analyses of the trial. The final manuscript is often the best platform from which the results of the trial can be broadcast. Therefore, it is no surprise that clinical trialists work hard to have this

---

[12] Design manuscripts have the additional advantages of (1) engaging the clinical trial investigators in the publishing process, an activity that can help to improve morale in a long trial, and (2) conserving space in the final manuscript that is published when the clinical trial has been completed by describing the trial's methodology in complete detail in the earlier appearing design manuscript.

[13] This "final" manuscript is the manuscript that reports the clinical trial's results for the primary endpoints of the study. This is the only thing final about this paper. There are many manuscripts which appear after the final manuscript, e.g., manuscripts that describe in detail findings from the clinical trial for secondary endpoints, subgroup analyses, exploratory analyses, and other subsidiary findings.

summary manuscript accepted in the most prestigious and highly respected clinical journals.

The groundwork for this important paper is laid during the design phase of the trial. It may seem somewhat premature to map out the final manuscript during this early planning phase of the study. After all, the clinical trial now being designed may not be concluded for several years, and much can happen (and commonly does) during that period of time. However, limiting the impact of unforeseeable events that may plague the study's execution is one of the primary reasons for the time-consuming, careful, and thoughtful development of the experimental plan. The design, execution, and analysis phases of a well-designed clinical experiment are so tightly linked, with the design embedding itself into and guiding the execution of the study, that the designers of the trial can see the skeleton of the final manuscript well before the study execution begins.

The motivation for executing the clinical trial is clearly known to the trial planners while they design the study. These experimentalists know the scientific question the study will address because they must repeatedly reexamine this question as they tailor the study's design to answer it. Both the motivation for this question and the question itself comprise the introduction section of the final manuscript. Since the designers constantly refer to this information during the planning phase of the clinical trial, these workers can easily complete most of this first, important section of the final manuscript during the design phase of the study.

The methods section of the final manuscript can probably not be written in its entirety during the design phase of the study, but certain of its fundamental sections can be completed. In addition to other points, the methods section should answer the following questions: What was the process of patient selection for the trial? What are the inclusion criteria patients must have to enter the study? What are the demographic and comorbidity criteria that will exclude patients from the trial? How should the investigators decide what therapeutic interventions the patient should receive? Since these issues must be addressed during the design phase of the study, the answers to these questions have been identified, collected, and entered into the trial's protocol during this planning stage and are now available for inclusion into the methods section of a final manuscript draft.

In addition, the choices for the primary endpoints and the secondary endpoints of the study are completed during the experiment's planning phase. Once these endpoints have been selected and triaged, the trial epidemiologists and biostatisticians will quickly identify what analysis tools they require in order to evaluate the effect of the trial's intervention on them. These statements are also available to the trial designers, and can be entered into a preliminary draft of the methods section of the final manuscript.

One of the most important sections of the final manuscript is the results section. Although one might think this is one of the last sections of the manuscript to be written, critical components of it can be outlined during the design phase of the study. Since the endpoints and the endpoint analyses have been chosen prospectively, the trial designers are cognizant of both the format for the analyses and the clearest way to present the data. In fact, table shells can be mocked up, requiring only the data to complete them.

By thinking the study methodology issues out carefully and in detail during the clinical trial's design phase, it is easy to incorporate their resolution into a preliminary draft of the final manuscript. The idea is to tightly bind the design of the study to the final analysis, not just on paper, but within the thought processes of the investigators. This tight link between the analysis plan (developed during the clinical trial's design phase) and the analysis itself (carried out at the conclusion of the study) will require concordant trial execution, thereby producing interpretable results.

4.8 Multiple Primary Endpoint Interpretations

The evaluation of hypothesis tests and significance testing as initially developed by Jersey Neyman and Egdon Pearson, was straightforward. One merely computed the test statistic that was calculated from the data of the experiment and compared the resulting p-value to the α level that had been prospectively determined from the experiment. Unfortunately, the interpretation of these p-values has become more complex when multiple analyses are poorly planned.[14] The goal of this section is to demonstrate the ease of clinical trial interpretation when the appropriate prospective foundation for multiple analyses in clinical trials has been laid.

Consider the work of the investigator during the design phase of her study. She has completed the endpoint triage system, and has prospectively determined the K primary endpoints for which significance testing will be executed. The study is initially designed to have a familywise error level of ξ; this rate is dispersed among the K primary endpoints with the jth endpoint having test-specific α α_j such that either $\xi = 1 - \prod_{j=1}^{K}(1 - \alpha_j)$ or, using Boole's inequality, $\xi \leq \sum_{j=1}^{K} \alpha_j$. At the conclusion of the study, the investigator produces a p-value for each of these hypothesis tests. Let p_j be the p-value which is computed for the jth primary endpoint, j = 1, 2, 3,..., K. Then, just as a familywise error level ξ is computed during the design phase of the trial the observed familywise error level at the conclusion of the trial, or posterior familywise error level, E is computed based on the K different p-values produced, either as

$$E = 1 - \prod_{j=1}^{K}\left(1 - \min\left(\alpha_j, p_j\right)\right) \tag{4.7}$$

or, using Boole's inequality,

$$E \leq \sum_{j=1}^{K} \min\left(\alpha_j, p_j\right). \tag{4.8}$$

We need to be able to link comparisons of the *a priori* and posterior familywise error levels to the individual p-values of the K primary endpoints. The study is positive (or negative)[15] when the posterior familywise error level E is less than the *a*

---

[14] See Chapter 2 and Moyé, L.A. (2000). *Statistical Reasoning in Medicine. The Intuitive P-Value Primer*. New York. Springer.

[15] These comments assume that the clinical trial has been concordantly executed.

priori familywise error level ξ, or $E < \xi$. An alternative formulation is that the study is positive when

$$1-\prod_{j=1}^{K}\left(1-\min\left(\alpha_{j},\,p_{j}\right)\right)<1-\prod_{j=1}^{K}\left(1-\alpha_{j}\right), \qquad (4.9)$$

where $\min(a,\,b)$ is the minimum of the numbers a and b. The application of Boole's inequality to each side of the inequality (4.9) leads to the declaration that a concordantly executed clinical trial is positive if

$$\sum_{j=1}^{K}\min\left(\alpha_{j},\,p_{j}\right)<\sum_{j=1}^{K}\alpha_{j}. \qquad (4.10)$$

Inequalities (4.9) and (4.10) are satisfied when, for at least one of the K primary endpoints, $p_j < \alpha_j$. Thus, the familywise error level is conserved when the p-value for at least one of the primary endpoints is less than its prospectively specified type I error level. This inequality has important consequences, allowing investigators to broaden the circumstances under which clinical trials are judged to be positive (or negative).

 If for each of the K primary endpoints, the p-value is less than the pre-specified α error rate, then the minimum function is not necessary and we may write $\sum_{j=1}^{K}p_{j}<\sum_{j=1}^{K}\alpha_{j}$. However, if the p-value for at least one of the test statistics is greater than its α level, that analysis is judged as null (or uninformative, depending on the power) and the type I error rate that accrues is the α level, not the p-value.

> Example: A clinical trial investigator is interested in demonstrating the effectiveness of a therapy in reducing the effect of early senile dementia on cognition. After much discussion, she settles on three primary endpoints (1) Boston Naming Task, (2) Digit Symbol Substitution, and (3) quality of life. She decides to allocate the type I error rate equally to each of these endpoints. Setting the prospective familywise α level $\xi = 0.05$ and using Boole's inequality, she settles on $\alpha_j = 0.05/3 = 0.0167$. At the conclusion of the concordantly executed experiment, she reports the results (Table 4.2).

Table 4.2. Primary endpoint findings for
cognition study

Endpoints	Prospective alpha	P Value
Boston naming task	0.0167	0.044
Digit symbol substitution	0.0167	0.100
Quality of life	0.0167	0.001

The positive finding for the quality-of-life
primary endpoint makes this study positive.

For each of the Boston Naming Task and the Digit Symbol Substitution, the p-value is greater than prospective α allocation. However, for the quality of life component, the p-value is less than the prospective type I error rate allocated for that endpoint. By the criteria of this section this study is positive. We know from the design phase of the study, $\xi = 0.05$. We may now compute the posterior familywise error level E as

$$
\begin{aligned}
E &= \sum_{j=1}^{K}\left(\min \alpha_j, p_j\right) \\
&= \min(0.0167, 0.044) + \min(0.0167, 0.100) \\
&\quad + \min(0.0167, 0.001) \\
&= 0.0167 + 0.0167 + 0.0010) = 0.0344.
\end{aligned}
\tag{4.11}
$$

Thus, $E < \xi$, and the study is positive.

The approach outlined in this section is a very effective procedure to both control the familywise error level and allow for the possibility that a trial can be considered to be positive on more than one endpoint. The literature has provided additional examples [9], [10].

4.9 Tactic 2: Differential α Allocation

Sections 4.5 to 4.7 discussed in detail the first of two tactics to be employed in controlling the familywise error level ξ in clinical trials where there are multiple endpoints to be analyzed. This first tactic required the investigators to first visualize the endpoints which would be of great value in answering the scientific question that was the primary motivation for the trial. These predefined endpoints will be specified in the clinical trial's protocol or rulebook. This prospective affirmation requires that the investigators commit themselves to the task of measuring these endpoints with great accuracy and attention to detail. These predesignated endpoints will themselves be prospectively classified as either primary endpoints or secondary endpoints. Primary endpoints will have type I error rate allocated prospectively to each one. The secondary endpoints provide support for the primary endpoints' findings in the clinical trial. Additional, nonprospectively defined exploratory endpoints are only remotely supportive of the findings of the primary endpoints, and serve mainly to raise new questions to be addressed in future research efforts.

This triaging system reduces the number of endpoints prospectively identified in the clinical trial to the small number of primary endpoints on which the trial will be judged as positive, negative, null, or uninformative. The second tactic that will now be developed focuses on the allocation of type I error rate probability among the small number of primary endpoints. For this discussion, we will continue to assume that the primary endpoints are independent one from the other.

After selecting the K primary endpoints for which the α error level is to be prospectively allocated, the only tool that we have developed thus far, to allocate a type I error level across these endpoints is that of equal allocation. Recall that, under this assumption, the familywise error level ξ may be written as

$$\xi = 1 - (1 - \alpha)^K. \qquad (4.12)$$

Alternatively, we have involved the following result from Boole's inequality

$$\xi \leq K\alpha \qquad (4.13)$$

or

$$\alpha \leq \frac{\xi}{K}. \qquad (4.14)$$

We will now explore the possibilities provided by the unequal α rate allocation.

4.9.1 Differential α Rate Allocation

There is no mathematical or statistical theory embedded in biology, pathophysiology, or therapeutics which requires that the test-specific α be equal across all K primary endpoints in a clinical trial. Consider the consequences of allowing each of the K primary endpoints in a clinical trial to have its own prospectively allocated α error level. Under this rubric, α_1 is prospectively allocated for the first primary endpoint, α_2 is prospectively allocated for the second endpoint, α_3 for the third endpoint, proceeding to α_K for the Kth primary endpoint. Then we may write ξ, the probability of a familywise error level as

$$\xi = 1 - (1 - \alpha_1)(1 - \alpha_2)(1 - \alpha_3) \dots (1 - \alpha_K)$$
$$= 1 - \prod_{j=1}^{K}(1 - \alpha_j). \qquad (4.15)$$

Example: If in a clinical trial there are three primary endpoints, with test-specific α levels of $\alpha_1 = 0.02$, $\alpha_2 = 0.01$, and $\alpha_3 = 0.005$, then the family-wise error level may be computed exactly as

$$\xi = 1 - (1 - 0.02)(1 - 0.01)(1 - 0.005) = 0.0345. \qquad (4.16)$$

Boole's equality may be evoked successfully within this paradigm of differential α allocation as

$$\xi \leq \alpha_1 + \alpha_2 + \alpha_3 + \cdots + \alpha_K = \sum_{j=1}^{K} \alpha_j \qquad (4.17)$$

We may apply this result to the previous example. This reveals that an upper bound for ξ is $0.02 + 0.01 + 0.005 = 0.035$.

As discussed in Chapter 3, both (4.12) and (4.13) have been commonly used since the 1960s as the basis for the adjustment of hypothesis testing results for multiple analyses and multiple endpoints. However, the criticisms raised by [11] and [12] remain valid to this day. The unavoidable result of spreading the type I error rate equally across several endpoints is the production of test-specific type I errors that are often too small to be useful. In the context of judging the merits of a new medication, type I errors levels that are too low offer a particular danger. Consideration of the benefit component in the risk–benefit evaluation of the clinical trial's intervention requires a realistic measure of the likelihood that the population will not see the advantages offered by the clinical trial's intervention. Small test-specific p-value thresholds that block a positive conclusion in the face of a clinically relevant effect size can prove to be just as much of a disservice to the medical community in their risk–benefit calculation as the absence of any p-value requirement at all.

This threat of inappropriately small test-specific α error rate thresholds continues to be an obstacle to a clinical trial's ability to contribute to the fund of knowledge about disease and its treatment, even if investigators follow tactic one and reduce the number of endpoints for which statistical hypothesis tests will be carried out. As an illustration, if in a clinical trial, the application of the first tactic produces 5 of 15 prospectively defined endpoints as primary endpoints (for convenience we number these primary endpoints as 1 to 5), then from (4.14) we see that each of these endpoints will be assessed at the $\xi/K = 0.05/5 = 0.01\,\alpha$ error level. Thus, the test-specific α level rates will be $\alpha_1 = \alpha_2 = \alpha_3 = \alpha_4 = \alpha_5 = 0.01$. Since sample sizes increase as the type I error level decreases (assuming everything else about the comparison, e.g., event rates, type II error levels, etc., remain constant), then the sample size required to be able to carry out the statistical hypothesis test for an α error rate of 0.01 may be prohibitive for the investigators.[16]

---

[16] Simple sample size computation examples and results are provided in Appendix D.

However, as an alternative, consider the possibility of $\alpha_1 = 0.03$, $\alpha_2 = 0.01$, and $\alpha_3 = \alpha_4 = \alpha_5 = 0.0033$. In this situation, there are three separate α levels. Since $\alpha_1 + \alpha_2 + \alpha_3 + \alpha_4 + \alpha_5 = 0.0499$, this test-specific α allocation conserves the family-wise error level. Once we designate different α level thresholds for each endpoint, we introduce a distinction between the trial's primary endpoints. The specific differential allocation of α introduced in this paragraph permits a greater risk of a type I error for primary endpoint 1, less risk of a type I error for primary endpoint 2, and even a smaller type I error level for primary endpoints 3 to 5. As (4.15) and (4.17) demonstrate, there is no mathematical obstacle to this alternative allocation of α. However, once the choice of an unequal allocation is made, the inequity of the allocation must be justified. This justification is a necessary step, and in my view, a worthwhile exercise in which investigators and statisticians should jointly engage.

The statistical literature does provide the suggestion for allocating α differentially across several endpoints. For example, Cook and Farewell [13] had suggested that the test-specific α be constructed based on the use of arbitrary weights. The underlying mathematics are briefly described as follows: let there be K primary endpoints, and the familywise error level is to be controlled at level ξ. Let w_j be the weight for the jth primary endpoint. Then we assign α_j, the test-specific α for the jth endpoint as

$$\alpha_j = \frac{w_j}{\sum_{J=1}^{K} w_j} \xi. \tag{4.18}$$

Example: Let a prospectively designed clinical trial have five prospectively defined endpoints. Let $\xi = 0.05$, and the test-specific endpoints have the weights $w_1 = 2$, $w_2 = 1$, $w_3 = 1$, $w_4 = 3$, $w_5 = 6$. Then $\sum_{j=1}^{5} w_j = 2+1+1+3+6 = 13$. Begin the test-specific type I error rate computation

$$\alpha_1 = \left(\frac{2}{13}\right)(0.05) = 0.00769.$$

Analogously, find that $\alpha_2 = \alpha_3 = 0.00385$, $\alpha_4 = 0.01154$, $\alpha_5 = 0.02308$. A quick check reveals that $\sum_{j=1}^{K} \alpha_j = \xi = 0.050$, thereby preserving the familywise error level.

This is a useful procedure but its implementation begs the question of how to choose the weights for the test-specific α error levels. Formal mathematical arguments to optimize the choice of the test-specific α error levels should be shunned in favor of developing the clinicians' *a priori* intuitions for the choice of these weights. This intuition should be built upon (1) a foundation of understanding of the disease process, (2) the relative persuasive power of the endpoints to convince the medical community of the effect of therapy, and (3) the need to keep the sample size of the trial small enough for the study to be executable.

Clinicians should be involved in the decision to allocate the type I error rate across the primary endpoints of the study because α allocation is a community protection device. As discussed in Chapter 3, the type I error probability in clinical trials makes an important contribution to the assessment of benefit in the eventual risk–benefit evaluation at the trial's conclusion. This is clearly the realm of the physician.

4.9.2 Clinical Decisions in Allocating α

Decisions concerning the allocation of test-specific α level rates for the K primary endpoints in a clinical trial are decisions about the statistical assumptions governing the hypothesis test for the endpoints at the conclusion of the study. The ability of the hypothesis test to permit conclusions about the effect of the intervention on a primary endpoint must take into account the sample size of the trial, the cumulative control group event rate of the study, the expected efficacy of the clinical trials intervention on reducing the endpoint's event rate, and the statistical power.

Thus, the decision to allocate type I error levels for primary endpoints are not made in a vacuum, but will have important implications for the sample size of the study. Since multiple primary endpoints are involved in this process, several different sample size computations must be simultaneously assessed. This will involve consideration of the control group event rate, the expected efficacy of the intervention being studied, and the statistical power of the evaluation for each of the primary endpoints.[17]

One useful strategy to follow in allocating α differentially across the prospectively specified primary endpoints of a clinical study is to first have the investigators carefully consider the clinical/epidemiologic determinants of the sample size formulation, i.e., the control group event rate and the proposed efficacy of the clinical trial intervention. Investigators should choose measures of event rates which are both accurate and allow for enough events to occur in the research sample, since the greater the cumulative control group event rate, the smaller the sample size, and the more flexibility there is in choosing a test-specific α of a reasonable level. Investigators should also carefully select efficacy levels. Advice for this can be found in several sources, notably [10], [14], [15], Although it is commonly assumed that efficacy levels should be the same across endpoints, this is not the only justifiable assumption.

After the endpoint control group event rates have been carefully selected, and the efficacy levels chosen, the investigator along with his statisticians and epidemiologists should examine different test-specific α error levels in combination with different power assumptions to provide the best control of the familywise error level and appropriate power for the hypothesis test. The remainder of this chapter is devoted to developing the skill to choose the relative levels of α error rates, and the skill in interpreting the results. In developing this concept and the process by which type I error levels are allocated prospectively, we will go through several different design scenarios for a single clinical trial's coprimary endpoints until we discover the correct combination of design parameters and statistical errors that allows us to

---

[17] A brief primer on sample size computations is provided in Appendix D.

consistently work within the principles of prospective design and confirmatory statistical hypothesis testing, all the while remaining relevant to the waiting medical and regulatory communities.

4.9.3 Example 1: Different Community Standards

As stated earlier, clinical investigators should be involved in the a priori α error level allocation decisions in a clinical trial. This is because the type I error level is an important consideration in determining the benefit patients will receive from the randomly allocated intervention. The likelihood that the intervention may not be effective in the patient population (which is measured by the type I error rate) is an important ingredient in the risk–benefit evaluation of the intervention when weighed by regulatory agencies in particular and the medical community in general.

However, it must also be acknowledged that some endpoints are more persuasive than others. An endpoint can be so influential that the medical community is willing to accept an increased risk of a type I error (keeping in mind that the magnitude of the effect size and its standard error must also be jointly considered in drawing a conclusion about the therapy's effect). Other less persuasive endpoints require a smaller type I error level before the result of the study is accepted.

Consider the following situation. An investigator is interested in conducting a clinical trial to determine the effectiveness of a medication for the treatment of patients with moderate to severe CHF. She thinks she will be able to recruit 4500 patients for this study. During the design phase of the study, numerous discussions take place concerning the endpoints to be measured in this clinical trial. Upon completion of the endpoint triage process, she settles on two primary endpoints, (1) the combined endpoint of total mortality or hospitalization for CHF and (2) the increase in patient activity level.

In this clinical trial, the total mortality/hospitalization primary endpoint will be rigorously collected. Relevant information for all deaths will be amassed. For each patient who is hospitalized during the course of the study, hospitalization records will be obtained and reviewed by a team of specialists in the treatment of CHF. These specialists will review this information to determine if the principal reason for the hospitalization episode was CHF.

It is expected that most of the patients who are recruited into the study and followed until the study's completion will not present paperwork describing a hospitalization during the course of the trial. In these circumstances, the clinical trial investigators will contact the patients to assure themselves that in fact no hospitalization took place that the investigators may have missed. This additional step will avoid undercounting the number of patients who were hospitalized for CHF during the study. These determined efforts by the trial investigators will produce a precise estimate of the incidence rate[18] of CHF hospitalizations during the course of the trial.

---

[18] The incidence rate is the number of new cases of the event of interest for a specified time period divided by the number of patients at risk of having the event. This is distinguished from the prevalence rate, a quantity that integrates both the new cases (incident cases) with the old cases (background cases). In the example being discussed, the prevalence measure of

The second primary endpoint relies on the patient's own measurement of their self-perceived change in activity level over the course of the study. Patients at the beginning of the trial will first measure their own activity level using a specially developed questionnaire, then measure it again at the study's conclusion when the patient's exposure to the study medication (active or placebo) is completed. The investigator believes changes in activity level are very important to patients with CHF, and that this measure of change as assessed by the questionnaire's metric is an important tool for estimating the effectiveness of the therapy from the patient's perspective.

After initial discussions about endpoint event rates in the control group and the effectiveness of the intervention being studied in the clinical trial, the investigators are able to compute an initial estimate of the sample size required (Table 4.3). This reflects no attempt to control the familywise error level. The computations for sample sizes for each of the endpoints in this table merely mark the starting point for the computations that will reflect alterations in the test-specific α levels. The trial designers have determined that the cumulative event rate for the combined endpoint of total mortality/CHF hospitalization in the control group is 25%, and that the reduction that they believe will be the minimum reduction that justifies the use of the therapy in the population of patients with CHF is 20%. The investigators then divide type I error levels equally between the two primary endpoints (Table 4.4).

Table 4.3. Alpha allocation, Example 1: First design scenario.

Endpoints	Cumulative control group event rate	Efficacy	Alpha (two-tailed)	Power	Sample size
Total mortality or CHF hosp	0.25	0.20	0.05	0.90	2921
Activity level increase	0.20	0.20	0.05	0.90	3867

With no concern for the family wise error rate, the maximum sample size is less than 3900.

Their first attempt at this allocating the type I error is based on a simple Bonferroni computation. With $K = 2$ endpoints, the type I α to be prospectively allocated to the two analyses is 0.025. This allocation will increase the sample size for each of the statistical hypothesis tests, assuming that there is no simultaneous change in the cumulative control group event rate, or the efficacy. At this point in the sample size computations and from this point forward, the event rates and hypothesized effectiveness of the intervention are fixed. All remaining changes in the sample size parameters are based on the statistical error rates.

CHF hospitalizations would include those patients in the study who were hospitalized during the study (new hospitalization) plus those who had been hospitalized in the past for heart failure before the study. Incidence cases are the more relevant to measure in a clinical trial because only the occurrence of incident cases would be influenced by the study intervention.

Table 4.4. Alpha allocation, Example 1: Second design scenario.

Endpoints	Cumulative control group event rate	Efficacy	Alpha (two-tailed)	Power	Sample Size
Total mortality or CHF hosp	0.25	0.20	0.025	0.90	3450
Activity level increase	0.20	0.20	0.025	0.90	4567

The result of the equal apportionment of alpha error rates across the two primary endpoints of the clinical trial.

The notion that the test-specific type I error should be equal between the two endpoints must now be addressed. There are important differences between these two primary endpoints. The second primary endpoint that measures the change in activity over time for patients with CHF, while informative, may be less widely accepted. Its implications are less clear, and it may not be measured very precisely. Thus, the medical community may require a smaller type I error level (everything else being equal) before they are persuaded that the medication has a beneficial effect on this less dominant primary endpoint.

We should note that the smaller type I error probability for the activity level endpoint is not useful in and of itself; it is useful only for what it implies. With everything else about the design of the study being the same, a smaller type I error probability indicates a greater effect size. It is this larger magnitude of effect that the medical and regulatory community require from this new endpoint. The less experience that these communities have with the endpoint, the greater the effect of the randomly allocated therapy on that endpoint must be in order to carry important persuasive weight. The smaller p-value is just a reflection of this observation.

To the contrary, the total mortality/hospitalization for CHF endpoint has been established as an influential endpoint by regulatory agencies. It is easy to understand. Even though the criteria for hospitalization may be regional, there is no doubt that a hospitalization for CHF is serious and something to be avoided. In addition, the investigators will go to great lengths to assure that the CHF hospitalization endpoint will be measured accurately, working patiently and diligently to ensure that both overcounts or undercounts are avoided. The traditional upper bound for a primary endpoint in clinical trials is 0.05[19] and the medical community would not require a lower level as an upper bound for acceptable type I error level. The investigators therefore chose to allocate a greater type I error level to this combined endpoint (Table 4.5).

---

[19] See the discussion in Chapter 1.

Table 4.5. Alpha allocation, Example 1: Third design scenario.

Endpoints	Cumulative control group event rate	Efficacy	Alpha (two -tailed)	Power	Sample Size
Total mortality or CHF hosp	0.25	0.20	0.03	0.90	3312
Activity level increase	0.20	0.20	0.02	0.90	4790

First attempt at differentially allocating type I error.

Continuing this development, the investigators consider allocating an even greater type I error level to hospitalization for CHF (Table 4.6).

Table 4.6. Alpha allocation, Example 1: Fourth design scenario.

Endpoints	Cumulative control group event rate	Efficacy	Alpha (two-tailed)	Power	Sample Size
Total mortality or CHF hosp	0.25	0.20	0.04	0.90	3093
Activity level increase	0.20	0.20	0.01	0.90	5476

The community is willing to bear a greater type I error for the hospitalization primary endpoint than for the exercise tolerance primary endpoint.

This further reduction in the α error level for the increased activity primary endpoint has increased the sample size for its hypothesis test to more than the 4500 subjects the investigator believes she will be able to recruit for the clinical trial. However, since the minimum power for the primary endpoints is 80%, she chooses to reduce the power for this second primary endpoint (Table 4.7).

Table 4.7. Alpha allocation, Example 1: Fifth design scenario.

Endpoints	Cumulative control group event rate	Efficacy	Alpha (two-tailed)	Power	Sample Size
Total mortality or CHF hosp	0.25	0.20	0.04	0.90	3093
Activity level increase	0.20	0.20	0.01	0.80	4298

A prospective decrease in power to 80% for the exercise tolerance endpoint keeps the power at an acceptable level but reduces the sample size to less than 4500.

At this point, each of the design criteria for these two analyses have been satisfied. The endpoints will be interpreted at their own test-specific α levels, conserving the familywise error level at no more than $0.04 + 0.01 = 0.05$. In addition, the sample sizes for each of the evaluations allow a statistical test for each primary endpoint with adequate power. The trial will be considered positive if the intervention has a statistically significant effect on either the combined endpoint or the measurement of activity level.

4.9.4 Example 2: The Underpowered Environment

One easily anticipated scenario for the allocation of type I error levels among several different primary endpoints is the situation in which one of those primary endpoints retains much clinical interest but suffers from a statistical power shortage. Managing familywise error levels in this setting is especially useful since it can produce not only confirmatory statistical hypothesis testing for the highly powered primary endpoints but, in addition, also ensure that a surprisingly strong effect of the intervention for the underpowered endpoint can be interpreted in a confirmatory and not exploratory light.

In this example, a clinical trial investigator is interested in carrying out a clinical trial to demonstrate the effect of a new "superaspirin" on patients who are at risk of having a future myocardial infarction (MI). The known risks of this medication (rash, diarrhea, ulcers, rare neutropenia) are well known to the regulatory and medical community. The benefits of this drug have not yet been assessed. The investigators wish to recruit patients into the study who are at risk of future ischemic cardiovascular disease, anticipating that they will be able to recruit 4000 patients for this study. The inclusion criteria for the study are patients who have a documented history of either (1) a prior MI, (2) a prior stroke, (3) peripheral vascular disease, (4) diabetes, or (5) hypertension.[20]

After completing the endpoint triaging process, the investigator settles on two primary endpoints for this clinical trial: (1) fatal and nonfatal MI and (2) total mortality. The familywise error level for the study $\xi = 0.05$. Since these are each primary endpoints, the investigator must now allocate an α error probability to each one. He begins with a preliminary examination of the sample sizes required for each (Table 4.8). For this preliminary evaluation, the two-sided type I error rate allocation for each hypothesis test is at the 0.05 level, and the power is set at 80%. The investigator recognizes that Table 4.8 does not preserve the familywise error level ξ at 0.05; he just wants to begin the evaluation of the implications of α allocation for each of the two primary endpoints. He is comfortable with the choice of 25% efficacy for each of the endpoints. The required sample size for the fa-

---

[20] Choosing patients with a risk factor for future ischemic cardiac disease will produce a cohort with a relatively higher rate of endpoint occurrence than would be seen from a cohort of patients with no risk factor for ischemic disease. This higher cumulative incidence endpoint rate will decrease the required sample size and the cost of the study (Appendix D). A criticism of this useful approach is that if the study is positive and the superaspirin is approved by the FDA, the indication for the drug will most likely not include the large target population of all adult patients regardless of the presence of ischemic disease, but the smaller population of those with a documented risk factor for future ischemic cardiovascular disease.

tal/nonfatal MI component is 4004, while that for the second co-primary endpoint of total mortality is 14,262. This large difference in the sample sizes is due to the difference in the cumulative event rates of the two primary endpoints.[21] The required sample for the fatal/nonfatal endpoint is one that the investigator believes can be achieved. However the sample size required for the total mortality endpoint greatly exceeds his ability to recruit patients.

Table 4.8. Alpha allocation, Example 2: First design scenario.

Endpoints	Cumulative control group event rate	Efficacy	Alpha (two-tailed)	Power	Sample size
Fatal/nonfatal MI	0.10	0.25	0.05	0.80	4004
Total mortality	0.03	0.25	0.05	0.80	14,262

Substantially more patients are required for the total mortality endpoint then for the fatal/nonfatal MI endpoint even without conservation of family wise error rate.

If the investigator were to allocate α based on (4.14) each of two endpoints would have a type-specific error level of $0.05/2 = 0.025$. Computing the required sample for size for each of the two primary endpoints can be recomputed using this α error level (Table 4.9).

Table 4.9. Alpha allocation, Example 2: Second design scenario.

Endpoints	Cumulative control group event rate	Efficacy	Alpha (two-tailed)	Power	Sample Size
Fatal/nonfatal MI	0.10	0.25	0.025	0.80	4848
Total mortality	0.03	0.25	0.025	0.80	17,271

Even allocation, of the type I error.

From Table 4.9, ξ is preserved at the 0.05 level. However, the sample size for the fatal/nonfatal MI has increased from 4004 to 4878, a sample size that the investigator cannot achieve. The sample size for total mortality has increased to 17271 when the α-specific error level decreased from 0.05 in Table 4.8 to 0.025 in Table 4.9.

From Tables 4.8 and 4.9, the investigator sees that either nominal testing or ξ conservation allows him to carry out a hypothesis test with adequate power for

---

[21] Since the cumulative mortality rate is low for this trial, deaths will occur infrequently. Therefore, more patients will be required to get sufficient events in order to keep the type I error level at the 0.05 level.

the fatal/nonfatal MI endpoint. However, the total mortality endpoint is completely underpowered for either a test-specific α of 0.05 or one of 0.025. The investigator desires to be able to test each of the primary endpoints with sufficient power but clearly has no real opportunity in either scenario to have appropriate power for the total mortality endpoint. Allocating α equally for each of two endpoints allows him to test neither with appropriate power with the attainable sample of 4000.

The investigator can retain the ability to have an adequate sample size to carry out a hypothesis test for the fatal/nonfatal MI component however, and still retain some ability to execute a hypothesis test for total mortality as demonstrated in the next computation (Table 4.10). In this case, the α error level is allocated unequally with the preponderance of the 0.05 rate assigned to the fatal/nonfatal MI component, and only 0.005 assigned to the total mortality endpoint. The sample size required for the fatal/nonfatal MI primary endpoint is 4132, close to the 4000 patients that the investigator believes can be recruited for the study. With this computation, the investigator acknowledges that he has no opportunity to carry out an appropriately powered evaluation of the total mortality endpoint (Table 4.10).

Table 4.10. Alpha allocation, Example 2: Third design scenario.

Endpoints	Cumulative control group event rate	Efficacy	Alpha (two-tailed)	Power	Sample Size
Fatal/nonfatal MI	0.10	0.25	0.045	0.80	4132
Total mortality	0.03	0.25	0.005	0.80	24,187

Evaluation of the total mortality component will be underpowered if 4132 patients will be recruited into this study

The medical community would be satisfied with an α specific error probability of 0.05 or less for the fatal/nonfatal MI component. In its view, this level of α error is sufficient to provide evidence of benefit of the intervention for this clinical consequence.

However, several comments must be made about the total mortality evaluation. First, it will clearly be underpowered if it is based on the assumptions from Table 4.10. Under this setting, if the hypothesis test for total mortality was carried out but did not fall in the critical region (i.e., the test was neither positive nor negative), then the finding cannot be considered null, but uninformative—the clinical trial did not exclude the possibility that in the population of patients (from which the sample of 4000 patients was obtained) there may be an effect on mortality, but through the play of chance a sample was provided that did not provide evidence of an effect on total mortality.[22] The hypothesis test on total mortality only contributes to the fund of knowledge about the benefit of the medication if the finding is positive.[23]

---

[22] This would be a beta, or type II error.

[23] The hypothesis test for total mortality would also be confirmatory if it was negative, indicating harm.

However, the possibility of a positive finding must also be examined carefully. According to Table 4.10, the finding for the total mortality endpoint would only be considered positive if the p-value at the study's conclusion for the hypothesis test for total mortality is less than 0.005. This might at first glance appear to be an exceedingly high threshold for a positive finding. However, this low p-value is not unreasonable for this particular clinical trial setting. Although of the two primary endpoints, the total mortality endpoint is the most persuasive, this persuasive power is sapped by a tepid beneficial mortality effect in this relatively small sample. The risk reduction for total mortality must itself be overwhelming in this relatively small sample size. If the investigator's prediction for the occurrence of mortal events is accurate, and the trial were to recruit 14,362 patients (from Table 4.8), then we could approximate the number of deaths to occur in the trial as $0.03(14,362) = 430$ deaths. This is a substantial number of deaths, and the regulatory and medical communities have demonstrated that conclusions based on this large number of deaths is sufficient evidence on which to base a confirmatory conclusion for total mortality.

However, if instead of 14,362 patients, only 4000 patients are randomized, then the expected number of deaths would be $(0.03)(4,000) = 120$ deaths. This is not many deaths at all on which to base a finding for total mortality. Stated another way, the total mortality risk reduction produced by the medication would have to be huge for the regulatory and medical community to draw a confirmatory conclusion from the positive total mortality hypothesis test based on only 120 deaths. This is the message the investigators convey by choosing an α-specific level of 0.005.

Taken to another level, the investigators can allocate all but a negligible fraction of α error level on the fatal/nonfatal MI endpoint (Table 4.11). Here, the overwhelming portion of type I error rate is allocated to the fatal/nonfatal MI primary endpoint, with only 0.001 allocated for the total mortality endpoint. This keeps the sample size of the study in the achievable range, with adequate power for the fatal/nonfatal MI evaluation, but inadequate power for the total mortality endpoint.

Table 4.11. Alpha allocation, Example 2: Fourth design scenario.

Endpoints	Cumulative control group event rate	Efficacy	Alpha (two-tailed)	Power	Sample Size
Fatal/nonfatal MI	0.10	0.25	0.049	0.80	4028
Total mortality	0.03	0.25	0.001	0.80	31,020

Familywise error rate control retains the smaller sample size for fatal/nonfatal
MI and will conceed the low power evaluation for the total mortality endpoint.

A reasonable question to ask at this point is, if the total mortality endpoint is so dramatically underpowered (using the results from Appendix D, the power for the total mortality endpoint is only 4%!) what is the advantage of even declaring the total mortality endpoint as a primary endpoint? Why not instead leave it as secondary or even exploratory? The advantage is based in the investigator's belief that the medication may in fact demonstrate a benefit for total mortality that would be strong enough to make its presence known even with the small sample size. If the hypothesis test for total mortality were to be strongly positive but total mortality was a secondary or exploratory endpoint, the study could not be considered positive since no α was allocated prospectively.[24] However, prospectively declaring total mortality a primary endpoint and allocating a type I error level to its hypothesis test, permits the study to be considered positive when such an overwhelming total mortality benefit is observed. Allocating a small percentage of α to a persuasive but underpowered endpoint preserves the ability to draw a confirmatory, positive conclusion about the finding, an ability which is lost if no α is allocated prospectively.

4.9.5 Example 3: Efficacy Reconsideration

In the previous example there were only two primary endpoints to consider. However, the following, more complex clinical question involves the treatment of isolated systolic hypertension. The purpose of this clinical trial is to examine the effect of antihypertensive medications in patients with borderline elevations in systolic blood pressures but with diastolic blood pressure less than 90 mm Hg. The investigators have considerable resources for this study, and believe that they can recruit 15,000 patients and follow them for seven years. However, the candidate patients for this trial will be relatively risk free with few patients having a history of cigarette smoking, diabetes, prior MI or prior stroke. Thus, the event rates for these patients will be relatively low, prolonging the duration of patient follow-up.

In the design phase of this study, the investigators have many candidate endpoints for the study distributed among biochemical markers, clinical endpoints, and endpoints which measure changes in cognition. These clinical trialists intensively labor to settle on a small number of primary endpoints, but can agree in the end to no less than five primary endpoints. They are (1) fatal and nonfatal stroke, (2) fatal and nonfatal myocardial infarction (MI), (3) CHF, (4) coronary artery disease (CAD) death, and (5) total mortality. The major interest is in fatal/nonfatal stroke, but important attention will be focused on the remaining four primary endpoints as well. The daunting task before these investigators is to allocate type I error among these endpoints, taking advantage of other aspects of these endpoints that would make a 15,000 patient trial justifiable.

Each of these endpoints is important, and the investigators are anxious to be able to make confirmatory statements about the effect of isolated systolic blood pressure control for each of them. To begin the process, these investigators collect event rate information and perform some initial sample size computations making no initial attempt to control the familywise error level ξ (Table 4.12). The relatively low event rates for these endpoints have produced some fairly large sample sizes. The calculation for CAD death is particularly worrisome, since its preliminary sample size is over 22,000 patients without any adjustment yet for the familywise error level.

---

[24] See the discussion in Chapter 2.

Table 4.12. Alpha allocation, Example 3: First design scenario.

Endpoints	Cumulative control group event rate	Efficacy	Alpha (two -tailed)	Power	Sample Size
Fatal/nonfatal stroke	0.090	0.20	0.05	0.90	9649
Fatal/nonfatal MI	0.100	0.20	0.05	0.90	8598
CHF	0.080	0.20	0.05	0.90	10,963
CHD death	0.040	0.20	0.05	0.90	22,789
Total mortality	0.060	0.20	0.05	0.90	14,905

A first examination of the sample sizes for each endpoint without conservation of familywise error rate.

The investigators approach the ultimate α level adjustments in two phases. The first phase focuses on the clinical assumptions contained in Table 4.12 which will support the statistical hypothesis tests to be carried out at the trial's conclusions. There is no way of course to adjust the cumulative control group event rates once the population for which the research sample is to be obtained has been chosen. However, the examination of efficacy levels across these five primary endpoints does bear some examination during the design phase of the study.

A common assumption in carrying out sample size computations and comparisons across candidate endpoints during the design phase of the trial is that efficacy levels are equal for each of the endpoints. However, there is no theoretical justification for the assumption of efficacy uniformity. In this particular scenario, an argument can be made that the efficacy levels for CAD death and total mortality should be higher. The low cumulative control group event rate for each of these two mortal endpoints is very low, implying that few deaths are expected during the course of the trial. This small number of deaths suggests that if the trial is to demonstrate persuasive findings for the effect of antihypertensive therapy on a small number of endpoints, these findings must reflect a particularly potent reduction in the cumulative incidence of these endpoints. With this as justification, the investigators prospectively choose an efficacy level of 25% for each of the relatively rare mortal primary endpoints, recomputing their sample size (Table 4.13).[25]

---

[25] The decision to change efficacy levels during the design phase of the trial should not be taken lightly. This concept is discussed in detail in Chapter 11.

Table 4.13. Alpha allocation, Example 3: Second design scenario.

Endpoints	Cumulative control group event rate	Efficacy	Alpha (two -tailed)	Power	Sample Size
Fatal/nonfatal stroke	0.090	0.20	0.05	0.90	9649
Fatal/nonfatal MI	0.100	0.20	0.05	0.90	8598
CHF	0.080	0.20	0.05	0.90	10,963
CHD death	0.040	0.25	0.05	0.90	14,190
Total mortality	0.060	0.25	0.05	0.90	9,285

Decrease in CHD Death and total mortality endpoints by increasing efficacy from 20% to 25%.

The investigators are now ready to control the familywise error level for the five primary endpoints of this study. The investigators choose to place a greater type I error rate on the fatal/nonfatal stroke endpoint, as this has been the single primary endpoint of a previous study evaluating the effect of therapy on isolated systolic hypertension in the past [2]. The investigators also wish to place as much additional test-specific α error level on the statistical hypothesis test for the total mortality primary endpoint. Allocating a type I error level in this fashion has a predictable and dramatic effect on the sample sizes for each of the primary endpoints. Leaving all other considerations the same, decreasing the type I error level will increase the sample sizes for each of the primary endpoints, inflating the sample size to profound levels for some of them (Table 4.14). However, sample sizes for the fatal/nonfatal stroke primary endpoint, fatal/nonfatal MI endpoint, and the total mortality endpoint, although larger, are still within the 15,000 patient sample size which is the sample size the investigators will be able to recruit. However, sample sizes for the remaining three primary endpoints exceed this cap.

Table 4.14. Alpha allocation, Example 3: Third design scenario.

Endpoints	Cumulative control group event rate	Efficacy	Alpha (two -tailed)	Power	Sample Size
Fatal/nonfatal stroke	0.090	0.20	0.0250	0.90	11,954
Fatal/nonfatal MI	0.100	0.20	0.0050	0.90	13,678
CHF	0.080	0.20	0.0050	0.90	17,440
CHD death	0.040	0.25	0.0050	0.90	22,573
Total mortality	0.060	0.25	0.0100	0.90	13,147

Increase in sample size by conserving the familywise error rate.

One last additional prospective procedure that can be used to provide an acceptable sample size for each of these five primary endpoints is an adjustment in the power. The minimal acceptable power in clinical trials is 80%. Since this is a minimum, and the investigators desire the maximum power possible, only the power for each of CHF, CAD death, and total mortality are each reduced (Table 4.15).

Table 4.15. Alpha allocation, Example 3: Fourth design scenario.

Endpoints	Cumulative control group event rate	Efficacy	Alpha (two -tailed)	Power	Sample Size
Fatal/nonfatal stroke	0.090	0.20	0.0250	0.90	11,954
Fatal/nonfatal MI	0.100	0.20	0.0050	0.90	13,678
CHF	0.080	0.20	0.0050	0.80	13,887
CHD death	0.040	0.25	0.0050	0.80	17,974
Total mortality	0.060	0.25	0.0100	0.80	10,318

Final reduction in sample sizes by selectively decreasing the power.

We are now at the conclusion of this process. Each of these endpoints is evaluated in such a fashion that the familywise error level is preserved. For four of these endpoints, there is adequate power for a sample size of 15,000. For the CAD death endpoint, power is reduced.[26] In doing so, the contribution of each of the primary endpoints was considered. The type I error level for the three endpoints fatal/nonfatal MI, CHF, and CAD death are each low (0.005 level). However, since the investigators insisted on five endpoints, this low level on some of the five endpoints was required. The investigators also insisted on increasing the efficacy for CAD death and total mortality to 25%, being motivated by the low cumulative control group event rate for each of these mortal endpoints.

The proposed solution in Table 4.15 is not the only solution. As an alternative, the investigators could have chosen the strategy of decreasing the power for the fatal/nonfatal MI component, permitting a smaller fatal/nonfatal MI test-specific α error level. This maneuver would permit a greater α level error level for the CAD mortality endpoint, thereby increasing the power to the 80% level for this mortal endpoint. The point of these exercises is to demonstrate that the use of design parameters of the experiment can be implemented to allow confirmatory hypothesis tests of several different primary endpoints. There may be many prospective paths to this goal. Arguments have been voiced to increase the familywise error level in clinical trials as well [16].

One undeniable observation in this scenario is that these five endpoints are not independent, and that information about the result of one hypothesis test will provide new information about another hypothesis test. If taken into account, these hypothesis test dependencies could produce a substantial reduction in the family-wise error level expended. The implications of these dependencies is the topic of Chapter 5.

---

[26] The actual power for the CAD death endpoint with the cumulative endpoint event rate, efficacy α, and in Table 4.9 for a sample size of 15,000 is 70%.

4.9.6 Example 4: Multiple Endpoints

The idea of allocating α differentially across a selection of primary endpoints can at first appear to be an unwarranted burden. However, it must be recognized that investigators, by taking the more customary tack of choosing a single primary endpoint on which the entire type I error level is to be placed, have the burden of choosing the single best endpoint on which they will pin all of their hopes for a successful study. This is a very difficult decision; however, the *a priori* design of an experiment requires precisely this level of prospective thought. Unfortunately, even when the best efforts of clinical scientists lead to the prospective selection of a clinical trial's sole primary endpoint, the investigators can still get it wrong in the end. Consider the circumstance of the Assessment of Treatment with Lisinopril and Survival (ATLAS) trial [17].

One of the therapies for the treatment of CHF is the use of ACE-i therapy. These therapies had been demonstrated to reduce the incidence of total mortality in randomized controlled clinical trials [18], [19]. However, while these clinical trials studied ACE inhibitor therapy at relatively high doses, practicing physicians have chosen to use ACE inhibitor therapy at lower doses for their patients. No clinical trial had ever tested the wisdom of this approach. The ATLAS trial was designed to test the efficacy of low-dose ACE inhibitor therapy (Lisinopril) when compared to high-dose Lisinopril therapy. Patients with either NYHA class II–IV heart failure and LVEFs of less than 30% despite treatment with diuretics for more than two months were eligible for the study.

There are many candidate endpoints to measure in patients with heart failure. Possible variables include a plethora of echocardiographic measures, cost effectiveness measures, quality of life measures, clinical measures of morbidity, and mortality. The investigators were accomplished physician-scientists who were skilled in the treatment of heart failure, and worked diligently to settle on the endpoints of the study. These researchers chose the cumulative incidence of all-cause mortality as the primary endpoint of ATLAS. In addition the ATLAS investigators chose four secondary endpoints: (1) cardiovascular mortality, (2) cardiovascular hospitalization, (3) all-cause mortality combined with cardiovascular hospitalization, and (4) cardiovascular mortality combined with cardiovascular hospitalization.

The trial commenced in October 1992, and recruited 3164 patients who were randomly assigned to either the low-dose or the high-dose therapy. An independent DSMB was constituted at the start of the study to periodically examine the interim results of the trial. This board was authorized to suggest that the trial be prematurely terminated if the treatment effect demonstrated either greater than anticipated benefit or hazard in the two treatment arms. However, during the course of the trial, the Steering Committee reopened the issue of endpoint selection for ATLAS. This committee chose to make a midcourse change in the endpoints selected for the trial, by adding a single endpoint; all-cause mortality and all-cause hospitalization.[27] However, a midtrial examination of the data suggested that the cumulative mortality rate was lower than anticipated. The steering committee now

---

[27] A patient is considered to have met this endpoint if they either (1) die or (2) survive and are hospitalized.

considered changing the primary endpoint, replacing the prospectively specified primary endpoint of cumulative total mortality with the new all-cause mortality/all-cause hospitalization combined endpoint. However, they instead chose to designate this new endpoint as a special secondary endpoint, one that would receive priority over prospectively selected secondary endpoints. These discussions point out the difficulty of choosing the "best" single primary endpoint.

With this change in endpoints, ATLAS proceeded until its conclusion, at which time the results of the study were announced. ATLAS reported a null finding for the primary endpoint of the study (Table 4.16). The finding for the primary endpoint of total mortality was null. There was no (nominal) statistical significance for the secondary endpoint of cardiovascular mortality. However, the findings for the prospectively defined secondary endpoint of total mortality/cardiovascular hospitalization and for the a priori secondary endpoint cardiovascular mortality/cardiovascular hospitalization was nominally positive. The added endpoint of all-cause mortality/all-cause hospitalization had a nominal p-value of 0.002.

How should this trial be interpreted? From a strictly α error level point of view, ATLAS is null. This is because a type I error rate was allocated only to the single primary endpoint of total mortality and the p-value for the effect of therapy exceeds the prospectively allocated 0.05 α error level. If one argues, alternatively, that the study should be considered positive for the added endpoint of all-cause mortality and all-cause hospitalization, then how could we unambiguously compute the type I error rate for this beneficial effect?

Table 4.16. Results of the ATLAS study.

Endpoints	Prospective Alpha allocation	Risk reduction	P value
Primary endpoint			
Total mortality	0.05	8%	0.128
Secondary endpoints			
Cardiovascular mortality		10%	0.073
Cardiovascular hosp.		16%	0.050
Total mortality / CV hosp.*		8%	0.036
CV mortality / CV hosp.		9%	0.027
Added endpoint			
All-cause mort / all-cause hosp.		12%	0.002

*CV=Cardiovascular: Hosp = Hospitalization
A priori distibution of alpha across the prospectively specifid endpoints could have been useful.

There is no question about the strong finding of the effect of therapy for this added endpoint in the sample. The important question is can this finding be generalized to the population from which the sample was obtained? It is not as simple as reporting $p = 0.002$, a reasonable strategy only if the endpoint and its α level had been chosen prospectively.[28] If we instead invoke (4.10), we would see that $E = 0.05 + 0.002$ which is greater than 0.05.

The unfortunate fact is that the investigators gained nothing by adding this endpoint to ATLAS during the course of the trial—it might as well have been added as exploratory endpoint at the end of the study, requiring confirmation from a later trial. This trial is a null trial despite even the findings for the prospectively specified secondary endpoints because all of the prospective type I error rate were placed in the single primary endpoint of total mortality.

Of course it is easy to look back over the course of ATLAS and envision an α allocation scheme that would have produced a clearly positive trial; such a retrospective glance is helpful to no one. However, one only need appreciate the struggle the ATLAS investigators had in choosing their endpoints to appreciate the difficulty in the traditional α allocation process of one primary endpoint/α allocation decision. The angst in ATLAS was caused by the perceived failure to choose the correct single primary endpoint prospectively. This task was itself exceedingly difficult to accomplish in ATLAS since each of the candidate endpoints were related to one another. The ATLAS investigators did the best job they could, even going to the extraordinary lengths of adding a mid trial "priority endpoint" only to have their results as null at the conclusion of the trial. If α had been allocated across several primary endpoints prospectively, there may very well have been concern about the α allocation midway through the ATLAS program as well. However, the investigators would have had some assurance that they did not have to put all of their α "eggs" into a single "basket." Making a decision as to what apportionment of α should be allocated to each endpoint is easier than having to decide which important endpoints to ignore in the α allocation.

4.10 Multiple Analyses

Although the discussion in this chapter has thus far focused on an investigator who must choose from a selection of endpoints, the selection process in reality is more complex. Investigators who design clinical trials are engaged not just in a multiple endpoint selection process but are actually choosing from among multiple analyses. Multiple analyses are composed of not only endpoint choices but of classes of different and alternative examinations of the same endpoint. It is the multiple analysis issue that appears commonly in clinical trials (Figure 4.3).

---

[28] While it might be argued that the new endpoints of all-cause mortality and all-cause hospitalization were not added to the trial after looking at the data for this endpoint, the data was examined and demonstrated that the total mortality cumulative event rate was low. If the investigators had not examined the data, they, in all likelihood, would not have added the new endpoint in the middle of the trial.

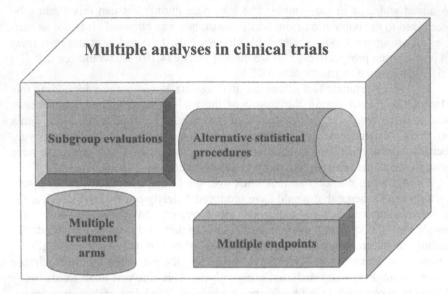

Figure 4.3. Different types of multiple analytic scenarios in clinical trials.

For example, a clinical trial may have chosen one endpoint—total mortality. However, the clinical trial may have more than two arms, such as a control arm and two treatment group arms. In this case, the evaluation of total mortality will include its cumulative incidence rate comparisons between the control group and each of two active groups. In this situation, there is one endpoint, but two analyses. As a second example, a clinical trial with a control group and a treatment group may have only one prospectively chosen endpoint. However the investigators may wish to compare the effect of the intervention on that endpoint not just in the entire research cohort, but also in a subcohort or subgroup of special interest, e.g., in women. Again, a clinical trial with only one endpoint has produced two different analyses. Finally, in the Glidel example discussed in Chapter 2[29], the issue taken up by the advisory committee was not the concern of which endpoint to consider as primary. The topic was which analysis of that endpoint would be accepted, the adjusted analysis or the unadjusted analysis.

4.10.1 Example

One of the consequences of a heart attack that patients commonly face is left ventricular remodeling. Ventricular remodeling is the process by which the left ventricle of the heart becomes distorted, misshapen, and dilated because of damage to the cardiac muscle. Nitrate therapy had been known to prevent left ventricular dilation. This change in the heart's architecture can lead to left ventricular dysfunction. In the early 1990s, attention focused on the use of a transdermal nitroglycerin

---

[29] Pages 65–66.

delivery system to provide nitrate therapy in a continuous drug delivery system. The NitroDur trial was designed to investigate the effects of intermittent, transdermal nitroglycerin patch therapy on left ventricular remodeling [20]. The study was a prospective, randomized double-blind placebo controlled multi-center trial, with a single placebo group and three active treatment groups. The three treatment groups delivered nitrate therapy by patch for six months in three doses: 0.4, 0.8, and 1.6 mg/hr respectively.

The endpoints of this study were complex, reflecting the investigators' interests in the global effects of this therapeutic intervention. The primary endpoint of the study was end systolic volume index. The secondary endpoints included end-diastolic volume index and LVEF. In addition, the NitroDur investigators wished to measure mean exercise time at three months of follow-up, as well as a combined endpoint that included recurrent MI, development of unstable angina, or the development of heart failure requiring revascularization. Each of these endpoints would be measured in each of the three treatment groups and the control group.

In addition to these endpoint-treatment comparison combinations, a special dose response analysis was to be performed for the radionuclide angiographic volume measures (y) of each of the end systolic volume and the end diastolic volume. The mathematical model that was prospectively chosen was

$$y = \beta_0 + \beta_1 X + \beta_2 X^2,$$ (4.19)

where X represents the dose of nitroglycerin delivered in mg/hr. For each of the two volume endpoints, two analyses were to be performed: (1) an analysis that included patients in each of the three treatment arms and the placebo group, and (2) an analysis with the placebo group removed. Several subgroup analyses were prospectively specified, namely (1) the evaluation of the effect of therapy in patients with >40% versus <40% ejection fraction, (2) patients taking or not taking ACE-i therapy, (3) patients on or off beta blocker therapy at baseline, and (4) patients with an anterior infarction versus patients with an inferior infarction.

Finally, the investigators were interested in determining whether the effect of transdermal nitroglycerin on left ventricular volume measurements was transient or sustained after the therapy's discontinuation. Therefore, they intended to measure end systolic volume, both at the conclusion of the study when nitroglycerin patch therapy was discontinued, as well as 2 weeks post nitroglycerin discontinuation. This final post therapy measurement, when compared to the last volume measurements while the patient was on therapy, would provide an evaluation of the sustainability of the nitroglycerin-induced effect on end systolic volume.

Thus, in NitroDur the issue of multiple analyses was not limited solely to multiple endpoints, but focused equally on alternative analyses of these endpoints, comparisons across multiple treatment arms, and subgroup analyses.

In reality, clinical trial investigators do not choose just primary, secondary, or exploratory endpoints, but instead chose primary, secondary, or exploratory analyses. The discussion from this point forward will focus on not just multiple endpoints in clinical trials, but multiple analyses.

4.11 Theory Versus Reality

The philosophy of the prospective selection of endpoints with the differential allocation of type I error rates, in concert with concordant trial execution, is a useful, if not indispensable, theoretical assembly. Its product is an interconnected, cohesive experimental unit that guides the conduct of the clinical trial's analysis. In doing so, it also guides the conduct of the trial. However, the executability of this theory is commonly threatened by the exigencies of reality.

Consider the following example[30] of a clinical trial that is designed to evaluate the effect of a novel intervention in patients with symptomatic coronary CAD. In a randomized, prospective, double-blind clinical trial format, the clinical trial investigators plan to assess the effect of injections of a new compound on the heart's ability to utilize oxygen in patients with ischemic cardiac disease. Eligible patients are to be selected from a population of patients who suffer from symptoms of angina pectoris despite the optimal use of antianginal medication, but who are not eligible for immediate percutaneous transluminal coronary angioplasty (PTCA) or coronary artery bypass surgery (CABG).

Once selected, patients will be randomized to receive either placebo infusion, low-dose infusion, or high-dose infusion of the intervention, with an equal number of patients being randomized to each of the 3 groups. These patients will then be followed for at least 12 months, and will have clinic visits at 12 weeks and 12 months. After 12 months of follow-up, the patients will be contacted by telephone to assess the occurrence of significant adverse events every 6 months until the last patient randomized completes their 12 month visit. Thereafter, patients will be contacted to update their clinical status every year for up to 5 years.

The analysis of this clinical trial was prospectively described in detail. The investigators designed two primary analyses, for which an α level was assigned to each a priori. The first of these primary analyses is an assessment of the patient's quality of life. Each patient completes a quality of life measure at baseline, and then at 12 weeks post randomization. The change in quality of life is to be measured for each patient; from these changes, a mean change in quality of life will be computed for each of the three therapy groups which will then be compared to each other. The total type I error rate to be expended upon these comparisons is prospectively set at 0.035. This analysis we will designate as primary endpoint P_1.

The second primary analysis of this clinical trial was designed to compare the percent of patients who had a 20% increase in their quality of life from baseline across the three randomized groups. This analysis will be described as primary endpoint P_2. A prospectively set α error level of 0.015 was allocated for this comparison.

Additionally, in a secondary analysis, the investigators prospectively specified an evaluation of the incidence of the composite endpoint of coronary events/all-cause mortality. The incidence of this clinical endpoint was to be compared across the three treatment groups. The criterion for statistical significance for

---

[30]The author served as a paid consultant to the sponsor in this example. He has altered some of the facts (the nature of the intervention, endpoints) to maintain confidentiality.

this endpoint was set at 0.05 (nominal significance), as its role was to be only supportive. We will refer to this evaluation as the clinical endpoint analysis.

This protocol was given to the FDA to review. However, the review was not completed until after the trial was well under way. In that review, the FDA stated that it was not very comfortable with the second primary endpoint P_2. It recommended that the sponsor change the type I error rate allocation from 0.035 for P_1 and 0.015 to P_2 to 0.05 for P_1; analysis P_2 would be reduced to a secondary analysis. In addition, the FDA recommended that the clinical analysis should have its status raised from that of a secondary endpoint. While the FDA did not specifically state that the type I error rate for the clinical endpoint analysis should be chosen so that the familywise error rate was conserved, it did suggest that the sample size of the trial should be increased in order to provide more clinical events in the study.

The investigators are faced with a dilemma here. They want to comply with the FDA's requests, given that the FDA will be the final arbiter of whether the investigators' efforts will result in an intervention that will receive approval. In all fairness, the FDA was only trying to be helpful and to provide the best guidance it could to the investigators; nevertheless, the FDA's recommendations were received after the trial had started. Effectively, the FDA was asking the investigators to do precisely what so many clinical trial investigators have been criticized for doing—changing the endpoint analysis after the trial was under way.

There are several issues that had to be addressed as the investigators carefully considered this delicate matter. One was the issue of timing. As we pointed out in Chapter 2, there are critical problems that arise when the incoming data stream is allowed to determine the endpoint analysis. But is that the case here? Is the study badly damaged if an endpoint is changed for an administrative reason early in the trial?

The first of two concerns that arise when considering an endpoint change for administrative reasons is logistical. The final selection of endpoints for a trial is not the end but the beginning of an intensely demanding process. Sample size estimates for the trial are based on the characteristics of the primary endpoints that are finally selected. Decisions have to be made about the quantity and quality of information to be collected, so that the investigators can satisfactorily document that an endpoint has occurred. Sometimes, expensive equipment must be purchased and calibrated, and the training session initiated to in order to provide assurance to the medical community that the endpoint was measured uniformly under a commonly occurring set of conditions. Human, logistical, and financial resources must be supplied for this effort. If a decision is made to change the endpoint very early in the trial, investigators can divert resources to its measurement. The investigators' flexibility is a direct consequence of the fact that these resources have not yet been expended. However, the later in the trial that the endpoint event changes are made, the less resilience the investigators have, and the more logistically problematic the new endpoint's implementation becomes.

The second problem is perceptual. The investigators, support staff, DSMB, and sponsor of a clinical trial are united in their desire for the trial to persuade the medical and regulatory community of the benefit–risk ratio of the clinical trial's intervention. These workers understand that, while it is common for amendments to be added to the protocol that guides the conduct of the trial, nonprospectively planned changes in the analysis plans must be avoided. Such serious perturbations raise the suspicions in the medical community about the propriety of the study's conduct. The greater the number of these perturbations, the greater the concern about the interpretability of the trial's results. The medical community understand both the temptation that can sometimes drive investigators to change endpoints based on incoming data and the resulting confusion that surrounds the trial's interpretation; the motivations for administrative endpoint changes are somewhat more difficult to discern by an outsider who is not intimately familiar with the intricate intratrial decision apparatus. Thus, a change in the analysis plan is viewed by outsiders as an important change that occurred presumably because of the appearance of an interesting new pattern in the trial's data stream regardless of whether this is the case or not.

In addition, the later in the trial the endpoint change is made, the greater this perception can become. This is because the longer the trial runs, the greater the trial's experience and the larger its repository of endpoint information. Since, in general, large datasets are more persuasive than smaller ones, endpoint changes that occur late in the trial, when they can be logistically difficult to achieve, engender the perception that they must have been propelled by powerful findings in a large and convincing dataset. Thus, the later the endpoint change is made the deeper the perception can be that the endpoint change is being driven by the incoming data (Figure 4.4). Thus, while an endpoint change after the trial commences may seem to be administratively justified, its convincing power is transmitted through a prism of perception. In the world of perceptions, it is not enough to be right—one must also appear to be right. It is difficult for a late endpoint change to appear to be right.

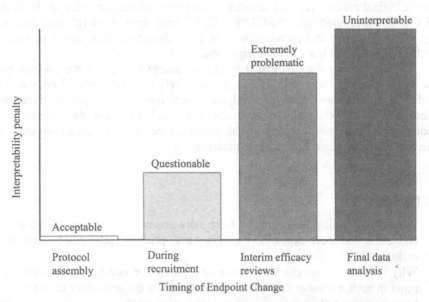

Figure 4.4. Interpretability difficulties increase with late endpoint changes

Another option to be considered would be to start the study again. While this maneuver would remove the concern about the late endpoint change (since the new study would incorporate the regulatory recommendations prospectively) other obstacles instantly emerge. New patients must be found to replace those subjects who had already been randomized. Also, much of the financial commitment to the first study could not be recouped. If the study had just started (with only 1% of the total number of patients randomized), these concerns would be minor.

Returning to our initial example, when the FDA provided their advice, approximately one-third of the total number of patients required for the trial had been recruited, and 15% of the total required cohort had been followed for at least 3 months. Thus, 15% of patients had or were preparing to have both of the two primary endpoints measured. In fact, the FDA has received information concerning the execution of the trial before they offered their advice. However, the data that the FDA had reviewed had only been safety data and not data that revealed any patterns of effectiveness. This close examination reveals that the FDA recommendation was not based on an evaluation of any efficacy data, i.e., the data were not driving the decision. Therefore, since the data from the trial are not being used to make the endpoint change, one could technically argue that the analysis plan could be altered without converting the planned confirmatory analysis of the primary endpoints to an exploratory one.

However, such a decision would be tightly nuanced at best. Certainly any endpoint change made after the trial had commenced should be viewed with suspicion by the medical community even if the FDA approved (or authorized) the change. In addition, while an administrative change in the endpoint may appear to be commendable by the current FDA reviewers, future FDA analysts may have a different point of view, and a future FDA advisory committee convened to evaluate the trial's final results may look askance at the proposed endpoint change. Both the US Carvedilol program and the CAPRICORN[31] trial serve as useful counterexamples to the argument that an adjustment in the endpoint selection and type I error levels is justified and leads to an interpretable result.

The sponsor decided that it would not accept the FDA's suggestions and that it should instead stay with its own prospectively delineated plan. Very careful, prudent decisions about the trial's endpoints were correctly and prospectively decided; these would be undone by midtrial alterations. The clinical trial was studying a complicated and new intervention and should not be clouded with a new analysis plan that would produce a murky interpretation.

Problems

1. Why does a clinical trial typically have more secondary endpoints than primary endpoints, and more exploratory analyses than primary endpoints or secondary endpoints?
2. Why does the prospective allocation of type I error rate to a secondary endpoint in such a manner that ξ is conserved convert the secondary endpoint to a primary endpoint?
3. Why does the absence of a prospective allocation of type I error allocation to a primary endpoint that is prospectively defined convert the primary endpoint to a secondary endpoint?
4. Are there any circumstances in which ξ the could be allowed to exceed the 0.05 level?
5. A clinical trial is designed with two primary endpoints. The test-specific type I error rate for the first primary endpoint P_1 is 0.045. Demonstrate that, if the ξ for the entire study is 0.05, then the remaining type I error rate for the second primary endpoint P_2 is 0.0052.
6. How does the assumption of independence directly effect the distribution of a type I error rate among the K different primary endpoints in a clinical trial?
7. A clinical trial is designed to have four primary endpoints. Without using the Bonferroni inequality, devise two different α allocation schemes that conserves the familywise error rate at the 0.05 level but provide different test-specific type I error rates.
8. A clinical trialist is troubled by the fact that analyses that are not prospectively determined will produce p-values that are uninterpretable. He suggests the following plan. During the design phase of the trial, the familywise error rate is divided into a component for the primary endpoints α_p, and a component for the exploratory analyses, α_x such that the familywise error rate is conserved. The type I error α_x is distributed among three exploratory analyses to be identified at the trial's conclusion. Does this approach produce confirmatory interpretations for the three exploratory analyses?

---

[31] These were discussed at length in Chapter 2.

References

1. Senn, S. (1997). *Statistical Issues in Drug Development*, Chichester, John Wiley, Section 15.2.1
2. The SHEP Cooperative Research Group. (1991). Prevention of stroke by antihypertensive drug therapy in older persons with isolated systolic hypertension: Final results of the systolic hypertension in the elderly program (SHEP). *Journal of the American Medical Association* **265**:255–3264.
3. The SHEP Cooperative Research Group. (1988). Rationale and design of a randomized clinical trial on prevention of stroke in isolated systolic hypertension. *Journal of Clinical Epidemiology* **41**:1197–1208.
4. Davis, B.R., Cutler, J.A., Gordon, D.J., Furberg, C.D., Wright, J.T., Cushman, W.C., Grimm, R.H., LaRosa, J., Whelton, P.K., Perry, H.M., Alderman, M.H., Ford, C.E., Oparil, S., Francis, C., Proschan, M., Pressel, S., Black, H.R., Hawkins, C.M. for the ALLHAT Research Group. (1996). Rationale and design for the antihypertensive and lipid lowering treatment to prevent heart attack trial (ALLHAT). *American Journal of Hypertension* **9**:342–360.
5. Moyé, L.A. for the SAVE Cooperative Group. (1991). Rationale and design of a trial to assess patient survival and ventricular enlargement after myocardial infarction. *American Journal of Cardiology* **68**:70D–79D.
6. Pratt, C.M., Mahmarian, J.J., Morales-Ballejo, H.,Casareto, R., Moyé, L.A. for the Transdermal Nitroglycerin Investigators Group. (1998). The long–term effects of intermittent transdermal nitroglycerin on left ventricular remodeling after acute myocardial infaction: Design of a randomized, placebo controlled mulitcenter trial. *American Journal of Cardiology* **81**:719–724.
7. Moyé, L.A., Richardson, M.A., Post-White, J. Justice, B. (1995). Research Methodology in Psychoneuroimmunology: Rationale and design of the IMAGES–P (imagery and group emotional support study-pilot) clinical trial. *Alternative Therapy in Medicine* **1**:34–39.
8. Pfeffer, M.A., Sacks, F.M., Moyé, L.A. et al. for the Cholesterol and Recurrent Events Clinical Trial Investigators. (1995). Cholesterol and Recurrent Events (Cholesterol and Recurrent Events Clinical Trial) trial: A secondary prevention trial for normolipidemic patients. *American Journal of Cardiology* **76**: 98C–106C.
9. Moyé, L.A. (1998). *P*-value interpretation and alpha allocation in clinical trials *Annals of Epidemiology* **8**:351–357.
10. Moyé, L.A. (2000). *Statistical Reasoning in Medicine: The Intuitive P-Value Primer*. New York. Springer.
11. Rothman, R.J. (1990). No adjustments are needed for multiple comparisons. *Epidemiology* **1**:43–46.
12. Pocock, R.J., Geller, N.L., Tsiatis, A.A. (1987). The analysis of multiple endpoints in clinical trials. *Biometrics* **43**:487–498.
13. Cook, R.J., Farewell, V.T. (1996). Multiplicity consideration in the design and analysis of clinical trials. *Journal of the Royal Statistical Association*. **159**:93–110.

14 . Meinert, C.L. (1986). *Clinical Trials Design, Conduct, and Analysis*. New York.Oxford University Press.
15. Friedman, L., Furberg, C., DeMets, D. (1996) *Fundamentals of Clinical Trials. 3rd Edition*. New York. Springer.
16. Moyé, L.A. (2000). A Calculus in Clinical Trials: Considerations and Commentary for the New Millenium. *Statististics in Medicine* **19**:767–779.
17. Packer, M., Poole-Wilson, P.A., Armstrong, P.W., Cleland, J.G.F., Horowitz, J.D., Massie, B.M., Rydén, L., Thygesen, K., Uretsky, B.F. on behalf of the ATLAS Study Group. (1999). Comparative Effects of Low and High Doses of the Angiotensin–Converting Enzyme Inhibitor, Lisinopril, on Morbidity and Mortality in Chronic Heart Failure. *Circulation* **100**:2312–2318.
18. Pfeffer, M.A., Braunwald, E, Moyé, L.A. et al. on behalf of the SAVE Investigators (1992). Effect of Captopril on mortality and morbidity in patients with left ventricular dysfunction after myocardial infarction – results of the Survival and Ventricular Enlargement Trial. *New England Journal of Medicine* **327**:669–677.
19. The SOLVD Investigators. (1991). Effect of enalapril on survival in patients with reduced left ventricular ejection fractions and congestive heart failure. *New England Journal of Medicine* **325**:292–302.
20. Pratt, C.M., Mahmarian, J.J., Borales–Ballejo, H., Casareto, R., Moyé, L.A. for the Transdermal Nitrogen Investigators Group. (1998). Design of a randomized, placebo–controlled multicenter trial on the long-term effects of intermittent transdermal nitroglycerin on left ventricular remodeling after acute myocardial infarction. *American Journal of Cardiology* **81**:719–724.

Chapter 5

Introduction to Multiple Dependent Analyses I

This is the first of two consecutive chapters that develop the concept of multiple hypotheses testing in a clinical trial when the primary analyses are related to each other. In this chapter, the problem of allocating a type I error level across a collection of dependent hypothesis tests within a clinical trial is developed from first principles. The concept of a dependency parameter is introduced, and examples are provided from the medical literature concerning the prospective development of dependent hypothesis tests. Realistic scenarios are presented that allocate α error levels in this circumstance. Guidelines and cautions are provided in estimating the degree of dependence between the hypothesis tests; concerns about the presence of too much dependence (hyperdependence) is addressed. Chapter 6 continues this development, and Appendix E provides several more advanced results of this approach to the problem of multiple dependent statistical analyses.[1]

5.1 Rationale for Dependent Testing

While there are several important, almost irresistible benefits that occur from taking advantage of the natural relationships between statistical hypothesis tests that are prospectively embedded into clinical trials, several traps are present as well. We will need to carefully examine this concept of dependence before we can fully and safely implement dependent hypothesis testing in clinical trials.

5.1.1 Review

Chapter 4 developed the principle of α allocation among a subset of endpoint analyses in a clinical trial. A series of endpoint selection steps was offered to guide the investigator who must choose from many different candidate endpoints during the design phase of a clinical trial. Throughout that process, we have insisted that investigators should be permitted "the desire of their hearts"; they should be allowed to measure all of the endpoints that they believe to be relevant and wish to evaluate. This includes the acknowledgment that the investigator will encounter new endpoints during the course of the execution and the analysis of the clinical trial. There are only two considerations that should discipline and restrain the investigator in this endpoint collection process. The first is that the endpoint should add to the scientific strength of the study. The second consideration is one of logistical

---

[1] Silvia Maberti was very helpful in her review of the content of this chapter.

constraints. The clinical trial must be able to measure the endpoint with sufficient quality so that the evaluation can be firmly fitted between the twin pillars of accuracy and precision.

After choosing these endpoints, we then required the investigators to triage the endpoints into prospectively determined categories of primary, secondary, and exploratory endpoints. The exploratory or hypothesis-generating endpoints serve not to answer questions but to raise them for evaluation in future research efforts. Secondary endpoints are determined prospectively and play a supportive role. The primary endpoints are endpoints for which α allocation rates are prospectively set. The principle results of the clinical trial will be based on the findings from these primary endpoints. The balance of Chapter 4 provided examples of how type I α rates should be allocated differentially among the primary endpoints of the study to conserve the familywise error level, ξ.

5.2 The Notion of Dependent Analyses

Each of the examples of the distribution of type I error levels among analyses in clinical trials in Chapter 4 has provided an allocation under the assumption that the hypothesis tests for each of the prospectively selected primary endpoints were independent.[2] However, in many circumstances these analyses are related to each other. This is a concept that will require some discussion.

5.2.1 The Nature of Relationships

Most of us have a general understanding of the concepts of dependence versus independence. However, although these two properties are somewhat intuitive, we need to elaborate on their fundamental characteristics. The descriptors "independence" or "dependence" are properties of a relationship. We don't ask if the occurrence of a cerebrovascular accident was "independent." We do ask if the occurrence of the stroke was related to (i.e., dependent) or independent of the patient's prior use of crack cocaine. The property of independence/dependence describes the state of the relationship between events.[3]

Specifically, at its most fundamental level, independence describes a relationship between two events that is characterized by the fact that the occurrence of one of these events provides no information about the occurrence of the other. An observer who notes the occurrence of one event learns nothing about the occurrence of the second event if the two events are independent. Consider the thought process of a doctor who is examining a patient who may or may not be suffering from lumbar nerve root compression. During his examination, the doctor may notice the patient's eye color. However, the observation that the patient's eyes are brown does not influence the likelihood that the patient has sustained a nerve root compression

---

[2] It was the independence assumption that permitted us to write $\xi = 1 - (1 - \alpha)^K$ in Chapters three and four.

[3] Even when words and expressions such as sovereign, autonomous, self-determination, or self-rule are used to describe independence, there is a relationship implied, e.g., sovereign from what?

injury. Eye color is uninformative about the occurrence of the nerve root injury, and knowledge of the patient's eye color does not affect one way or the other the doctor's assessment of the patient's chances of suffering from a nerve root compression. We say that the two events of eye color and the appearance of compression of the nerve root are independent of one another.

Dependent relationships are quite a bit more complicated. When two events are dependent, the observer can gain useful knowledge about the possibility that the second event occurred by knowing the first event's occurrence status. Dependent relationships can be very informative—however, the observer must understand the nature of the dependency. Specifically, she must know how to apply her knowledge of the first event's occurrence to update, re-evaluate, and thereby improve her assessment of the likelihood of the occurrence of the second event.

Dependencies between relationships can very rapidly become complicated because they can include more than just two events. For example, whether a passenger in a taxi arrives at his destination on time can depend on whether the taxi driver knows the route. We can say that the likelihood of an on-time arrival depends on (or is conditional on) whether the taxi driver knows the way to the destination. However, if the taxi driver does not know the way, the chance of the taxi's on-time arrival can depend on whether the passenger knows the route. Therefore, a more realistic assessment of the likelihood that the passenger arrives on time depends on both the taxi driver's knowledge and the knowledge of the passenger. As the number of events that are "conditioned on" increases, the evaluation of the probability of the occurrence of the event of interest improves; however, the complexity of the assessment also increases.[4]

While clinicians in their day-to-day practice may not formally think of events as being dependent, we nevertheless learn to link events in helpful ways. For example, a patient admitted to an emergency room complaining of chest pain will undergo a diagnostic evaluation that will provide information about the likelihood that the patient has suffered an MI. This information includes a complete history of the symptoms of the chest pain (e.g., Where is the pain located? Is the discomfort a pressure sensation? Is there associated pain in the jaw or the arms? Was there sweating with the discomfort? Was there any nausea or vomiting associated with the episode?) This is followed by a complete medical and family history, leading to a thorough physical exam and evaluation of the patient's blood assays and electrocardiogram.

Each of these procedures is designed to reveal useful information about the cause of the patient's chest pain and, based on these evaluations, the treating physician will come to a conclusion and make treatment recommendations. If the diagnostic workup of the patient reveals her to be a 20-year-old female whose chest pain (associated with contusions, soft tissue pain and swelling) occurred shortly after falling from a horse onto a fence, then the likelihood that the cause of the chest pain is a heart attack is dramatically reduced. Of course, substernal crushing chest

---

[4] Of course, traffic density, the presence of construction detours, and local weather conditions can all affect the probability that the taxi arrives at the desired time as well. Consideration of these events also increases the complexity of the assessment of the taxi's arrival.

pressure–pain in a 59-year-old obese male with a long history of cigarette smoking and hyperlipidemia who has sustained a heart attack in the past and who currently has ST-T segment elevations on his electrocardiogram is a set of circumstances that is easily recognized as being highly predictive of a heart attack. In each case, the events that the patient experienced before and during the emergency room visit were not independent of whether the patient was experiencing a heart attack. In fact, these events were evaluated precisely because they shed important light on the likelihood of a heart attack.[5] The dependence between the diagnostic findings and the assessment of the likelihood of a heart attack was used to advantage by permitting the findings of the diagnostic testing to change the emergency room doctor's assessment of the likelihood that the patient was having an MI.

Thus, when planned carefully, the relationships between dependent events can help the observer to draw appropriate conclusions about events of interest not yet observed. We will evaluate the utility of this concept of dependence to help us in planning and carrying out multiple analyses in clinical trials.

5.2.2 Endpoint Coincidence and Correlation

The preceding review of the general concepts of independence and dependence has placed us in the position to discuss these properties within the context of statistical hypothesis testing. Just as the emergency room physician in the preceding section took advantage of the dependent relationship between his diagnostic tests and the likelihood that a patient was experiencing an MI, we will now take advantage of the relationship between statistical hypothesis tests of primary endpoints (i.e., primary analyses) in clinical trials to compute a priori α levels.

Let's first set up a very simple paradigm as an instructive aid. Let's assume that an investigator is in the design phase of his clinical trial, and he has settled on two and only two primary endpoints, P_1 and P_2. The statistical hypothesis test for P_1 that will test the effect of the randomly allocated intervention on P_1 is H_1. H_1 is assigned an *a priori* type I error level α_1. Analogously, the statistical hypothesis test for the effect of the intervention on the endpoint P_2 is H_2, and the type I error level for hypothesis test H_2 is α_2. We developed this paradigm in Chapter 4.

What does "independent hypothesis testing" mean in this circumstance? Specifically, independence means that execution of hypothesis test H_1 neither educates us about nor predicts for us the result of H_2. It would be useful to examine the nature of the relationship between H_1 and H_2 in terms of the type I error rate, since ultimately this is the error whose level we seek to control. In the end, we hope to learn the likelihood that we will commit a type I error in drawing conclusions from both H_1 and H_2 since this is the information that we need to control the familywise error level ξ.

If this is the investigator's goal, then, specifically, independence tells us that knowledge about the commission of a type I error for hypothesis test H_1 reveals

---

[5] On the other hand, part of the diagnostic workup of a patient with a possible MI does not include interrogating the patient about their rate of fingernail growth. Rapid fingernail growth provides no useful information about the occurrence of a heart attack, and we say that rapid fingernail growth and the occurrence of an MI are independent events.

nothing about the occurrence of a type I error for hypothesis test H_2—it does not inform us one way or the other about the commission of a type I error for the second hypothesis test. Before any hypothesis test proceeds, the best estimate of the likelihood of a type I error for H_2 is α_2. If H_1 and H_2 are truly independent, then after the evaluation of the hypothesis test for the primary endpoint P_1, our best estimate for the type I error level for the execution of H_2 remains α_2.

How would the result be different? Consider the following demonstration. Allow P_1 and P_2 to be the primary endpoints from a clinical trial evaluating the effect of a therapy in patients with coronary artery disease. Let P_1 be the cumulative incidence of total mortality and P_2 be the cumulative incidence of death due to a CAD death.[6] In this hypothetical clinical trial, the entry criteria for the study are such that only patients with advanced coronary artery disease are recruited for the study. Thus, in this circumstance, the overwhelming majority of deaths that occur in the study will be from CAD death. Let's say that 99% of the deaths in the trial are from fatal MI.

Our intuition tells us that the effect of therapy for each of these endpoints is going to be very similar. If the therapy produces an important reduction in the cumulative total mortality rate in the research sample, by necessity it must reduce the CAD death rate. Assume that the study demonstrates a 15% reduction in each of these two primary endpoints. If a type I error occurred for the total mortality event rate hypothesis, then the population that experiences no beneficial effect of the therapy on the cumulative incidence rate of total mortality produced a sample that demonstrated a 15% reduction in the total mortality rate. But if the therapy does not produce a reduction in total mortality in this population of patients in whom a death by and large means a CAD death, then the therapy will not produce a beneficial effect on the CAD death rate in this population either. In addition, if the research sample demonstrated a 15% reduction in total mortality, by necessity it must produce a similar effect for CAD death since, essentially, a death in this sample means a CAD death.

Thus, the joint occurrence of these two endpoints in the same patients implies that a type I error for the effect of therapy on the cumulative total mortality incidence rate H_1 all but guarantees a type I error for the hypothesis test for CAD death. The α error level for the CAD death endpoint has already been included in the α error level for the total mortality endpoint; it need not be counted again. By counting it twice, either through direct computation, $\xi = 1 - (1 - \alpha_1)(1 - \alpha_2)$, or by using upper bound of the Bonferroni approximation, $\xi \leq \alpha_1 + \alpha_2$, we overestimate the familywise type I error rate.

If we want to avoid double counting the type I error levels, then we should be able to adjust the value of α_2 given that we know both α_1 and the degree of dependence between a type I error for H_1 and a type I error for H_2. If we know the level of dependence between H_1 and H_2, this will be an easy calculation for us to complete.

Continuing, if we are to incorporate this notion of dependency between statistical hypothesis tests into clinical trial analyses, we need to determine pre-

---

[6] These deaths would be primarily fatal MI and sudden death.

cisely what features of the hypothetical trial described above led to the overestimation of the familywise error level. One characteristic of the trial that induced dependency was that the two primary endpoints (total mortality and CAD death) frequently occurred in the same patients. Recall that these endpoints are dichotomous endpoints (i.e., they either occur or not do not occur). We will call dichotomous endpoints that occur in the same patient *coincident endpoints*. In the previous illustration, the sample of patients was chosen such that patients who died during the clinical trial died of coronary artery disease, making death and CAD death coincident. Continuous endpoints (e.g., blood pressure) that occur in the predictable patterns in patients are called correlated endpoints. Since mixing dichotomous and continuous endpoints can be very problematic in their interpretation ([1], [2]), we will avoid this situation in our first treatment of dependent endpoints.

An example of a clinical trial with primary correlated endpoints is a study that is conducted to compare two blood pressure reducing therapies in patients for whom both the diastolic blood pressures (DBP) and the systolic blood pressures (SBP) are elevated. In this setting, allow P_1 to be the difference between the change in DBP over the follow-up period of the study between the two therapy groups. This analysis will address hypothesis H_1 with type I error rate α_1. Endpoint P_2 will be the analagous examination of SBP for hypothesis test H_2 and type I error rate α_2. In this circumstance, it is difficult to envision that the therapy would act differently on DBP than on SBP. Here, we might again expect a type I error for hypothesis H_1 to suggest that a type I error would also occur for hypothesis test H_2. This example suggests that a reasonable measure of the overlap in the α error events for the statistical hypotheses H_1 and H_2 would be measured by the correlation between DBP and SBP.

These first examinations seem to suggest that we simply need associated endpoints to be either coincident or correlated in order to conserve type I error levels for their hypothesis tests. Implementing correlation in this fashion as a tool in this endeavor has been suggested in the literature [3]. However, the use of the correlation between two endpoints as the only tool to gauge the degree of dependency between the two hypothesis tests presumes that the randomly allocated therapy will have the same effect on each endpoint. There are vexsome counter-examples to this idea.

One illustration of nonuniform treatment effects for separate but related endpoints is the joint consideration of exercise tolerance and total mortality in patients with CHF. It is very reasonable and plausible to assume that patients with CHF have a reduced ability to adequately perfuse skeletal muscle. As the disease progresses, the patient's ability to perfuse continues to fail, to the point where the patient becomes less and less active, is reduced to a bed rest existence, and finally dies. Clearly, the pathophysiology of CHF links the inability to exercise to the possibility of a death from CHF. Populations of patients characterized by diminished exercise tolerance would be expected to have a greater proportion of deaths due to CHF. We might then expect that if exercise tolerance and total mortality were two primary endpoints in a clinical trial, then these endpoints would be related. However, the effect of therapy on these two endpoints has been seen to be disparate within the same research sample. Holding aside the difficulty in generalizing the results of the US Carvedilol program,[7] its research sample demonstrated that although therapy reduced total mortality in the research sample of patients, it paradoxically and consistently failed to produce a benefit in the exercise tolerance endpoint.

In this circumstance of suspected paradoxical therapy effects, if one were designing a trial with exercise and total mortality as the prospectively defined primary endpoints of the study, then one could not use the correlation between the endpoints as the measure of type I error overlap between H_1, the hypothesis test for exercise tolerance and H_2, the hypothesis test for total mortality. This is because a population in which the intervention has no effect on exercise tolerance may demonstrate an effect of the intervention on the total mortality rate. Thus the occurrence of a type I error for the effect of the intervention on exercise tolerance may not be predictive of a type I error occurring for the effect of therapy on total mortality, despite the association between the two endpoints. Therefore, if endpoint correlation or coincidence is to be the measure of endpoint dependence, then that measure must be sharply discounted when the randomized intervention has a history of paradoxical effects (Figure 5.1).

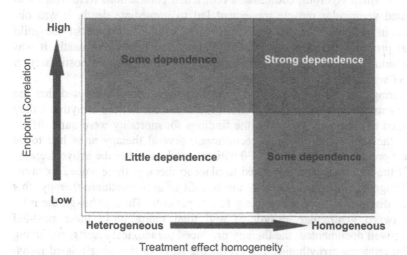

Figure 5.1. The strongest hypothesis testing dependence is when the endpoints are correlated and the treatment effect is the same for each of the endpoints.

The paradoxical effect of therapy on correlated endpoints has been seen in diseases other than CHF. In the late 1960s, the University Group Diabetes Program (UGDP) [4] evaluated the effects of phenformin, then a new medication to improve

---

[7] The US Carvedilol program was presented in Chapter 2.

the blood sugar control of type II diabetes. Elevated blood sugar levels had been linked to increased cumulative mortality rates in patients with type II diabetes. In the UGDP study, the randomized therapy did produce the expected reduction in blood glucose. However, the effect of the therapy was paradoxical because phenformin use was associated with an increase in the total mortality rate. The medication simultaneously produced a beneficial effect for blood glucose reduction, but a harmful effect on total mortality. The issue remains controversial to this day. Designing a study with the primary analysis of (1) the effect of the intervention on blood glucose reduction and (2) the effect of the therapy on the cumulative total mortality rate is reasonable. However, using the association between blood glucose level and cumulative total mortality rate as the sole gauge of statistical hypothesis testing dependency is not.

One final, shocking example of the difficulty posed by relying on endpoint correlation as the measure of dependency, is the paradoxical effect of therapy in the Cardiac Arrhythmia Suppression Trial (CAST) [5]. In the middle of the twentieth-century, cardiologists began to understand that there was a gradient among heart arrhythmias. Some of these dysrhythmias, such as premature atrial contractions and premature ventricular contractions, were in and of themselves benign. Others, such as ventricular tachycardia and ventricular fibrillation, were dangerous. Ventricular fibrillation, in which vigorous, coordinated ventricular contractions were reduced to uncoordinated ventricular muscle movement led to immediate death. It was observed that, in patients who had suffered an MI, the occurrence of the mild arrhythmias preceded the more severe arrhythmias and subsequent death. It was therefore assumed that treating the mild arrhythmias would prevent postinfarction death. CAST was designed to test this hypothesis.

During the course of the study, the investigators demonstrated that the randomized antiarrhythmic therapies reduced the occurrence of the arrhythmia they were designed to eliminate. However, the findings for mortality were quite different. Before the trial could complete recruitment, several therapy arms had to be discontinued prematurely. Out of the 730 patients randomized to the active therapy, 56 died. Of the 725 patients randomized to placebo therapy, there were 22 deaths. In a trial designed to demonstrate only the benefit of antiarrhythmic therapy, this therapy was discovered to be more likely to kill patients. Thus, although the relationship between ventricular arrhythmia and total mortality in these post-MI patients was well documented, the therapy produced paradoxical results, producing "benefit" by reducing arrhythmias, but producing harm in the other related measure—mortality.

5.2.3 Surrogate Endpoint Definition

At the heart of this difficulty is the concept of the surrogate endpoint. A surrogate endpoint is an intermediate endpoint that is itself associated with more important clinical events. For example, weight reduction in the morbidly obese is a surrogate endpoint for total mortality. It might naturally be assumed that the correlation between the surrogate endpoint and the outcome measure can automatically be used as the sole criteria for building statistical hypothesis test dependency into the analysis for the primary endpoints. The difficulty with this use of endpoint association is that it by no means guaranteed that the therapeutic effect of a randomized therapy on a surrogate endpoint will directly translate into a therapeutic effect on the final clinical endpoint of severe morbidity or mortality. UDGP and CAST are examples of clinical trial programs where the beneficial effect of therapy on the surrogate endpoint was translated into a harmful effect for the endpoint of total mortality.

Taking advantage of dependency between these endpoints is a procedure which holds promise for the conservation of type I error rates in these increasingly complicated clinical trial designs and analyses. However, hypothesis testing dependency will be more than a function of the correlation between the endpoints. We must have evidence that the therapy will work by the same or related mechanism for each of the endpoints. If this remains an issue in the design phase of the trial, then our ability to use dependence must be adjusted, and perhaps deemphasized. Understanding this principle will permit us to discount without ignoring the association between primary endpoints as we build in a more realistic measure of dependency between the associated statistical hypothesis tests.

5.3 Literature Review

Of the tremendous volume of literature written on the multiple analyses issue in clinical trials, much of it focuses on the need to take into account dependency among study endpoints. This has been a subfield of the multiple analyses issue and has evolved considerably. We will briefly survey that field here. Let us first return to our accustomed paradigm, in which there are K prospectively defined primary endpoints, with test-specific α error levels α_1, α_2, α_3, ..., α_K. Under the assumption of independence, then we know that if ξ is the familywise error level then

$$\xi = 1 - \prod_{k=1}^{K}(1-\alpha_k). \tag{5.1}$$

If we assume that $\alpha_k = \alpha$ for $k = 1 \ldots K$ then (5.1) reduces to $\xi = 1 - (1-\alpha)^K$. We can solve this equation easily for α,

$$\alpha = 1 - (1-\xi)^{\frac{1}{K}}, \tag{5.2}$$

an expression we have important experience with from Chapters 3 and 4.

5.3.1 Tukey's Procedure and Related Ad Hoc Computations

An adjustment that became popular for taking dependency between hypothesis tests into account was that recommended by Tukey [6]. He suggested that an adjustment for dependence between hypothesis tests may be simply computed by calculating the test-specific type I error probability as α, where

$$\alpha = 1 - (1 - \xi)^{\frac{1}{\sqrt{K}}}. \tag{5.3}$$

This computation produces larger values of the type I error rate than that produced from the Bonferroni procedure (Table 5.1).

Table 5.1. Comparison of test-specfic α levels.

K	Independence assumption	Dependence Tukey adjustment
1	0.050	0.050
2	0.025	0.036
3	0.017	0.029
4	0.013	0.025
5	0.010	0.023
6	0.009	0.021
7	0.007	0.019
8	0.006	0.018
9	0.006	0.017
10	0.005	0.016

There is a greater alpha error rate available under the Tukey computation for dependence ($\xi = 0.05$).

This is our first exposure to a direct computation of test-specific α error levels under the assumption of dependent hypothesis testing, and it permits a direct comparison of the test-specific α error levels between the independence and dependence assumptions. Note that the test-specific α under the assumption of dependence is larger than that under the independence assumption for all $K > 1$. As an illustration, for five primary endpoints ($K = 5$) the independence assumption leads to a test-specific α level of 0.010, while the Tukey dependence computation, by taking a measure of dependency into account, produces $\alpha = 0.023$. There is more than twice the test-specific α error level available under the independence assumption. This difference in test-specific α levels widens to more than a threefold increase for $K = 10$. The increase in test-specific α error level under the dependence assumption satisfies our intuition developed in previous sections, where we said that dependence between the hypothesis tests should allow us to increase the test-specific α error level, since the familywise error level will be much less than the sum of the test-specific α error levels.

Having satisfied our intuition about the test-specific α error levels under the dependent hypothesis-testing scenario, we can't help but notice some limitations of (5.3). One limitation is that the test-specific α is computed under the assumption that the test-specific α level is the same for each of the K primary hypothesis tests. This is a step backward from our work in Chapter 4, in which we justified the use of unequal allocations of the type I error rate among the K prospectively identified hypothesis tests. In addition, it is difficult to see the degree of dependency between the endpoints from an examination of formula (5.3). Consider two hypothetical clinical trials, each examining the effect of a randomly allocated intervention. Each of these two trials has three prospectively chosen primary endpoints, but no primary endpoint is common to the two trials. For the first trial, the simultaneous circumstances of high endpoint correlation among the three primary endpoints and a history of treatment homogeneity[8] suggest that the level of dependency between the endpoints is high (Figure 5.2). The second trial has three prospectively determined primary endpoints, but the endpoints are not as highly correlated as in the first trial, and, in addition, there is a more heterogeneous effect of the therapy across the endpoints. Based on the discussion in the previous section, the measure of dependence across the three hypothesis tests should be smaller in the second trial than in the first trial. However, (5.3) does not permit different levels of dependency, so it is unclear which trial should use this equation to compute the test-specific α for its individual primary endpoint hypothesis tests. It is hard to know the level of dependency embedded in Tukey's equation, and therefore it is a challenge to know when to use it.

The work of Dubey [7] and of O'Brien [8] have provided other related procedures for computing the test-specific α levels when the statistical hypothesis tests are correlated. If there are K hypothesis tests to be evaluated, each for a separate endpoint, then the calculation they suggest for the test-specific α level, α, is

$$\alpha = 1 - (1 - \xi)^{\frac{1}{m_k}} \tag{5.4}$$

and

$$m_k = K^{1-r_k} \text{ and } r_k = \frac{\sum_{j \neq k}^{K} r_{jk}}{K-1} \tag{5.5}$$

where r_k is the average of the correlation coefficients reflecting the association between the K endpoints to be evaluated. An advantage of this method over Tukey's is that the actual correlations are built into the computation.[9] However, in simulation analyses, Sankoh [9] points out that the Tukey procedure still works best when there are large numbers of highly correlated endpoints. Sankoh also noted that the procedure suggested by Dubey and O'Brien required additional adjustment at all correlation levels despite its specific inclusion of endpoint correlation. Finally, we note in passing that there is no consideration of therapy heterogenity, the topic of the previous section.

There is other relevant literature on this issue. Hochberg and Westfall discuss an important subset of multiplicity problems in biostatistics in general [10]. James uses multinomial probabilities when dealing with the issue of multiple end-

---

[8] Treatment homogeneity is the observation that the effect of the randomly allocated intervention will be the same across the endpoints.

[9] Treatment homogeneity, however, is not considered in these calculations. This concept will be addressed later in this chapter.

points in clinical trials [11]. Neuhauser discusses an interesting application of multiple clinical endpoint evaluation in a trial studying patients with asthma [12]. Reitmeir and Wasmer discuss one-sided hypothesis testing and multiple endpoints [13], and Westfall, Ho, and Prillaman engage in a deeper discussion of multiple union-intersection tools in the evaluation of multiple endpoints in clinical trials [14]. Closed testing is discussed by Zhang [15]. Weighted α-partitioning methods are available for the Sime's test as well [16]. These procedures, while appropriate and useful, are not the focus of this text. We will turn instead to the development of a procedure that can (1) be easily implemented by nonstatisticans, and (2) provide the physician–investigator with good control of the level of inter-statistical hypothesis dependence as well as prospective control of the familywise error level for dependent hypothesis testing in clinical trials.

5.4 Hypothesis Test Dependency: Notation

In this section we will develop some notational devices that will be useful in the development of a constructive incorporation of dependency among several statistical hypothesis tests in a clinical trial. Let's return to our by now familiar paradigm of a clinical trial in which there are K primary hypothesis tests H_1, H_2, H_3, ... H_K. Let H_j denote the jth hypothesis test. For each of these K hypothesis tests we have the prospectively specified type I error levels α_1, α_2, α_3, ... α_K. Now, let's define T_j, for $j = 1, 2, 3, ..., K$ as a variable that captures whether a type I error has occurred for the jth hypothesis test. We will let each of the T_j's take on only one of two possible values, 0 or 1. For example, consider the first hypothesis test. Let $T_1 = 0$ if no type I error occurred for this first hypothesis test, and we will assign T_1 the value 1 if a type I error has occurred. We will proceed in this fashion for each of the remaining $K - 1$ prospectively identified hypothesis tests. Thus, we have K pairs, (H_1, T_1), (H_2, T_2), (H_3, T_3), ..., (H_K, T_K), where H_j identifies the statistical hypothesis test and T_j denotes whether a type I error has occurred for that test. From this development, we already know the probability that T_j will be one; this is simply the probability of a type I error on the jth hypothesis test, or α_j, i.e., $P[T_j = 1] = \alpha_j$.

We can now expand this concept to the familywise error level. Using our usual notation of ξ as the familywise error level, let T_ξ denote whether a familywise type I error level will occur, an event that we recall means that there is at least one type I error among the K prospectively defined primary analyses. That event will be denoted by $T_\xi = 0$. Continuing then, we may write that $P[T_\xi = 0]$ is the probability that there were no type I errors among the K hypothesis tests, and analogously, that $P[T_\xi = 1]$ is the probability that there was at least one type I error among these K endpoints. Thus $\xi = P[T_\xi = 1]$.

We only need to add one notational device. Let the symbol $\cap$ connect events that can occur together. Then the event $A \cap B$ simply means "the joint occurrence of event A and event B."

We can now proceed. We know that no familywise error occurs if there is not a single type I error among each of the K prospectively defined primary endpoints, or

$$P(T_\xi = 0) = P(\{T_1 = 0\} \cap \{T_2 = 0\} \cap \{T_3 = 0\} \cap .... \cap \{T_K = 0\}). \qquad (5.6)$$

We may therefore easily write

$$P(T_\xi = 1) = 1 - P(\{T_1 = 0\} \cap \{T_2 = 0\} \cap \{T_3 = 0\} \cap ... \cap \{T_K = 0\})$$

$$= 1 - P\left(\bigcap_{j=1}^{K} T_j = 0\right). \qquad (5.7)$$

This is the fundamental equation that produced the results in Section 3.3. The last line of (5.7) now becomes the focus of our attention. When the individual hypotheses are independent of one another, then the expression

$$P\left(\bigcap_{j=1}^{K} T_j = 0\right)$$

is simply the product of the probabilities or

$$P\left(\bigcap_{j=1}^{K} T_j = 0\right) = \prod_{j=1}^{K} P(T_j = 0) = \prod_{j=1}^{K} (1 - \alpha_j). \qquad (5.8)$$

However, if the K prospectively specified hypothesis tests are dependent, then the evaluation of the expression $P\left(\bigcap_{j=1}^{K} T_j = 0\right)$ will become much more complicated to evaluate. We will proceed with our evaluation of this in stages. The first evaluation will be the simplest paradigm of all to assess, i.e., independence. We will develop and sharpen our intuition as we move from the familiar situation of independence between statistical hypothesis tests to the more complex settings in which the hypothesis tests are dependent.

5.5 The Independence Scenario

We will begin with the simplest scenario. Consider a clinical trial that is designed to have two and only two primary analyses. Using the notion developed thus far in this chapter, we can denote these hypothesis tests as H_1 and H_2 and, furthermore, identify the corresponding variables that reflect whether a type I error has occurred as T_1 and T_2, where as before $P[T_1 = 1] = \alpha_1$, and $P[T_2 = 1] = \alpha_2$. We can without any loss of generality order these two tests prospectively such that the α associated with the first hypothesis test is greater than or equal to that of the second hypothesis test, or $\alpha_1 \geq \alpha_2$ (we will see that this ordering will make no difference in our conclusions, nor will it require us to carry out the hypothesis tests in any particular order). In this situation, there are four possible events involving the occurrence of a type I error, namely,

$$\{T_1 = 0 \cap T_2 = 0\},$$
$$\{T_1 = 0 \cap T_2 = 1\},$$
$$\{T_1 = 1 \cap T_2 = 0\},$$
$$\{T_1 = 1 \cap T_2 = 1\}.$$

Assuming the hypothesis tests are independent of each other, we can calculate the probabilities of each of these events (Table 5.2).

Table 5.2. Probability table for joint type I error rates: Independence assumption.

	$T_1 = 0$	$T_1 = 1$	Total
$T_2 = 0$	$(1 - \alpha_2)(1 - \alpha_1)$	$\alpha_1(1 - \alpha_2)$	$1 - \alpha_2$
$T_2 = 1$	$\alpha_2(1 - \alpha_1)$	$\alpha_1 \alpha_2$	α_2
Total	$1 - \alpha_1$	α_1	1

To compute the probability of each of these joint events involving T_1 and T_2 under the independence assumption, we merely multiply the probabilities of the event involving T_1 and T_2. For example, to compute the probability that $T_1 = 1$ and $T_2 = 0$ we compute

$$P[T_1 = 1 \cap T_2 = 0] = P[T_1 = 1]P[T_2 = 0] = \alpha_1(1 - \alpha_2). \tag{5.9}$$

In order to calculate ξ where $\xi = P[T_\xi = 1]$, we only need to consider the joint event of $P[T_1 = 0 \cap T_2 = 0] = (1 - \alpha_1)(1 - \alpha_2)$ and find

$$\xi = P\left[T_\xi = 1\right]$$
$$= 1 - P\left[T_\xi = 0\right] \tag{5.10}$$
$$= 1 - (1 - \alpha_1)(1 - \alpha_2).$$

This expected result relates the familywise error probability ξ to the test-specific error rates α_1 and α_2 in the familiar setting of independence that we discussed in Chapter 4.

We can use this scenario of independence to compute some probabilities that will be very helpful as we consider the scenario of statistical hypothesis test dependence. We begin by asking what is the probability that there is no type I error committed on hypothesis test H_2 given that there is no type I error for hypothesis test H_1? This is the measure of dependence that gets to the heart of the matter, since, if there is dependence, we would specifically want to know how to update our estimate of the probability of type I error for the second hypothesis test given the result of the first hypothesis test. Recall that the conditional probability of no type I error on H_2 given that there has been no type I error for hypothesis test H_1 can be written as $P\ [T_2 = 0|T_1 = 0]$ and is defined (using the basic definition of conditional probability) as

$$P[T_2 = 0\,|\,T_1 = 0] = \frac{P[T_1 = 0 \cap T_2 = 0]}{P[T_1 = 0]}. \tag{5.11}$$

Thus, the conditional probability can be computed if we know the joint probability $P[T_1 = 0 \cap T_2 = 0]$ and the test-specific α error level for the first primary hypothesis test. Note however that we can also rewrite (5.11) as

$$P[T_1 = 0 \cap T_2 = 0] = P[T_2 = 0\,|\,T_1 = 0]P[T_1 = 0] \tag{5.12}$$

essentially formulating the joint probability of the event $\{T_1 = 0\}$ and $\{T_2 = 0\}$ as a function of the conditional probability. This will be a very useful equation for us as we develop the notion of dependency in hypothesis testing, since the key to computing the probability of a familywise error $P\ [T_\xi = 0]$ is the computation of the joint probability $P\ [T_1 = 0 \cap T_2 = 0]$. This calculation is easy in the independence scenario. Our intuition tells us that, in the case of independence, knowledge of whether a type I error has occurred on the first hypothesis test should tell us nothing about the occurrence of a type I error on the second hypothesis test H_2.

These computations confirm this intuition. Without knowing anything about the occurrence of a type I error for H_1, we know that the probability of no type I error on hypothesis test H_2 is simply $1 - \alpha_2$. To compute this probability using knowledge of H_1 we see

$$P[T_2 = 0\,|\,T_1 = 0] = \frac{P[T_1 = 0 \cap T_2 = 0]}{P[T_1 = 0]} = \frac{(1-\alpha_1)(1-\alpha_2)}{(1-\alpha_1)} = 1 - \alpha_2 \tag{5.13}$$

and the "update" has, as anticipated, provided no useful information.

We will see that the presence of dependence complicates the identification of the joint probability $P\ [T_1 = 0 \cap T_2 = 0]$. Fortunately, (5.12) tells us that we can rewrite the joint probability $P\ [T_1 = 0 \cap T_2 = 0]$ as a function of the conditional probability $P\ [\ T_2 = 0|T_1 = 0]$. It will be easier for us to supply this conditional probability under the circumstances of dependence than it will be to supply the joint probability. Equation (5.12) tells us how to convert this conditional probability into the necessary joint probability, and thereby permits the computation of $P\ [T_1 = 0 \cap T_2 = 0]$, and then the calculation of $P\ [T_\xi = 1]$, the familywise error level.

5.6 Demonstration of Perfect Dependence

The situation that we examined in Section 5.5 was the state of independence between two prospectively specified statistical hypothesis tests within a clinical trial. From that examination, we developed the principle of assessing the conditional probability of a type I error on the second hypothesis test given that a type I error occurs on the first hypothesis test, or $P\ [T_2 = 0|T_1 = 0]$. We will now examine the opposite extreme—that of perfect dependence—using the conditional probability as our principle evaluation tool.

We have already discussed the meaning of hypothesis testing dependence in Section 5.2. Perfect dependence denotes that state between two statistical hypothesis tests in which the occurrence of a type I error for H_1 automatically produces a type I error for statistical hypothesis test H_2. In this situation, the two tests are so intertwined that knowledge that a type I error occurred for the first hypothesis test guarantees that a type I error will occur for the second hypothesis test. This is the opposite extreme of the independence setting.

An example of perfect dependence would be the illustration provided in Section 5.2.2 pushed to the extreme. In that original scenario, we had a hypothetical clinical trial in which there were two prospectively identified primary analyses. The first analysis tested the effect of the randomly allocated therapy on the total mortality rate, and the second evaluated the effect of this therapy on the cumulative incidence rate of CAD death. The population from which this research sample was obtained was one in which the overwhelming majority of patients in the trial died a CAD death. If we push this example to its extreme, then every single patient in the study who dies must have that death caused by CAD. Thus, patients who died in this study would be counted in both of these two primary analyses. We will also assume that the therapy will affect the event rates of each of these in the same manner. This combination of perfect endpoint coincidence and therapeutic homogeneity represents perfect dependence.

We will now evaluate the implications of this trial design on the familywise error level ξ, beginning with the conditional probability $P\ [T_2 = 0|T_1 = 0]$. When we assumed that the two tests were independent in the previous section, we saw that the conditional probability $P\ [T_2 = 0|T_1 = 0] = P\ [T_2 = 0] = 1 - \alpha_2$. In this new setting, what would the probability of a type I error for H_2 be, given we know that no type I error occurred for first hypothesis test H_1? Perfect dependence dictates that this conditional probability should be one, or

$$P[T_2 = 0 \mid T_1 = 0] = 1.\qquad(5.14)$$

In order to see how the value of this conditional probability helps us to compute the familywise error level ξ, recall the last comments in Section 5.5. There, we said that, given knowledge of the conditional probability $P\ [T_2 = 0|T_1 = 0]$, we could compute the joint probability $P\ [T_1 = 0 \cap T_2 = 0]$. This is precisely the quantity we need to calculate the familywise error level $\xi = 1 - P\ [T_1 = 0 \cap T_2 = 0]$. We begin this process by computing

$$P[T_1 = 0 \cap T_2 = 0] = P[T_2 = 0 \mid T_1 = 0]P[T_1 = 0]$$
$$= (1)(1 - \alpha_1) = 1 - \alpha_1.\qquad(5.15)$$

Just as we computed the joint probabilities for the events $\{T_1 = 0\}$ and $\{T_2 = 0\}$ for the independence scenario of Section 5.5, we may compute an analogous table for the perfect dependence scenario (Table 5.3). Since we know what the sum of each row and column must be, it is easy to complete this table from knowledge of P $[T_1 = 0 \cap T_2 = 0]$.

Table 5.3. Probability table for joint type I error rates: Dependence assumption.

	$T_1 = 0$	$T_1 = 1$	Total
$T_2 = 0$	$1 - \alpha_1$	$\alpha_1 - \alpha_2$	$1 - \alpha_2$
$T_2 = 1$	0	α_2	α_2
Total	$1 - \alpha_1$	α_1	1

Recalling that $\xi = 1 - P[T_1 = 0 \cap T_2 = 0]$ and using the result of (5.15), we easily compute that

$$\xi = 1 - P[T_1 = 0 \cap T_2 = 0] = 1 - (1 - \alpha_1) = \alpha_1. \tag{5.16}$$

Note that the familywise error level for this problem ξ is the same as the prospectively set a type I error rate for H_1, namely α_1. We have demonstrated that in the state of perfect dependence between two statistical hypothesis tests, setting α_1 and then choosing $\alpha_2 = \alpha_1$ leads to a value of $\xi \neq 1 - (1 - \alpha_1)(1 - \alpha_2)$, but simply $\xi = \alpha_1$. This also satisfies our intuition. Thus, in this setting of complete dependence, one can maintain ξ at its desired level by simply choosing $\alpha_2 \leq \alpha_1 = \xi$. Since the occurrence of a type I error on the first statistical hypothesis test implies that a type I error has occurred on the second hypothesis test, the joint occurrence is reflected by the one occurrence.

5.7 Scenario Contrasts

We had two purposes in mind when we examined the impact of different degrees of dependence between statistical hypothesis tests on prospectively allocated α error levels. The first purpose was to develop additional notation that would be useful as we quantitate the degree of dependence. Our evaluation allowed us to settle on the conditional probability, $P[T_2 = 0|T_1 = 0]$ as the quantity that contains within it the measure of dependence between the two hypothesis tests.

Our second purpose was to explore the extremes of the dependence property and its effects on the relationship between the familywise error level, ξ, and the test-specific α rates α_1 and α_2. Since dependent hypothesis testing can be a useful design feature, we need to know how dramatic the savings (at least in theory) in the type I error levels of the hypothesis tests can become. In this evaluation, we demonstrated that, in the setting of perfect dependence between two hypothesis tests H_1 and H_2 (with test-specific α rates α_1 and α_2 such that $\alpha_1 \geq \alpha_2$), the probability of at least one type I error is substantially less than in the case of independence. In the case of independence, ζ is as large as $1 - (1 - \alpha_1)(1 - \alpha_2)$. In the setting of perfect dependence it is as small as α_1. We can therefore bound or trap ξ between these extremes, writing

$$\alpha_1 \leq \xi \leq 1 - (1 - \alpha_1)(1 - \alpha_2). \tag{5.17}$$

A specific example would be useful to crystallize the difference in the α error levels under these two assumptions. Consider the case of a clinical trial in which there are two prospectively defined primary hypothesis tests H_1 and H_2 with associated test-specific α error levels α_1 and α_2. Choose $\alpha_1 = \alpha_2 = 0.05$. In the familiar case of independence, we have demonstrated that $\xi = 1 - (0.95)(0.95) = 0.0975$. However, under the assumption of perfect dependence $\xi = 0.05$.

This difference in the value of ξ has important implications for the design of the clinical trial. As we saw in Chapter 3, in order to control the familywise error level, ξ, at a level less than 0.05, then each of α_1 and α_2 must have a value less than 0.05. For example, using the Bonferroni approximation, each test-specific α error probability could be set at 0.025. However, in the case of perfect dependence, limiting ξ to a value ≤ 0.05 requires only that $\alpha_1 \leq 0.05$ and that $\alpha_2 \leq \alpha_1$. In fact, we can set $\alpha_1 = \alpha_2 = 0.05$ and keep $\xi = 0.05$. Since there is complete overlap in the occurrence of type I error for H_1 and H_2, we do not use additional type I error for the second hypothesis test. In a sense, the second hypothesis test "comes for free," a result that seems intuitive if we recall that in this example of extreme dependence, type I error for hypothesis test 1 ensures that a type I error will occur for hypothesis test 2.

We are not suggesting here that the circumstance of perfect dependence is a goal toward which investigators should work as they design clinical trials. Clearly, in the scenario where there is complete overlap in the occurrence of type I errors between two hypothesis tests H_1 and H_2, H_2 would not be executed at all since it provides no useful new information about the effect of therapy. In that study, the execution of the statistical hypothesis test on total mortality provides all of the useful information about the effect of therapy on the two primary endpoints. In reality, there would be only one primary endpoint, total mortality. However, spending time evaluating the properties of the perfect dependence scenario reveals the maximum savings in α_2 that dependent statistical testing can produce. We will discuss the potential implications of "hyperdependence" for labeling indications at the regulatory level later in this chapter.

5.8 Creation of the Dependency Parameter

The previous section developed the range of the familywise error level as the level of dependence between the statistical hypothesis tests increased. Our goal in this section is to construct a quantitative measure D that will measure the degree of dependence between the statistical hypothesis tests. If we can construct D

appropriately, then knowledge of D would allow us to compute ξ from the values of the test-specific α levels α_1 and α_2, or, alternatively, compute α_2 from knowledge of ξ and α_1.

Recall from the previous section that in the circumstance of the design of a clinical trial in which there are two prospectively determined primary analyses H_1 and H_2 with test-specific α error levels α_1 and α_2, respectively, we were able to determine the full range of values of ξ, i.e., $\alpha_1 \leq \xi \leq 1 - (1 - \alpha_1)(1 - \alpha_2)$. However, this is not the only quantity that can be so bounded. We can also compute a range of values within which the conditional probability, $P\,[T_2 = |T_1 = 0]$ should fall. We saw that the value of this conditional probability was $1 - \alpha_2$ in the independence scenario; in the scenario of perfect dependence, $P\,[T_2 = 0|T_1 = 0] = 1$. Since these two extremes reflect the full range of dependence, we can write

$$1 - \alpha_1 \leq P\big[T_2 = 0\,|\,T_1 = 0\big] \leq 1. \tag{5.18}$$

If, for example we assume that α_1 has the value of 0.05, then inequality (5.18) reveals[10] that $0.95 \leq P\,[T_2 = 0|T_1 = 0] \leq 1$. If the strength of the dependence between the two statistical hypothesis tests lies between the extremes of independence and full dependence, then the conditional probability $P\,[T_2 = 0|T_1 = 0]$ will assume a value that falls within this interval denoted by $[1 - \alpha_1, 1]$. We will now develop a measure, termed D, that will reflect this level of dependence. We would like D to have *a minimum* of zero and a maximum of one. The instance when D is zero should correspond to the condition of independence between the statistical hypothesis tests, and identify the situation in which $P\,[T_2 = 0|T_1 = 0] = 1 - \alpha_2$. Analogously, $D = 1$ will denote perfect dependence, i.e., the case in which the conditional probability of interest $P\,[T_2 = 0|T_1 = 0]$ attains its maximum value of one. We can then extend the inequality reflected in (5.18) as follows:

$$\begin{aligned} 1 - \alpha_1 &\leq P\big[T_2 = 0\,|\,T_1 = 0\big] \leq 1, \\ 0 &\leq \quad\quad D^2 \quad\quad \leq 1. \end{aligned} \tag{5.19}$$

If we are to choose a value of D that will have the aforementioned properties, then we can write D in terms of the conditional probability

$$D = \sqrt{1 - \frac{\big(1 - P[T_2 = 0\,|\,T_1 = 0]\big)}{\alpha_2}}. \tag{5.20}$$

To see if (5.20) meets our criteria, assume first that the statistical hypothesis tests for the two prospectively defined primary analyses H_1 and H_2 are independent. In

---

[10] Note that this range for the conditional probability is not very broad. The upper bound on this probability can of course be no greater than one. Because we insist on a small type I error probability (0.05), the lower bound is also quite high, at 0.95.

this case $P[T_2 = 0 | T_1 = 0] = 1 - \alpha_2$ and D becomes 0. When H_1 and H_2 are perfectly dependent, then (5.20) produces $D = 1$.

In general, we will not use (5.20) to compute D. Our ultimate goal is to supply the value of D, and then write the familywise error level in terms of D. To do that, we will first need to write the conditional probability that a type I error does not occur on the second statistical hypothesis test H_2 given that there is no type I error on the first hypothesis test H_1 as a function of D. This task follows easily from (5.20):

$$
\begin{aligned}
P[T_2 = 0 \,|\, T_1 = 0] &= (1 - \alpha_2) + D^2 [1 - (1 - \alpha_2)] \\
&= 1 - \alpha_2 (1 - D^2).
\end{aligned}
\tag{5.21}
$$

We may now proceed by expressing $P[T_2 = 0 \cap T_1 = 0]$ in terms of this dependence parameter D.

$$
\begin{aligned}
P[T_2 = 0 \cap T_1 = 0] &= P[T_2 = 0 \,|\, T_1 = 0] P[T_1 = 0] \\
&= \left[1 - \alpha_2 (1 - D^2) \right](1 - \alpha_1).
\end{aligned}
\tag{5.22}
$$

Thus, the familywise error level for the two statistical hypothesis tests H_1 and H_2 may be written as

$$
\begin{aligned}
\xi &= 1 - P[T_2 = 0 \cap T_1 = 0] \\
&= 1 - \left[1 - \alpha_2 (1 - D^2) \right](1 - \alpha_1).
\end{aligned}
\tag{5.23}
$$

Therefore, the familywise error is formulated in terms involving the test-specific α error rates α_1, α_2 and the dependency parameter D where $\alpha_1 \geq \alpha_2$.

Equation (5.23) may be rewritten to reflect more clearly the relationship between the familywise error level ξ and the dependency parameter D. Write (5.23) as

$$
\begin{aligned}
\xi &= 1 - \left[1 - \alpha_2 (1 - D^2) \right](1 - \alpha_1) \\
&= 1 - \left[(1 - \alpha_1) - (1 - \alpha_1) \alpha_2 (1 - D^2) \right] \\
&= 1 - 1 + \alpha_1 + (\alpha_2 - \alpha_1 \alpha_2)(1 - D^2) \\
&= \alpha_1 + \alpha_2 - \alpha_1 \alpha_2 - D^2 (1 - \alpha_1) \alpha_2.
\end{aligned}
\tag{5.24}
$$

Thus,

$$
\xi = \alpha_1 + \alpha_2 - \alpha_1 \alpha_2 - D^2 (1 - \alpha_1) \alpha_2.
\tag{5.25}
$$

Now recall, that under the assumption of independence between the statistical hypothesis tests H_1 and H_2, $\xi = 1 - (1 - \alpha_1)(1 - \alpha_2)$. If we denote the familywise error under the independence assumption as ξ_I, then we can write

$$\xi_I = 1-(1-\alpha_1)(1-\alpha_2)$$
$$= 1-(1-\alpha_1-\alpha_2+\alpha_1\alpha_2) \qquad (5.26)$$
$$= \alpha_1+\alpha_2-\alpha_1\alpha_2,$$

we note that the last line in expression (5.26) is contained in (5.25). If we now denote the familywise error under the assumption of dependence as ξ_D, we may now substitute the last line of expression (5.26) into (5.25) to compute

$$\xi_D = \xi_I - D^2(1-\alpha_1)\alpha_2. \qquad (5.27)$$

Constructing D as we have, we see that the familywise error level decreases as D increases. When D is equal to 0, H_1 and H_2 are independent and $\xi_D = \xi_I$. When D is one and the state of perfect dependence between the statistical hypothesis tests H_1 and H_2 exists, then $\xi_D = \alpha_1$. The relationship between ξ, the familywise error level and D can be easily illustrated (Figure 5.2).

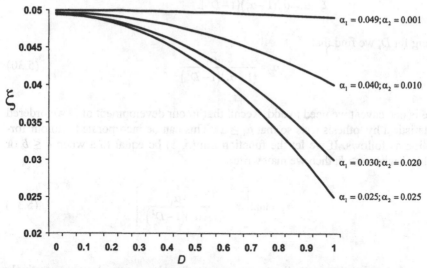

Figure 5.2. For any combination of α1 and α2, increasing hypothesis test dependence D reduces the family wise error rate ξ.

Figure 5.2 demonstrates that, as the dependency parameter D increases, the familywise error level ξ decreases, which is the result our intuition led us to expect. The reduction in ξ demonstrated in this figure is a function of the test-specific type I error levels α_1 and α_2. This is because the familywise error level expended must be at least α_1, the amount allocated for H_1. The smaller the value of α_1, the greater the difference between ξ and α_1, and the greater the potential decrease in ξ that can be achieved by increasing the dependency parameter D. A discussion of how to select D is provided in Section 5.12.

5.9 Solving for α_2 as a Function of D

The previous section provided a computation for ξ, the familywise error level as a function of α_1 and α_2 in a clinical trial with two prospectively chosen primary endpoints. The procedure that was followed there was to (1) choose α_1 and α_2 such that $\alpha_1 \geq \alpha_2$, (2) select D, and then (3) compute

$$\xi = \alpha_1 + \alpha_2 - \alpha_1\alpha_2 - D^2(1-\alpha_1)\alpha_2. \tag{5.28}$$

However, during the design phase of the trial, as the investigators work to select the appropriate levels of the test-specific α error levels for the study, they will first fix ξ, and then choose α_1 and D, moving on to compute the acceptable range of α_2. This is easily accomplished. We need only solve (5.28) for α_2.

$$\begin{aligned}
\xi &= \alpha_1 + \alpha_2 - \alpha_1\alpha_2 - D^2(1-\alpha_1)\alpha_2, \\
\xi - \alpha_1 &= \alpha_2 - \alpha_1\alpha_2 - D^2(1-\alpha_1)\alpha_2, \\
\xi - \alpha_1 &= \alpha_2(1-\alpha_1) - D^2(1-\alpha_1)\alpha_2, \\
\xi - \alpha_1 &= \alpha_2(1-\alpha_1)(1-D^2).
\end{aligned} \tag{5.29}$$

Solving for D, we find that

$$\alpha_2 = \frac{\xi - \alpha_1}{(1-\alpha_1)(1-D^2)}. \tag{5.30}$$

There is one caveat we need to add. Recall that in our development of D we ordered the statistical hypothesis tests so that $\alpha_1 \geq \alpha_2$. This can be incorporated into our formulation as follows. If we let the function $\min(a, b)$ be equal to a when $a \leq b$ or equal to b when $a > b$, then we may write

$$\alpha_2 = \min\left[\alpha_1, \frac{\xi - \alpha_1}{(1-\alpha_1)(1-D^2)}\right]. \tag{5.31}$$

This is an equation that we will return to repeatedly when we wish to prospectively incorporate dependent hypothesis testing into clinical trial analysis plans.

It would be useful to check this computation when $D = 0$. We know from Chapter 3 that, in this setting of independence between statistical hypothesis tests H_1 and H_2, we can directly compute

$$\xi = 1 - (1-\alpha_1)(1-\alpha_2). \tag{5.32}$$

Therefore, we can find α_2 in terms of ξ and α_1 as

$$\xi = 1 - (1 - \alpha_1)(1 - \alpha_2),$$

$$(1 - \alpha_1)(1 - \alpha_2) = 1 - \xi,$$ (5.33)

$$(1 - \alpha_2) = \frac{1 - \xi}{(1 - \alpha_1)},$$

and thus,

$$\alpha_2 = 1 - \frac{1 - \xi}{1 - \alpha_1} = \frac{\xi - \alpha_1}{1 - \alpha_1}.$$ (5.34)

This is the computation that results from the direct computation of α_2 in the setting of independence. What is the result from (5.31) when D is zero? This is easily seen by rewriting (5.31) as follows:

$$\alpha_2 = 1 - \frac{1 - \xi}{1 - \alpha_1}$$

$$= \frac{1 - \alpha_1}{1 - \alpha_1} - \frac{1 - \xi}{1 - \alpha_1} = \frac{1 - \alpha_1 - 1 + \xi}{1 - \alpha_1}$$ (5.35)

$$= \frac{\xi - \alpha_1}{1 - \alpha_1}.$$

(5.34) is produced from (5.31) by setting $D = 0$. Thus, the result from (5.31) reproduces the α error level for H_2 in the setting of independence.[11]

5.10 Example 1: Implantable Cardiac Devices

The purpose of this chapter's preceding efforts was to develop a parameter D that reflected the degree of dependence between two prospectively specified statistical hypotheses, H_1 and H_2. The measure D would then be used to compute the test-specific α levels α_2 from α_1 and ξ, allowing for conservation of the familywise error level. We will now show how this procedure can be implemented in the design of a clinical trial with the following illustration.

A group of investigators are interested in designing a clinical trial to detect the effect of an implantable ventricular defibrillating device in patients who have CHF. The clinical hypothesis is that this electromechanical device will detect whether the heart has shifted its rhythm to a destabilizing (and perhaps fatal) ventricular tachycardia or ventricular fibrillation. When this shift has been detected, the device will automatically provide an electric shock to the heart, converting the destabilizing rhythm to a more stable (hopefully sinus) rhythm.

---

[11] We can match the result for perfect dependence as well. When $D = 1$, the denominator of $\alpha_2 = \xi - \alpha_1 \Big/ (1 - \alpha_1)(1 - D^2)$ becomes zero, implying that α_2 is infinite. However, the minimum function in equation (5.31) chooses $\alpha_2 = \alpha_1$, the result we demonstrated in Section 5.6.

The clinical trial will have two groups of patients, all of whom will receive standard medical care for their chronic CHF. There are 1000 patients available for this study. In addition, these patients will be randomly selected to have either the defibrillator device implanted or to receive standard antiarrhythmic therapy for their arrhythmias. Since both the physician and the patient will know whether the patient has received a defibrillator, this clinical trial cannot be blinded. For this reason, along with the investigators' desire to build the most convincing case possible for the benefit of this defibrillation therapy, they choose two persuasive primary endpoints: (1) total mortality incidence rate and (2) total hospitalization incidence rate. Each of these endpoints can be determined unambiguously and should not have their ascertainment influenced by the knowledge of the treatment group to which the patient was assigned. With this information, the sample size computation begins (Table 5.4). As was our practice in Chapter 4, the first computations do not attempt to adjust for the familywise error level.

Table 5.4. Alpha allocation, Example 1: First Design Scenario.

Primary analyses	Cumulative control group event rate	Efficacy	Alpha (two-tailed)	Power	Sample size
Total mortality	0.20	0.35	0.05	0.90	1171
Total hospitalizations	0.35	0.45	0.05	0.90	324

The expected high efficacy keeps the sample sizes for the two primary endpoints low.

Patients in this clinical trial will be followed for 15 months. The lower control group event rate for total mortality, in addition to the somewhat lower efficacy, produces a minimum sample size for the analysis of the effect of the intervention on the total mortality rate that is greater than that of the total hospitalization primary endpoint.[12] The investigators then divide the α error level between the two endpoints, so that the familywise error level is conserved at 0.05.

The decision as to how to divide the type I error was a difficult one. More type I error was allocated to the total mortality endpoint because it was the most persuasive of the two endpoints. Therefore, everything else being equal, the medical community was more willing to accept the smaller effect size associated with the larger p-value as a positive finding.

---

[12] Appendix D provides a brief primer on sample size computations.

Table 5.5. Alpha allocation, Example 1: Second Design Scenario.

Primary analyses	Cumulative control group event rate	Efficacy	Alpha (two-tailed)	Power	Sample size
Total mortality	0.20	0.35	0.035	0.90	1281
Total hospitalizations	0.35	0.45	0.015	0.90	426

Differential alpha allocation, has increased the sample sizes.

Now the investigators are ready to come to grips with the issue of dependence between the two statistical hypothesis tests. In this population of subjects with CHF, most patients who will be hospitalized during the course of the clinical trial will be hospitalized for CHF. In addition, most patients who die will have heart failure as the cause of death. Furthermore, those who die from heart failure will have been hospitalized for heart failure in all likelihood. While this does not mean that all patients who are hospitalized for heart failure will die of CHF, it does imply some coincidence between these two primary endpoints. This association, in turn suggests that the measure of dependence between the two statistical tests for the effect of the intervention on these primary endpoints will be great.

However, this point of view must be moderated by concern for the homogeneity of the treatment effect. As discussed in Section 5.4, one of the criteria for strong dependence between two statistical hypothesis tests must be that the intervention has the same effect on each of them. In the case of the implanted defibrillator, this homogeneity of effect remains an open question. Patients who have had the device implanted often have to return to the hospital to have the device recalibrated. In the commonly used intent to treat analysis,[13] these hospitalizations would be accumulated and counted as primary endpoints in the treatment group. While there is no suggested increase in the risk of death due to this calibration procedure, there is an attenuating effect on the intervention–hospitalization relationship. Specifically, the reduction in hospitalizations produced by the beneficial effect of the implanted defibrillator on heart rhythms would be overshadowed by the short-term increase in hospitalizations due to the calibration. This suggests that we need to attenuate our estimate of dependence. D was chosen as 0.40.[14] The test-specific α error level was recomputed using (5.31) (Table 5.6).

$$\alpha_2 = \min\left[\alpha_1, \frac{\xi - \alpha_1}{(1-\alpha_1)(1-D^2)}\right]$$

---

[13] This was covered in Chapter 1.

[14] A discussion of how to choose the value of D is covered in Section 5.12.

Table 5.6 follows the format of Tables 5.4 and 5.5 with the exception of one change. That alteration is the addition of the line that provides the measure of dependence. The primary analyses are listed so that the dependence measure is reflected in the test-specific type I error level below it. Thus, in Table 5.5, $\alpha_1 = 0.035$, $D = 0.40$, and α_2 is 0.019, reflecting a 27% increase over the initial estimate of α_2 of 0.015. Of course, larger choices for D would lead to larger increase in α. For example, selecting $D = 0.70$ produces $\alpha_2 = 0.30$. However, the recognition of potential therapy effect heterogeneity requires moderation of the selection for D.

Table 5.6. Alpha allocation, Example 1: Third Design Scenario.

Primary analyses	Cumulative control group event rate	Efficacy	Alpha (two-tailed)	Power	Sample size
Total mortality	0.20	0.35	0.035	0.90	1281
			$D = 0.40$		
Total hospitalizations	0.35	0.45	0.019	0.90	408

The prospectively set alpha level for total hospitalizations has increased from 0.015 to 0.019.

Reducing the power to 80% for the total mortality endpoint results in the final sample size computation for the study (Table 5.7).

Table 5.7. Alpha allocation, Example 1: Fourth Design Scenario.

Primary analyses	Cumulative control group event rate	Efficacy	Alpha (two-tailed)	Power	Sample size
Total mortality	0.20	0.35	0.035	0.80	970
			$D = 0.40$		
Total hospitalizations	0.35	0.45	0.019	0.90	408

The sample size for each analysis is less than 1000.

One important feature in our derivation is that we chose the "first" hypothesis test as the one for which the prospectively selected type I error level is the greatest. It is important to note that this ordering of the hypothesis tests such that $\alpha_1 \geq \alpha_2$ does not imply that the hypothesis tests themselves must be executed in any order. Once the α level probabilities have been selected, the order in which the hypothesis tests for these two primary endpoints are executed does not affect the conclusions of the study.

Finally, it would be informative to examine the relationship between α_2, α_1, and D for a familywise error level of 0.05. This evaluation will mirror the use of the measure of dependency between statistical hypothesis tests derived in this chapter. The investigator first chooses the level of α_1, and D. From this, the investigator then computes the test-specific probability for the second hypothesis test, α_2.

For each level of α_1 there is a value of D beyond which there can be no additional savings in the type I error level α_2 for statistical hypothesis H_2 This is the perfect dependence threshold. As α_1 decreases, this threshold decreases as well, finally reaching 0.60 for $\alpha_1 = 0.030$.

Table 5.8. Dependency relationships: α_2 as a function of D and α_1*

	α_1				
D	0.049	0.045	0.040	0.035	0.030
0.00	0.0011	0.0052	0.0104	0.0155	0.0206
0.05	0.0011	0.0052	0.0104	0.0156	0.0207
0.10	0.0011	0.0053	0.0105	0.0157	0.0208
0.15	0.0011	0.0054	0.0107	0.0159	0.0211
0.20	0.0011	0.0055	0.0109	0.0162	0.0215
0.25	0.0011	0.0056	0.0111	0.0166	0.0220
0.30	0.0012	0.0058	0.0114	0.0171	0.0227
0.35	0.0012	0.0060	0.0119	0.0177	0.0235
0.40	0.0013	0.0062	0.0124	0.0185	0.0245
0.45	0.0013	0.0066	0.0131	0.0195	0.0259
0.50	0.0014	0.0070	0.0139	0.0207	0.0275
0.55	0.0015	0.0075	0.0149	0.0223	0.0296
0.60	0.0016	0.0082	0.0163	0.0243	0.0300
0.65	0.0018	0.0091	0.0180	0.0269	0.0300
0.70	0.0021	0.0103	0.0204	0.0305	0.0300
0.75	0.0024	0.0120	0.0238	0.0350	0.0300
0.80	0.0029	0.0145	0.0289	0.0350	0.0300
0.85	0.0038	0.0189	0.0375	0.0350	0.0300
0.90	0.0055	0.0276	0.0400	0.0350	0.0300
0.95	0.0108	0.0450	0.0400	0.0350	0.0300
0.99	0.0490	0.0450	0.0400	0.0350	0.0300

* Familywise error is 0.05.

5.11 Example 2: The CURE Trial

The illustration in the previous section presented how the incorporation of dependency between two prospectively declared statistical endpoints in a clinical trial could be embedded into its design. A second example of this type of effort is that of the CURE trial [17]. CURE (Clopidogrel in Unstable Angina to Prevent Recurrent Events) examined the role of thienopyridine derivatives in preventing death and cardiovascular events in patients with unstable angina pectoris or acute coronary syndrome. Before this study, there was no evidence available that supported the notion that this type of anticoagulation therapy would produce a long-term benefit for patients who were in immediate danger of having a heart attack. To test the benefit of these thienopyridine derivatives, a clinical trial was designed to examine the effect of the oral anticoagulation agent clopidogrel when compared to standard care for patients at risk of acute coronary syndrome.

CURE was a randomized, double-blind, placebo-controlled trial with two arms. Patients who had been hospitalized with acute coronary syndromes within 24 hours of their symptoms but who did not demonstrate evidence of ST segment elevation on their electrocardiograms were recruited. All of these patients received the standard care for this condition including the administration of aspirin. In addition, patients randomized to the active arm of the study received clopidogrel, while patients in the control group arm received placebo therapy.

The investigators prospectively designed this study for the analysis of two primary endpoints. The first primary endpoint was a combination of death from cardiovascular causes, nonfatal MI or stroke.[15] Thus, a patient reaches this first primary endpoint if they (1) die from a cardiovascular cause, or (2) die from a noncardiovascular death but have a nonfatal MI or a stroke, or (3) survive but have an MI or a stroke. The second primary endpoint consisted of the first primary endpoint or refractory ischemia.[16] Thus, a patient meets the criteria for this second prospectively defined primary endpoint if (1) they meet the criteria for the first, or (2) they do not meet the criteria for the first primary endpoint, but they have refractory ischemia. Secondary outcomes included severe ischemia, heart failure, and the need for revascularization.

The idea of dependency between the two primary endpoints is an admissible one. However, the level of dependence requires some discussion. Certainly, if there are very few patients with recurrent ischemia, then the second primary endpoint is the same as the first one and we would expect strong dependence. However if there are many patients who have recurrent ischemia, knowledge of a type I error for the first primary endpoint will provide less information about the probability of a type I error for the second primary endpoint, and the measure of dependency is reduced.[17]

The CURE investigators provided the information to reproduce the sample size computations (Table 5.9). While the investigators do not tell us the degree of dependency between these two primary endpoint analyses, they do state that "parti-

---

[15]The analysis and interpretation of combined endpoints is the topic of Chapter 6.

[16] Refractory ischemia was defined as recurrent chest pain lasting more than 5 minutes with new ischemic electrocardiographic changes while the patient was receiving "optimal" medical therapy.

[17] For example, there could be a strong beneficial effect of therapy for the first primary endpoint. However, a large number of patients with recurrent ischemia and the absence of a beneficial effect of this therapy on recurrent ischemia could produce a different finding for this second primary endpoint. The occurrence of a type I error for the first primary endpoint would shed no light on the probability of the type I error for the second primary endpoint in this circumstance.

tioning the α maintains an overall level of 0.05 after adjustment for the overlap between the two sets of outcomes."

The sample size analysis follows (Table 5.9)[18]. However we can use Table 5.7 to see the level of dependency that corresponds to the CURE investigator's correction for dependency between the two hypothesis tests. Table 5.7 demonstrates that $\alpha_1 = 0.45$ and $\alpha_2 = 0.010$ corresponds to a value of D of between 0.65 and 0.70. Thus, the CURE investigators assume a moderate level of dependency between the two primary endpoints for their study design.[19]

Table 5.9. CURE primary analysis design

Primary analyses	Cumulative control group event rate	Efficacy	Alpha (two-tailed)	Power	Sample size
CV death/MI/Stroke	0.10	0.169	0.045	0.90	12568
CV Death/MI/Sroke/Ischemia	0.14	0.164	0.010	0.90	12630

Differential type I error rate allocation and an adjustment for overlap.

An alternative analysis plan has also been provided in the literature [18].

5.12 Example 3: Paroxysmal Atrial Fibrillation

As a final example of an application of the methodology developed in this chapter for building hypothesis test dependency between two statistical tests, consider the design of the following study to help reverse paroxysmal atrial fibrillation (PAF). Recognizing the difficulties presented by standard pharmacologic antiarrhythmic therapy and DC cardioversion (shock therapy) to treat this difficult arrhythmia, a group of investigators has developed a novel intervention. Specifically, these investigators have acquired the ability to deliver a dose of medication through a catheter directly onto the nidus of the aberrant electrical pathway in the heart, stopping the arrhythmia. They would like to design a clinical trial to test this therapeutic innovation.

In this study, patients with PAF will be randomized to either the control or the active treatment group. The control group will receive standard therapy for their fibrillation. The treatment group will receive standard therapy and, at the time of randomization, have a catheter threaded into their heart and have medication delivered. These active group patients will receive the medication only once. The

---

[18] The size of CURE was increased from 9000 to 12,500 patients because of a lower than expected placebo event rate.

[19] The results of CURE were positive. There was a 20% reduction in the cumulative incidence rate of the primary endpoint with a p-value of < 0.001. Clopidogrel reduced the cumulative incidence of the second primary endpoint by 14% with a p-value of < 0.001.

investigators would be able to recruit between five and six hundred patients, and all patients will be followed for 1 year.

The investigators struggled with the selection of a primary endpoint. The cumulative total mortality rate for these patients was too small to be able to detect with any degree of reliability, and the investigators were not sure at all sure that the catheter-delivered intervention would even save lives. However, they did believe that the medication would reduce atrial fibrillation (AF). After these discussions, the investigators settled on two endpoints. The first endpoint was the recurrence of AF. In addition, they decided to include a second primary endpoint that would be described as "AF load." This second primary endpoint would measure the burden that AF places on the patients. This endpoint would include (1) total number of hospitalizations the patient experienced, (2) total number of days spent in the hospital, and (3) total number of shocks. By reducing the incidence of PAF, the investigators believed the active therapy would reduce these three measures of morbidity that patients with PAF experience. After these decisions, initial sample size estimates for each of the two primary analyses were obtained (Table 5.10).

Table 5.10. Atrial fibrillation study: First design scenario.

Primary analyses	Cumulative control group event rate	Efficacy	Alpha (two-tailed)	Power	Sample size
PAF* Recurrence	0.60	0.350	0.050	0.90	228
AF Burden	0.45	0.300	0.050	0.90	534

*PAF is paroxysmal atril fibrillation; AF is atrial fibrillation.

The high PAF rate in combination with the efficacy of 35% has helped to keep the sample size for the PAF recurrence rate small. However, even without controlling the familywise error level (which assuming independence is $1 - (0.95)^2 = 0.098$), the required sample size for the AF burden endpoint exceeds 500.

The investigators next control the familywise α rate by distributing the type I error level asymmetrically between the two endpoints and, by doing so, initially make the sample size situation worse for the AF burden endpoint (Table 5.11).

Table 5.11. Atrial fibrillation study: Second design scenario.

Primary analyses	Cumulative control group event rate	Efficacy	Alpha (two-tailed)	Power	Sample size
PAF* Recurrence	0.60	0.350	0.040	0.90	241
AF Burden	0.45	0.300	0.010	0.90	756

*PAF is paroxysmal atril fibrillation; AF is atrial fibrillation.

The sample size has increased for each of the two primary endpoints, but the increase is most remarkable for the AF burden analysis, driving the sample size to well above the maximum of 600. There are of course alternative allocations of the α error level. For example, one could reverse the type I error allocation, placing most of the α error level on the hypothesis test that examines the effect of the intervention on the PAF burden (Table 5.12) In this table, the reversal of the α error level allocation from Table 5.11 solves the sample size problem of this clinical trial at once. By providing a higher α error level for the AF burden primary endpoint analysis, the sample size required for this evaluation is 540 while, at the same time, the required number of patients for the PAF recurrence primary endpoint remains below 500. These results meet the goal of keeping the sample size for the trial between 500–600 patients.

Table 5.12. Atrial fibrillation study: Third design scenario.

Primary analyses	Cumulative control group event rate	Efficacy	Alpha (two-tailed)	Power	Sample size
PAF* Recurrence	0.60	0.350	0.002	0.90	414
AF Burden	0.45	0.300	0.048	0.90	540

*PAF is paroxysmal atril fibrillation; AF is atrial fibrillation.

However, this solution should be rejected because it flies in the face of the principle that type I error level allocation is a community protection procedure. First, consider the role of the AF burden analysis. AF burden is certainly a prospectively chosen primary endpoint for this clinical trial, but it is a relatively weak one. Its three multiple components could be differentially influenced by therapy (the first component was total number of hospitalizations, the second was the total number of days hospitalized, and the third was the total number of shocks)[20]. It is reasonable to expect that the medical community will require greater evidence of benefit (as measured by a larger effect size and a smaller p-value) for this new endpoint—an endpoint with which the community has limited experience in interpreting. They need to be sure that if the study is positive for this endpoint, this positive benefit is not just the product of sampling error. The medical community will require an α level well below 0.05 to provide an additional margin of comfort that the research findings are not just due to the random play of chance. This comfort margin is not provided in Table 5.12.

The more persuasive of the two primary analyses for this clinical trial to the medical community is the PAF recurrence. Its presence in a patient will be measured accurately, and the pathophysiology of PAF recurrence is directly linked to the effect of the medication. The medical community would be satisfied that the therapy effectively reduced the PAF recurrence rate at an α level of 0.05 and should not be required to discard the therapy because the hypothesis test did not meet the superrigorous threshold of 0.002. Just as for the AF burden analysis, the α error level for the PAF endpoint was not chosen with community protection in mind. The 0.002 level was chosen because it was the residual; only 0.002 was remaining after 0.048 had been devoted to "shoehorning" the AF burden analysis into the 500-600 sample size restraint.

Returning them to Table 5.12, the investigators determine a moderate level of dependence between the two primary endpoints to conserve α error level (Table 5.13).

Table 5.13. Atrial fibrillation study: Fourth design scenario.

Primary analyses	Cumulative control group event rate	Efficacy	Alpha (two-tailed)	Power	Sample size
PAF* Recurrence	0.60	0.35	0.040	0.90	241
		$D =$ 0.70			
AF Burden	0.45	0.30	0.020	0.90	659

*PAF is paroxysmal atril fibrillation; AF is atrial fibrillation.

Finally, adjustments in the power are made, keeping the power for each of the two prospectively declared analyses above the 80% minimum. We must be clear about the observation that Table 5.14 does not provide the only solution for this particular clinical trial with two primary endpoints. Other type I error allocation arguments are equally admissible. The central point here is that investigators can develop the necessary experience to allocate α levels prospectively and differentially, even in the presence of dependency between statistical hypothesis tests.

---

[20] For example, there may be many patients in this study who are hospitalized but not hospitalized for PAF. The therapy having no influence on the occurrence of these hospitalizations will be viewed as less effective in reducing total hospitalizations.

Table 5.14. Atrial fibrillation study: Fifth design scenario.

Primary analyses	Cumulative control group event rate	Efficacy	Alpha (two-tailed)	Power	Sample size
PAF* Recurrence	0.60	0.35	0.040	0.95	296
		$D = 0.70$			
AF Burden	0.45	0.30	0.020	0.80	508

*PAF is paroxysmal atril fibrillation; AF is atrial fibrillation.

5.13 Choosing the Dependency Parameter

One of the foundations of this chapter is the use of the dependency parameter D in making prospective determinations about the type I error allocation levels in clinical trials. Beginning in Section 5.8, the computations for α error levels have been predicated on the investigators knowing the parameter of D. For example, in the circumstance where there are two prospectively specified primary analyses in a clinical trial, once D has been identified, we can compute either the familywise error level ξ once we have chosen α_1 and α_2, or we can compute α_2 given ξ and α_1. However, how do we select D?

5.13.1 Overestimation of Dependency Parameter

Certainly, the choice of D is critical and its overestimation of D will not conserve the familywise error level. For example, consider the circumstance of a clinical trial with two prospectively determined primary analyses. The investigators in this study choose a familywise error level of 0.05, and then decide that the test-specific type I error α_1 is 0.04 for the first primary analysis. If the investigators assume that the dependency parameter for the two statistical hypothesis tests is 0.70, then (5.31) produces

$$\alpha_2 = \min\left[\alpha_1, \frac{\xi - \alpha_1}{(1 - \alpha_1)(1 - D^2)} \right]$$ (5.31)

This is all of the information that the investigators need in order to compute the test-specific type I error level, α_2 given the familywise error level ξ, the test-specific error level α_1 and the dependency parameter D. This calculation follows:

$$\alpha_2 = \min\left[0.04, \frac{0.05 - 0.04}{(1 - 0.04)(1 - 0.70^2)}\right]$$

$$= \min\left[0.04, \frac{0.01}{(0.96)(0.51)}\right] \tag{5.36}$$

$$= \min[0.04, 0.020] = 0.020.$$

However, if in reality D was not 0.70 but instead was 0.20 then we would find that the test-specific α error level for the second primary analysis was

$$\alpha_2 = \min\left[0.04, \frac{0.05 - 0.04}{(1 - 0.04)(1 - 0.20^2)}\right]$$

$$= \min\left[0.04, \frac{0.01}{(0.96)(0.96)}\right] \tag{5.37}$$

$$= \min[0.04, 0.011] = 0.011.$$

Thus, the α specific error level depends on D. Another way to state this is that the familywise error level is not well conserved when the value of D is overestimated. For example, we know that we can compute ξ given that we have the values of α_1, α_2, and D from (5.23) as $\xi = 1 - \left[1 - \alpha_2(1 - D^2)\right][1 - \alpha_1]$. Now if the investigators decide to let $\alpha_1 = 0.04$ and, assuming $D = 0.70$, computed $\alpha_2 = 0.02$, when in fact D was not 0.70 but was instead 0.02, then the true familywise error level ξ would be not 0.05 but instead

$$\xi = 1 - \left[1 - \alpha_2(1 - D^2)\right][1 - \alpha_1]$$

$$= 1 - \left[1 - 0.02(1 - 0.20^2)\right][1 - 0.04]$$

$$= 1 - \left[1 - 0.02(0.96)\right][1 - 0.04] \tag{5.38}$$

$$= 1 - [0.9808][0.96] = 0.058,$$

and we see that the familywise error level has not been conserved at 0.05. Therefore, any use of the dependency parameter requires vigilance against its overestimation, a topic that we now will address.

5.13.2 Guides to Choosing the Dependency Parameter

The development in the preceding section leads us to the conclusion that the most accurate specification of D is critical. However, this may seem like a daunting task, especially to investigators who have no experience in making any selection of D at all. Fortunately, it does not take long to gain useful intuition into choosing a realistic value for the required dependency parameter.

D, like α and the statistical power must be chosen prospectively, during the design phase of the trial. To select D, one should first understand the relationship between the primary analyses. Specifically, the two important questions whose answers will provide a range of values for D are (1) how closely coincident are the endpoints and (2) how homogeneous is the treatment effect for each of these endpoints?

This first question focuses on how coincident the analyses are. Perfect coincidence occurs when the contribution a patient makes to each of the endpoints is exactly the same. As a starting point, it is worthwhile for the investigators to work through the exercise developed earlier in Section 5.6 when we considered the appearance of perfect dependence. Consider the case of a clinical trial where there are two primary analyses in which each analysis evaluates the effect of therapy on a different, prospectively specified endpoint (e.g., the first primary endpoint is total mortality, and the second primary endpoint is fatal CAD death). If the inclusion and exclusion criteria for this trial were so restrictive that the two primary endpoints measured occurred in the same patients, then there would be perfect dependence and $D = 1$. How different are the inclusion and exclusion criteria in the actual trial from their counterparts in this hypothetical one? How much non-CAD mortality will there be? The smaller the degree of coincidence, the smaller the level of dependence between the hypothesis tests for the two primary endpoints. In this case, the investigators might start by approximating the coincidence as the proportion of all deaths in the trial that are CAD deaths.

The conclusion of this discussion should initiate a new conversation about the homogeneity of the therapy effect for the two endpoints. Is there evidence that the effect of the therapy will be different for the different primary analyses? Returning to the illustration of the previous example, there will almost certainly be heterogeneity of effect. Medications designed to reduce CAD death rate by and large will have little effect on deaths due to cancer, automobile accidents, emphysema, or other causes of non-CAD death. Thus, a useful starting approximation for the value of D would be to further reduce it in the presence of therapy heterogeneity. A useful formulation of this relationship is

$$D = c\left[1-(1-c)(1-h)\right], \tag{5.39}$$

where c is the coincidence level and h measures therapy homogeneity. In this circumstance, $h = 1$ denotes perfect therapy homogeneity, i.e., the therapy has the same effect in each of the analyses. Expression (5.39) was developed to demonstrate the different effect of the homogeneity of therapy and coincidence of subjects. When there is perfect heterogeneity, $h = 1$, and the dependency parameter is the measure of coincidence. However, when the therapy has a heterogeneous effect, the lack of homogeneity reduces the dependency parameter. In the example of the previous paragraph, if the proportion of deaths believed to be CAD death is equal to 0.75, and there is no effect of therapy in the patients who die a non-CAD death, then $c = 0.75$, $h = 0$ and

$$D = 0.75\left[1-(1-0.75)(1-0)\right] = (0.75)^2 = 0.56. \tag{5.40}$$

Thus, (5.39) demonstrates a relationship in which the degree of dependence is discounted by the absence of complete heterogeneity of therapy. This formulation permits a straightforward evaluation of the relationship between the dependency parameter D, and each of the determining factors coincidence (c) and homogeneity of therapy effect (h) (Figure 5.4).

There are some additional comments that we can make in the interest of being conservative in estimating D. Clearly overestimating D is to be avoided. The greatest impact on overestimating the dependency parameter D on the familywise error rate ξ is the assumption of strong dependence between the statistical tests for the primary analyses. Assume, for illustrative purposes, that in a clinical trial there are two prospectively planned primary analyses and $\alpha_1 = 0.04$. If the investigators assume a dependence level of $D = 0.90$ when D in reality is 0.50, then ξ will not be 0.05 but, instead, $\xi = 0.069$, representing a moderate level of α error level inflation. However, if in this same scenario the investigators assumed that $D = 0.50$ when D was in reality 0.10, then $\xi = 0.051$. This represents a much smaller increase in the familywise error level. Thus, if there is any doubt about the range of D, D should not be chosen to be at high levels (i.e., 0.70–1.00) but instead at moderate levels (0.30 - 0.70), since overestimation of D in these middle ranges will produce less ξ inflation above the prespecified level. For the rest of this text, a conservative approach will be taken for the selection of the dependence parameter.

Finally, if investigators, after considerable debate remain divided over how to choose the dependency parameter D, then there is no acceptable alternative to choosing $D = 0$, returning them to the more conservative Bonferroni approximation.

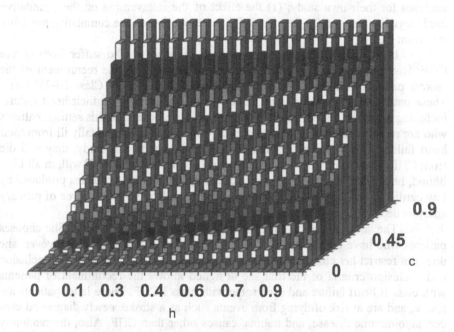

Figure 5.3. Relationship between the dependency parameter, D and the two factors (1) coincidence (c), and (2) homogeneity of therapy effect (h).

5.14 Hyperdependent Analyses

The foregoing discussions concerning the role of dependency between statistical hypothesis testing have perhaps further motivated clinical trial investigators to recognize the value of formally adjusting for analysis dependency during the design phase of their study. However, the implications of endpoint dependency go further than merely being able to observe the relationship between primary analyses already chosen for a research effort. Indeed, much as the discerning epidemiologist can see and take advantage of an "experiment in nature,"[21] the perspicacious investigator envisions that the careful incorporation of inclusion and exclusion criteria can affect the level of primary analysis dependence.

5.14.1 Hyperdependence as a Disadvantage

As an illustration of the use of this tool, consider the task of two investigators (Investigator 1 and Investigator (2) who are each designing their own trial to examine the effect of an intervention for the treatment of CHF. They are each interested in

---

[21] Discussed in Chapter 1, page 10.

determining if the intervention will have an effect on important clinical measures of the consequences of this disease. Each investigator chooses the same primary analyses for their own study: (1) the effect of the intervention on the cumulative total mortality rate and (2) the effect of the intervention on the cumulative mortality rate from CHF.

Investigator 1 chooses a population of patients who suffer from severe CHF. His inclusion and exclusion criteria will permit only the recruitment of the sickest patients with CHF, namely, those who have NYHA Class III–IV CHF. These patients must already be on maximal medical therapy for their heart failure, including diuretics, digitalis, ACE-i therapy, and β-blockers. In this setting, patients who are recruited into the study are already critically if not terminally ill from their heart failure. It is very likely that when a patient dies in this study, they will die from CHF. Even those very few patients who do not die from CHF will, in all likelihood, have their terminal course influenced by the clinical problems produced by low cardiac output. In this trial, one can expect a relatively high degree of primary analysis dependence.

The second investigator chooses a very different population. She chooses patients who have been diagnosed with CHF (as did Investigator I); however, she does not restrict her clinical trial to only the sickest of these patients. The inclusion and exclusion criteria of the trial she designed allows the recruitment of patients with class II heart failure and even some with class I CHF. These latter patients are active, and are at risk of dying from events such as a stroke, newly diagnosed cancer, autoimmune disease, and trauma, causes other than CHF. Also, the randomly assigned intervention in her trial is likely to have a smaller influence on patients who do not have severe CHF, suggesting some therapy heterogeneity. These factors combine to reduce the level of dependence between the primary analyses in this experiment.

In these examples, the degree to which the primary analyses were dependent itself was related to the inclusion/exclusion criteria for the trials. As we have demonstrated in previous sections of this chapter, the greater the primary analysis dependence, the greater the conservation of the familywise error level ξ. This purely mathematical argument would suggest that clinical trials that engender high levels of dependence among their prospectively planned primary analyses (as seen in the trial designed by Investigator (1) are preferred.

However, there is much more to good clinical trial design than α conservation. What has Investigator 1 gained by carrying out two statistical tests on mortality in patients with severe CHF? Because of the selection of the population for his clinical trial, an evaluation of the effect of the intervention on the cumulative incidence of mortality is effectively (in this example, almost precisely) an evaluation of the intervention's effect on mortality due to heart failure. Having carried out the assessment of the intervention-total mortality relationship, nothing new is learned about the effect of therapy on CHF-caused death. The conclusion from one evaluation serves as the conclusion from the other. The extreme dependence, or hyperdependence between the primary analyses of Investigator 1 makes them redundant—one of them is unnecessary. Such hyperdependence reduces the contribution the clinical trial makes to this body of knowledge about the effect of the intervention. After all, the purpose of measuring multiple endpoints is to gain an appreciation of the length and breadth of the disease's response to the randomly assigned intervention, not merely to measure the same disease consequences in different guises in the hopes of gaining dependence in hypothesis testing.

There are potential regulatory implications for the interpretation of a positive trial in the hyperdependence environment. Recall that it is the indication section of the label that describes the benefits of the drug that the FDA and the sponsor reasonably believed would occur in those patients who use the drug as directed.[22] Many times the sponsors of a new intervention express great interest in gaining as many approved indications for its use as possible. This is, in fact, one motivation for implementing a prospectively planned multiple primary analysis mechanism in the design of clinical trials. However, the relevant Code of Federal Regulations (CFR) requires that each indication "shall be supported by substantial evidence of effectiveness." Hyperdependence among primary analyses would undermine any claim that each of the primary analyses provides substantial evidence of effectiveness. It is therefore difficult to envision that the FDA would provide an indication for the positive findings among each of prospectively defined primary, but hyperdependent analyses produced from a clinical trial.

While dependence between prospectively specified primary endpoints can be both produced and wielded to reduce familywise error levels in clinical trials, this tool must be used carefully. Hyperdependence can serve no good purpose and in fact can be counterproductive to expanding the information about the effect of the intervention studied in the clinical trial. Investigators will perhaps serve better if they design the primary analyses of their clinical trials so that these evaluations provide substantial information about the independent effects of therapy. This is provided when the degree of dependence is moderate. When the degree of dependence is too great, the different measures of the intervention are not really so different at all.

5.14.2 Hyperdependence as an Advantage

The previous subsection outlined the disadvantages of the presence of hyperdependence in the evaluation of several prospectively defined primary analyses in a clinical trial. There it was pointed out that, while the evaluation of the effect of a randomly allocated therapy on each of two closely related prospectively defined primary endpoints may produce two statistically significant results, these two evaluations will probably not produce two new indications for the intervention that was tested. This is because the endpoints themselves are so closely related.

However, there are circumstances where the investigators would be willing to sacrifice one of the two possible indications. Such a situation might be when, during the design phase of a clinical trial, there is agreement among the investigators on the identity of the one endpoint that will be used as the primary analysis; however, the same investigators can reach no consensus on the analysis plan for this endpoint. The result of this situation may produce the same confusion that we saw in Chapter 2 when the assessment of the compound Glidel was considered be-

---

[22] The relevant code appears in Appendix C.

fore an FDA advisory committee. Recall from Chapter 2 that the effect of Glidel on the cumulative total mortality rate in patients with glioblastoma was controversial, not because of the choice of the endpoint, but because of confusion surrounding the specific analysis of this primary endpoint. The prospectively chosen analysis was an evaluation that was unadjusted for the effect of country, and was not statistically significant. However, the country-adjusted analysis was significant.

During the design of a clinical trial in which patients undergo randomized stratification within clinical centers,[23] there is often debate and discussion that is focused on which procedure (purely unadjusted analysis versus a center-adjusted analysis) is the most appropriate one to perform at the trial's conclusion. The findings of the clinical trial for Glidel can increase the anxiety level at these preclinical trial meetings in which analysis plans are discussed since, as was plainly demonstrated in the Glidel example, adjusted and unadjusted analyses can produce different and contrary conclusions. The situation can be tense, since the investigators often feel pressured to settle on one and only one analysis plan for the total mortality endpoint.

Consider the following alternative scenario. During the design phase of the study, the investigators choose one and only one endpoint—total mortality. However, the investigators also prospectively declare that they will execute two primary analyses for the effect of the randomly allocated intervention on the cumulative mortality rate of this endpoint. The first analysis is the unadjusted effect of the intervention on the total mortality rate. The second analysis is a center-adjusted evaluation of the effect of therapy on this same endpoint.

Each of these two analysis plans are announced prospectively, and type I error is allocated between them. Clearly, these analysis plans are dependent on each other. The endpoints are perfectly coincident. However, the effect of therapy may be different in the two analyses. If the joint consideration of coincident endpoints and heterogeneity of therapy produced a dependency parameter estimate of $D = 0.70$, one can compute test-specific α levels (Table 5.15).

In this circumstance, a type I error is allocated to each of the unadjusted and adjusted analysis. Since only one indication for the therapy is sought, the investigators would be pleased if either the unadjusted or the adjusted analysis was statistically significant.

---

[23]While simple randomization of the intervention in a clinical trial is most commonly carried out to assure that patients have the same probability of receiving the active versus the control therapy across the entire clinical trial, this procedure may produce imbalances within several clinical centers in a multicenter study. Randomized stratification within clinical center means that the randomization procedure is altered to ensure that patients are equally likely to receive active versus control therapy within each clinical center. This is discussed in Chapter 1.

Table 5.15. Allocating type I error levels
between two analyses one endpoint.

Primary analyses	Alpha (two-tailed)
Unadjusted analysis	0.040
$D = 0.70$	
Adjusted analysis	0.020

The dividend of this redundant testing however does not come without a cost. The price the investigators will pay for this ability to carry out each of these analyses as a primary analysis is the larger sample size required when testing occurs at the $\alpha_1 = 0.04$ level versus $\alpha_2 = 0.05$ level. However, in the scenario provided in Table 5.14, the sample size penalty is small,[24] if one permits the evaluation of the adjusted analysis to be underpowered.

Problems

1. Why can we intellectually and internally grasp the nature of dependence easily and naturally yet the mathematics of dependency rapidly becomes complicated?
2. What is the precise implication of the statement that two prospectively defined endpoints of a clinical trial are dependent?
3. What do we mean by the conservation of the familywise error rate?
4. Explain exactly how dependency between two endpoints in a clinical trial can produce statistical hypothesis tests that are dependent and should improve familywise error rate conservation?
5. How does the Bonferroni procedure overestimate the familywise error rate in the presence of dependent statistical hypothesis tests?
6. What characteristics of statistical analyses in clinical trials produce dependent statistical hypothesis tests?
7. What is the relationship between surrogate endpoints and dependent hypothesis testing?
8. In what circumstance is the joint occurrence of two prospectively defined primary endpoints in a clinical trial not sufficient to conclude that there is substantial dependency between statistical evaluations of the effect of therapy on these endpoints.

---

[24] Consider, for example, a clinical trial designed to detect the effect of an intervention on the cumulative total mortality rate. If the cumulative mortality rate in the control group of this trial is 30% then, in order to detect a 20% reduction in total mortality with 80% power requires 1711 patients for a two sided α error level of 0.05, and 1828 patients for a two-sided 0.04 evaluation.

9. Describe the advantages of using dependent hypothesis testing for the evalua-
    tion of the effect of therapy on multiple primary endpoints in a well-designed,
    well executed clinical trial.
10. What problems arise in the interpretation of clinical trials in which there is a
    great deal of dependency between the primary endpoints? What is the counter-
    argument to the claim that a benefit can be asserted for each of the dependent
    primary endpoints in this study that produced small p-values?
11. Describe one advantage and one disadvantage of Tukey's procedure for inter-
    preting results from dependent statistical hypothesis tests.
12. The computer is off line in a multi-floor treatment unit, and the resident physi-
    cian has forgotten on which floor his patient has been admitted. There are four
    floors. The resident can only guess on which floor his patient is located. A
    wrong guess leads to a futile search of that floor for his patient, after which he
    will have to guess again. (A)Show that the probability that the resident chooses
    the correct floor on his first guess is ¼?   (B) Using conditional probability
    show that the probability that the residence chooses the correct floor after a
    growing sequence of incorrect guess increases?
13. How does the assumption of independence between events simplify the compu-
    tation of probabilities concerning the events joint occurrences, while
    dependence, although perhaps a more realistic assumption, complicate the
    computation.
14. From Table 5.3, can you show why a critical assumption in the derivation of
    the dependency parameter is that $\alpha_1 \geq \alpha_2$? Why is the minimum function re-
    quired in 5.31
15. In the situation where there are two hypothesis tests, what are the implication
    of defining D as

$$D = 1 - \frac{\left(1 - P[T_2 = 0 \mid T_1 = 0]\right)}{\alpha_2}$$

    and not as the square root of this function, as defined in (5.19)?
16. What problems arise in the estimation of the familywise error ξ when the de-
    pendency parameter is overestimated? What are the safeguards that can be
    taken to avoid this overestimation?

References

1. Moyé, L.A., Davis, B.R., Hawkins, C.M. (1992). Analysis of a clinical trial
    involving a combined mortality and adherence dependent interval censored
    endpoint. *Statistisics in Medicine*.11:1705–1717.
2. Federal Food and Drug Administration Advisory Committee Transcript. Car-
    dioRenal Advisory Committeee. Captopril and Enalapril Session. February 18,
    1993.
3. Westfall, P.H., Young, S.S. (1993). *Resampling-Based Multiple Testing: Ex-
    amples and Methods for P-Value Adjustment*. New York John Wiley.

4. The UGDP Investigators. (1971). University group diabetes program: A study of the effect of hypoglycemic agents on vascular complications in patients with adult-onset diabetes. *Journal of the American Medical Association* **218**:1400–1410.
5. The CAST Investigators. (1989). Preliminary Report: Effect of encainide and flecainide on mortalithy in a randomized trial of arrhythmia suppression after MI. *New England Journal of Medicine* **212**:406–412.
6. Tukey, J.W., Ciminera, J.L., Heyse, J.F. (1985). Testing the statistical certainty of a response to increasing doses of a drug. *Biometrics* **41**:295–301.
7. Dubey, S.D. (1985). Adjustment of p–values for multiplicities of intercorrelating symptoms. *Proceedings of the VIth International Society for Clinical Biostatisticians*, Germany.
8. O'Brien, P.C. (1984). Procedures for comparing samples with multiple endpoints. *Biometrics* **40**:1079–1089.
9. Sankoh, A.J., Huque, M.F., Dubey, S.D. (1997). Some comments on frequently used multiple endpoint adjustment methods in clinical trials. *Statistics in Medicine* **16**:2229–42.
10. Hochberg, Y., Westfall, P.H. (2000). On some multiplicity problems and multiple comparison procedures in biostatistics. P.K. Sen and C.R. Rao eds., *Handbook of Statistics*, Vol 18, Elsevier Sciences B.B. pp. 75–113.
11. James, S. (1991) Approximate multinomial probabilities applied to correlated mutliple endpoints in clinical trials. *Statistics in Medicine* 1123–1135.
12. Neuhauser, M., Steinijans, V.W, Bretz, F. (1999). The evaluation of multiple clinical endpoints with application to asthma. *Drug Information Journal* **33**:471–477.
13. Reitmeir, P., Wassmer, G. (1996). One sided multiple endpoints testing in two-sample comparisons. *Communications in Statistics: Simulation and Computation* **25**:99–117.
14. Westfall, P.H., Ho, S.Y., Prillaman, B.A. (2001). Properties of multiple intersection–union tests for multiple endpoints in combination therapy trials. *Journal of Biopharmaceutical Stastistics* **11**:125–138.
15. Westfall, P.H., Wolfinger, R.D. (2000). Closed Multiple Testing Procedures and PROC MULTITEST. SAS Observations, July 2000.
16. Hochberg, Y., Liberman, U. (1994). An extended Simes' test, *Statistics and Probability Letters* **21**: 101–105.
17. The Clopidogrel in Unstable Angina to Prevent Recurrent Events Trial Investigators. (2001). Effects of clopidogrel in addiition to aspirin in patients with acute coronary syndromes without st–segment elevation. *New England Journal of Medicine* **345**: 494–502.
18. Berger, V.W. (2002). Improving the information content of categorical clinical trial data. *Controlled Clinical Trials* **23**:502–514.

Chapter 6

Multiple Dependent Analyses II

This chapter continues the development of multiple dependent analyses in clinical trials. It demonstrates in detail the formulations for the familywise type I error level when there are three dependent primary analyses, it then provides a general solution for the scenario of K dependent primary analyses. Several simplifications are available for the clinical investigator and are described in this chapter, the detailed derivations of which appear in Appendix E. If the reader is willing to accept the argument that the dependency parameter can be generalized to three or more primary endpoints, they may proceed directly to Chapters 7 to13.

6.1 Three Multidependent Analyses

Chapter 5's discussion of prospectively planned multiple dependent analyses focused on the evaluation of two and only two statistical hypothesis tests. However, the reality of modern clinical trial design and execution is more complex. We have demonstrated (indeed, have encouraged) investigators in clinical trials to have more than one primary analysis in their studies. In fact, as we have developed the notion of dependence, it is easy for us now to envision examples of a clinical trial where there are three primary analyses, each of them related to the other. Such an example would be a clinical trial that prospectively declares that there are three primary analyses: total mortality, fatal and nonfatal myocardial infarction, and fatal and nonfatal stroke. Patients drawn from such a population are likely to experience two or sometimes (sadly) all three of these events. If we are to embed dependency between these hypothesis tests for these prospectively chosen endpoints into the analysis plan, we will need the tools to expand the consideration from the $K = 2$ primary endpoint analyses case.

Fortunately, the case for $K = 3$ is a straightforward generalization of the consideration for two endpoints and we can carry forward the same nomenclature that we developed in Section 5.4. In our current situation, there are investigators who have three prospectively declared primary endpoints with corresponding statistical hypothesis tests denoted by H_1, H_2, and H_3. We define the variables T_1, T_2, and T_3 that take on the value of one when a type I error has occurred, and zero when no type I error has occurred. Then, as before, we have $P[T_1 = 1] = \alpha_1$, $P[T_2 = 1] = \alpha_2$, and $P[T_3 = 1] = \alpha_3$. We will also assume that $\alpha_1 \geq \alpha_2 \geq \alpha_3$. We may write the experiment wide type I error as

$$\xi = 1 - P[T_1 = 0 \cap T_2 = 0 \cap T_3 = 0]. \tag{6.1}$$

Recall how we proceeded for the $K = 2$ case. We first wrote

$$\xi = 1 - P\big[\{T_1 = 0\} \cap \{T_2 = 0\}\big], \tag{6.2}$$

then used conditional probability to write

$$P[T_1 = 0 \cap T_2 = 0] = P[T_2 = 0 \mid T_1 = 0]P[T_1 = 0]. \tag{6.3}$$

We then created a measure of dependency D,

$$D = \sqrt{1 - \frac{\big(1 - P[T_2 = 0 \mid T_1 = 0]\big)}{\alpha_2}}, \tag{6.4}$$

allowing us to write

$$
\begin{aligned}
P[T_2 = 0 \mid T_1 = 0] &= (1 - \alpha_2) + D^2\big[1 - (1 - \alpha_2)\big] \\
&= 1 - \alpha_2\big(1 - D^2\big).
\end{aligned}
\tag{6.5}
$$

Then we calculated

$$
\begin{aligned}
\xi &= 1 - P[T_1 = 0 \cap T_2 = 0] \\
&= 1 - P[T_2 = 0 \mid T_1 = 0]P[T_1 = 0] \\
&= 1 - \big[1 - \alpha_2\big(1 - D^2\big)\big][1 - \alpha_1].
\end{aligned}
\tag{6.6}
$$

The process proceeds analogously for the case of $K = 3$. Just as we could identify the joint probability $P[T_1 = 0 \cap T_2 = 0]$ for the case of $K = 2$, we must now identify $P[T_1 = 0 \cap T_2 = 0 \cap T_3 = 0]$. Begin with

$$P[T_3 = 0 \mid \cap\ T_1 = 0 \cap T_2 = 0] = \frac{P[T_1 = 0 \cap T_2 = 0 \cap T_3 = 0]}{P[T_1 = 0 \cap T_2 = 0]}. \tag{6.7}$$

This conditional probability is the probability that there is no type I error for the third hypothesis test H_3, given the results of the hypothesis tests H_1 and H_2. This means that

$$P[T_1 = 0 \cap T_2 = 0 \cap T_3 = 0] = P[T_3 = 0 \mid \cap\ T_1 = 0 \cap T_2 = 0]P[T_1 = 0 \cap T_2 = 0]. \tag{6.8}$$

Now we write the dependency measure

$$D_{3|1,2} = \sqrt{1 - \frac{\left(1 - P[T_3 = 0 \mid T_1 = 0 \cap T_2 = 0]\right)}{\alpha_3}}. \tag{6.9}$$

We write $D_{3|1,2}$ to denote the fact that it measures the dependence between H_3 given knowledge of H_1 and H_2. We can therefore write the dependency measure between two statistical hypothesis tests H_1 and H_2 as $D_{2|1}$ since that measure of dependency is the dependence measure for H_2 given that we know H_1 has occurred. We now solve (6.9) for the conditional probability

$$P[T_3 = 0 \mid T_1 = 0 \cap T_2 = 0] = (1 - \alpha_3) + D_{3|2}^2 [1 - (1 - \alpha_3)]$$
$$= 1 - \alpha_3 (1 - D_{3|1,2}^2). \tag{6.10}$$

We now insert the relationship expressed in (6.10) into (6.8) to find

$$\xi = 1 - P[T_1 = 0 \cap T_2 = 0 \cap T_3 = 0]$$
$$= 1 - P[T_3 = 0 \mid T_1 = 0 \cap T_2 = 0] P[T_1 = 0 \cap T_2 = 0] \tag{6.11}$$
$$= 1 - \left[1 - \alpha_3 (1 - D_{3|1,2}^2)\right] P[T_1 = 0 \cap T_2 = 0].$$

Finally, recalling that

$$P[T_1 = 0 \cap T_2 = 0] = \left[1 - \alpha_2 (1 - D_{2|1}^2)\right][1 - \alpha_1] \tag{6.12}$$

we write the familywise error level ξ,

$$\xi = 1 - \left[1 - \alpha_3 (1 - D_{3|1,2}^2)\right]\left[1 - \alpha_2 (1 - D_{2|1}^2)\right][1 - \alpha_1]. \tag{6.13}$$

Note that ξ is a function of the three test-specific α levels α_1, α_2, α_3 and the two dependency measures $D_{2|1}$ and $D_{3|1,2}$.

As was the case for two hypothesis tests, it will be useful for us to prospectively compute the test-specific α level α_3 for primary analysis 3 given the levels α_1 and α_2 for the other two hypothesis tests H_1 and H_2. Solving (6.13) for α_3 reveals

$$\alpha_3 = \min\left[\alpha_2, \frac{1 - \dfrac{1 - \xi}{[1 - \alpha_1]\left[1 - \alpha_2 \left(1 - D_{2|1}^2\right)\right]}}{1 - D_{3|1,2}^2}\right]. \tag{6.14}$$

If the value for the dependency measure is the same across the three prospectively planned, primary analyses, then $D_{2|1} = D_{3|1,2} = D$, and (6.14) becomes

$$\alpha_3 = \min \left[\alpha_2, \frac{[1-\alpha_1]\left[1-\alpha_2\left(1-D^2\right)\right]-(1-\xi)}{[1-\alpha_1]\left[1-\alpha_2\left(1-D^2\right)\right]\left(1-D^2\right)} \right]. \tag{6.15}$$

6.1.1 Example of Dependency Among Three Endpoints

As an example of how dependency among three endpoints can be used to design a clinical trial, consider the work of investigators who would wish to examine the effect of an intervention designed to reduce the morbidity and mortality of patients who have ischemic heart disease. The trial designers wish to demonstrate the effect of this therapy in patients who are at relatively low risk of death, MI, or stroke. With extensive experience in the field of atherosclerotic cardiovascular disease, these scientists recognize that since the number of clinical events that can be related to ischemic cardiovascular disease will be small, they anticipate that many thousands of patients will be required to complete this experiment.

After extensive discussions, the trial designers decide to choose three primary endpoints for the study. They are (1) total mortality, (2) fatal and nonfatal MI, and (3) fatal and nonfatal stroke. They recognize that there will be dependence among the hypothesis tests for these three analyses and wish to design these dependencies into their clinical trial. With this in mind they begin a sample size evaluation, computing the minimum sample size required for each of the three prospectively chosen primary analyses with, at this early stage, no concern for the conservation of the familywise type I error level ξ (Table 6.1).

Table 6.1. Alpha allocation for trial with three primary endpoints: First design scenario.

Primary analyses	Cumulative control group event rate	Efficacy	Alpha (two-tailed)	Power	Sample size
Total mortality	0.10	0.20	0.05	0.90	8595
Fatal/nonfatal MI	0.06	0.15	0.05	0.90	27,189
Fatal/nonfatal stroke	0.04	0.15	0.05	0.90	41,588

This initial examination of the required sample size confirms what the investigators expected. The combination of small event rates and relatively low efficacy produces sample sizes of between 8592 and 41,588. Partitioning type I error levels among the three endpoints increases the required sample sizes (Table 6.2).

Table 6.2. Alpha allocation for trial with three primary endpoints: Second design scenario.

Primary analyses	Cumulative control group event rate	Efficacy	Alpha (two-tailed)	Power	Sample size
Total mortality	0.10	0.20	0.03	0.90	9746
Fatal/nonfatal MI	0.06	0.15	0.01	0.90	38,502
Fatal/nonfatal stroke	0.04	0.15	0.01	0.90	58,893

The investigators are now interested in embedding the dependence between the statistical hypothesis tests. They have a population in which patients can have multiple morbidities. All of the available prior information suggests that the intervention will act homogeneously on each of these prospectively chosen endpoints. Using the subjective measures described in Chapter 5, the investigators choose for $D_{2|1}$ the value of 0.65 (Table 6.3).

Table 6.3. Alpha allocation for trial with three primary endpoints: Third design scenario.

Primary analyses	Cumulative control group event rate	Efficacy	Alpha (two-tailed)	Power	Sample size
Total mortality	0.10	0.20	0.03	0.90	9746
		$D_{2|1} = 0.65$			
Fatal/nonfatal MI	0.06	0.15	0.030	0.90	30,829
Fatal/nonfatal stroke	0.04	0.15	0.01	0.90	58,893

The exact computation for α_2 the test-specific α level for the fatal and nonfatal MI primary analysis, as computed from

$$\alpha_2 = \min\left[\alpha_1, \frac{\xi - \alpha_1}{(1 - \alpha_1)(1 - D^2)}\right], \tag{6.16}$$

and from the expression that we derived in section 5.9. This expression has two components. The first component requires the calculation of $(\xi - \alpha_1)\Big/(1 - \alpha_1)(1 - D^2)$, producing a candidate value $\alpha_2 = 0.036$. However, one of the conditions for the computation is that $\alpha_1 \geq \alpha_2$, so we start with the value of $\alpha_2 = \alpha_1 = 0.30$.

However, there is one additional consideration that we must make. A value for the type I α error level for the fatal/nonfatal MI primary analysis of 0.03 is the maximum value of α_2 permitted. If this value is actually selected, then the family-wise error level ξ will be 0.05, with no available type I error level for the third primary analysis for the cumulative incidence of stroke. The investigators therefore reduce α_2 from 0.03 to 0.02 and use (6.14) to compute α_3 with $D_{3|1,2} = 0.75$. The value computed from the following component of this equation,

$$1 - \frac{\dfrac{1-\xi}{\left[1-\alpha_1\right]\left[1-\alpha_2\left(1-D_{2|1}^2\right)\right]}}{1-D_{3|1,2}^2} \tag{6.17}$$

provides a value of $\alpha_3 = 0.021$. However, since this computed level exceeds the value of α_2, the value of α_3 is set as $\alpha_3 = \alpha_2 = 0.02$ (Table 6.4).

Table 6.4. Alpha allocation for trial with three primary endpoints. Fourth design scenario.

Primary analyses	Cumulative control group event rate	Efficacy	Alpha (two-tailed)	Power	Sample size
Total mortality	0.10	0.20	0.03	0.90	9746
		$D_{2|1} = 0.65$			
Fatal/nonfatal MI	0.06	0.15	0.020	0.90	33,683
		$D_{3|1,2} = 0.75$			
Fatal/nonfatal stroke	0.04	0.15	0.021	0.90	51,013

Finally, power is adjusted to minimum values for the fatal/nonfatal stroke primary analysis (Table 6.5). Power is increased for the total mortality analysis, since more patients will be required for the evaluation of the effect of the intervention on the cumulative incidence of fatal/nonfatal stroke permitting those same patients to contribute to the cumulative total mortality rate evaluation.

Table 6.5. Alpha allocation for trial with three primary endpoints: Fifth design scenario.

Primary analyses	Cumulative control group event rate	Efficacy	Alpha (two-tailed)	Power	Sample size
Total mortality	0.10	0.20	0.03	0.95	11,905
		$D_{2\|1} = 0.65$			
Fatal/nonfatal MI	0.06	0.15	0.020	0.90	35,561
		$D_{3\|1,2} = 0.75$			
Fatal/nonfatal stroke	0.04	0.15	0.020	0.80	39,723

6.2 The Solution for Four Dependent Analyses

The derivation for three prospectively identified, primary analyses in a clinical trial was provided in the previous section. This derivation developed in a straightforward manner because we were able to build on the intuition we gained from the analysis of the simplest of cases for dependency between statistical hypothesis tests in Chapter 5 (i.e., when there are two and only two dependent tests). Now that we have completed the solution for $K = 3$, it is possible for us to continue the evaluations for the computation of the familywise error level ξ and the test-specific α levels for the clinical trial's primary analyses.

For example, the same pattern of solution developed in Section 6.1 can be used as a blueprint for the construction of a solution for four dependent endpoints. In fact, these evaluations can be evaluated for successively larger values of K, the number of dependent primary analyses. However, the equations become more complex as K increases. The derivations for these solutions are each provided in Appendix E. We simply report the final results here.

If during the prospective design of a clinical trial, investigators decide on four primary analyses with levels of dependence $D_{2|1}$, $D_{3|1,2}$, and $D_{4|1,2,3}$, and test-specific α levels α_1, α_2, α_3, and α_4, the familywise error ξ is

$$\xi = 1 - \left[1 - \alpha_4\left(1 - D_{4|1,2,3}^2\right)\right]\left[1 - \alpha_3\left(1 - D_{3|1,2}^2\right)\right]\left[1 - \alpha_2\left(1 - D_{2|1}^2\right)\right]\left[1 - \alpha_1\right]. \quad (6.18)$$

If we let D_m be the minimum of the values of $D_{2|1}$, $D_{3|1,2}$, and $D_{4|1,2,3}$, then a conservative estimate for ξ is

$$\xi = 1 - \left[1 - \alpha_1\right]\prod_{j=2}^{4}\left[1 - \alpha_j\left(1 - D_m^2\right)\right]. \quad (6.19)$$

If ξ and α_1 are known, then the solutions for the test-specific α levels α_2, α_3, and α_4 are as follows:

$$\alpha_2 = \min\left[\alpha_1, \frac{\xi - \alpha_1}{(1-\alpha_1)(1-D_{2|1}^2)}\right] \tag{6.20}$$

$$\alpha_3 = \min\left[\alpha_2, \frac{1 - \dfrac{1-\xi}{[1-\alpha_1][1-\alpha_2(1-D_{2|1}^2)]}}{1-D_{3|1,2}^2}\right] \tag{6.21}$$

$$\alpha_4 = \min\left[\alpha_3, \frac{1 - \dfrac{1-\xi}{[1-\alpha_1][1-\alpha_2(1-D_{2|1}^2)][1-\alpha_3(1-D_{3|1,2}^2)]}}{1-D_{4|1,2,3}^2}\right] \tag{6.22}$$

Let D_m be the minimum values of $D_{2|1}$, $D_{3|1.2}$, and $D_{4|1,2,3}$, these estimates become

$$\alpha_2 = \min\left[\alpha_1, \frac{\xi - \alpha_1}{(1-\alpha_1)(1-D_m^2)}\right] \tag{6.23}$$

$$\alpha_3 = \min\left[\alpha_2, \frac{[1-\alpha_1][1-\alpha_2(1-D_m^2)] - [1-\xi]}{[1-\alpha_1][1-\alpha_2(1-D_m^2)][1-D_m^2]}\right] \tag{6.24}$$

$$\alpha_4 = \min\left[\alpha_3, \frac{[1-\alpha_1][1-\alpha_2(1-D_m^2)][1-\alpha_3(1-D_m^2)][1-D_m^2]-[1-\xi]}{[1-\alpha_1][1-\alpha_2(1-D_m^2)][1-\alpha_3(1-D_m^2)][1-D_m^2]}\right] \tag{6.25}$$

6.3 K Multidependent Analyses

For the general circumstance of K dependent hypothesis tests, a general solution for the familywise error level ξ_K can be found (the proof is in Appendix E).

$$\xi_K = 1 - \left[\prod_{k=2}^{K}\left[1 - \alpha_k\left(1 - D_{k|1,2,3,\dots,k}^2\right)\right]\right][1-\alpha_1] \tag{6.26}$$

and the computation of the test-specific α level for the kth hypothesis test is

$$\alpha_k = \min \left[\alpha_{k-1}, \ \frac{1 - \dfrac{1-\xi}{[1-\alpha_1]\prod\limits_{j=2}^{k-1}\left[1-\alpha_j\left(1-D^2_{j|1,2,3,\ldots,j-1}\right)\right]}}{1 - D^2_{k|1,2,3,\ldots,k-1}} \right] \tag{6.27}$$

If the level of dependency is the same across all hypothesis tests D, then (6.26) reduces to

$$\xi = 1 - \left[\prod_{k=2}^{K}\left[1-\alpha_k\left(1-D^2\right)\right]\right]\left[1-\alpha_1\right], \tag{6.28}$$

and (6.27) becomes

$$\alpha_k = \min \left[\alpha_{k-1}, \ \frac{1 - \dfrac{1-\xi}{[1-\alpha_1]\prod\limits_{j=2}^{k-1}\left[1-\alpha_j\left(1-D^2\right)\right]}}{1 - D^2} \right]. \tag{6.29}$$

6.4 Conservative Dependence

In Chapter 5, we discuss the problems that occurs by overestimating the dependency parameter when constructing type I error levels for prospectively chosen primary analyses in a clinical trial. Another useful procedure to follow, to help avoid overestimating the dependence parameter, may be invoked when there are at least three dependent primary analyses. In Section 6.3, we generalized the concept of D to the case of $K = 3$ hypothesis tests. In this circumstance, there is not just one parameter D, but two, namely, $D_{2|1}$ and $D_{3|1,2}$. While the formulations of Section 6.3 provided estimates for computing α_2 and then α_3, we had to specify the value of each of $D_{2|1}$ and $D_{3|1,2}$ to accomplish this. A conservative approach would be to compute each of $D_{2|1}$ and $D_{3|1,2}$ based on the guidelines previously provided in Chapter 5, and then choose a value D_m which is the minimum for each of these. If we define the $\min(a, b)$ equal to a when $a \leq b$ and equal to b when $b < a$, we then define

$$D_m = \min\left(D_{2|1}, D_{3|1,2}\right). \tag{6.30}$$

This provides not just a conservative estimate of the dependency between the prospectively defined statistical hypothesis tests, but it also provides some formula simplification. Recall that in the case of three primary analyses, we wrote

$$\alpha_3 = \min\left[\alpha_2, \ \frac{1 - \dfrac{1 - \xi}{[1 - \alpha_1]\left[1 - \alpha_2\left(1 - D_{2|1}^2\right)\right]}}{1 - D_{3|1,2}^2}\right]. \tag{6.31}$$

Taking the conservative approach of using the minimum value D_m allows this expression to be written as

$$\alpha_3 = \min\left[\alpha_2, \ \frac{[1 - \alpha_1]\left[1 - \alpha_2\left(1 - D_m^2\right)\right] - [1 - \xi]}{[1 - \alpha_1]\left[1 - \alpha_2\left(1 - D_m^2\right)\right]\left[1 - D_m^2\right]}\right]. \tag{6.32}$$

Analogously the familywise error level ξ, originally computed as

$$\xi = 1 - \left[1 - \alpha_3\left(1 - D_{3|1,2}^2\right)\right]\left[1 - \alpha_2\left(1 - D_{2|1}^2\right)\right][1 - \alpha_1] \tag{6.33}$$

can now be written as

$$\xi = 1 - \left[1 - \alpha_3\left(1 - D_m^2\right)\right]\left[1 - \alpha_2\left(1 - D_m^2\right)\right][1 - \alpha_1]. \tag{6.34}$$

In the circumstance of K hypothesis tests, there are degrees of dependence that vary across subsets of these hypothesis tests. Thus, $D_{2|1} \neq D_{3|1,2} \neq D_{4|1,2,3} \neq \ldots \neq D_{K|1,2,3,\ldots,K-1}$. In this circumstance, although (6.28) and (6.29) can be used to compute the familywise error level ξ_K, or to compute the test-specific α levels, these computations can be time consuming. However, one can make the following adjustment. Let D_m be the minimum of all of the measures of dependency, i.e.,

$$D_m = \min_{k=1,2,\ldots K} D_{k|1,2,3,\ldots,k-1} \tag{6.35}$$

which means that (6.28) and (6.29) can be rewritten as

$$\xi = 1 - \left[\prod_{k=2}^{K}\left[1 - \alpha_k\left(1 - D_m^2\right)\right]\right][1 - \alpha_1]. \tag{6.36}$$

The use of D_m permits us to write α_k as

$$\alpha_k = \min\left[\alpha_{k-1}, \; \frac{1 - \dfrac{1-\xi}{[1-\alpha_1]\prod\limits_{j=2}^{k-1}\left[1-\alpha_j\left(1-D_m^2\right)\right]}}{1-D_m^2}\right]. \tag{6.37}$$

This calculation using the minimum value D_m has the advantage of being somewhat protective of overly optimistic estimates of the dependency parameter. Rather than have to estimate each of the dependency parameters, one need only identify the minimum value above which all of the dependency parameters may be found. Using the minimum value of the dependency parameters we will describe as working within the environment of *conservative dependence*.

6.5 Generalization of the Bonferroni Inequality

Appendix E provides the derivation of other results that will be both useful and easy to implement. Simplifying some of the more complex results of the previous subsection will make the computations for the incorporation of type I error dependency into prospectively planned primary analyses of clinical trials easier and perhaps more intuitive.

Recall that ξ is the familywise error level for K primary analyses in a clinical trial. As we have defined previously, let the test-specific α level for the jth primary analyses be α_j, and let $D_{j|1,2,3,...,j-1}$ be the level of dependency between the jth primary analyses and the previous $j-1$ primary analyses. Finally we will, as before, let $D_m = \min\limits_{k=1,2,...K} D_{k|1,2,3,...,k-1}$. Then

$$\xi \leq \sum_{j=1}^{K}\alpha_j \qquad\qquad\qquad\qquad \textit{independence,}$$

$$\xi \leq \alpha_1 + \sum_{k=2}^{K}\alpha_k\left(1-D_{k|1,2,3,...,k-1}^2\right) \quad \textit{full dependence,} \tag{6.38}$$

$$\xi \leq \alpha_1 + \left(1-D_m^2\right)\sum_{k=2}^{K}\alpha_k \qquad \textit{conservative dependence.}$$

Expression (6.38) tells us how to compute the familywise error probability under the assumption of independence and under the two different conditions for dependence. These expressions are actually generalizations of the Bonferroni inequality. Full dependence assumes that all of the different levels of dependence are incorporated into the test-specific α levels. Conservative dependence uses only the minimum value of these levels of dependence.

If we assume that all of the test-specific type I error levels are to be equal then expression (6.38) can be further simplified to

$$\xi \le K\alpha \qquad\qquad\qquad independence,$$

$$\xi \le \alpha \sum_{j=1}^{K}\left(1-D^2_{j|1,2,3,\ldots j-1}\right) \quad full\ dependence, \qquad (6.39)$$

$$\xi \le K\left(1-D^2_m\right)\alpha \qquad conservative\ dependence.$$

Finally, we can provide a basic rule for computing test-specific α levels if they are all to be the same. It is

$$\alpha_j \le \frac{\xi}{K} \qquad\qquad independence,$$

$$\alpha_j \le \frac{\xi}{K\left(1-D^2_m\right)} \quad conservative\ dependence. \qquad (6.40)$$

These simplified computations for incorporating dependence into prospectively planned primary analyses will be utilized throughout the rest of this text.

6.6 Subclass Dependence

While dependence can be a useful tool to conserve the familywise error level for prospectively designed primary analyses in a clinical trial, the problem of computing appropriate values of the dependency parameters for each of the endpoints can be complicated. We know that if there are K prospectively defined primary analyses in a clinical trial, then there will be $K-1$ dependency parameters $D_{2|1}$, $D_{3|1,2}$, $D_{4|1,2,3}$, ..., $D_{K|1,2,3,\ldots,K-1}$ that require estimation. While it is possible to go down the list of the K primary analyses, first ranking them so that $\alpha_1 \ge \alpha_2 \ge \alpha_3 \ge \ldots \ge \alpha_K$, and then sequentially going through the thought process necessary to compute and defend each value $D_{j|1,2,3,\ldots,j-1}$ for $j=2$ to K, as we did in Chapter 5 for $K=2$ and the earlier part of this chapter for $K=3$, there is a more intuitive approach available.

6.6.1 Solutions for Two Subclasses

The process that is described in this section is the identification of primary analyses which are composed of dependent subclasses. The underlying idea is to group the K primary analyses into two or three groups or subclasses of analyses. Each primary analysis is categorized into only one subclass of analyses. What differentiates one subclass of analyses from another is that the primary analyses within one subclass of events all have the same dependency parameter. This process allows the investigator to quickly bring his or her own clinical intuition to bear on the problem of identifying values for dependency parameters. For example, if there are $K=5$ primary endpoints (1), (2), (3), (4), (5) and analyses (1) and (5) have the same level of dependency while analyses (2), (3), and (4) have a different level of dependency, then we may say that we have $S=2$ subclasses of primary analyses; {(1) (5)} and {(2) (3) (4)}. The conservatism of this procedure is improved by categorizing the subclass dependence measure as the minimum dependence measure among the events within that subclass. Thus, in the previous example, if in the second subclass $\{(2)\ (3)\ (4)\}$, $D_{3|2} < D_{4|2,3}$ then compute the α to be allocated among the subclass as the minimum value of D in the second subclass or $D_{m(2)} = D_{3|2}$.

No new concepts are required to compute type I error level allocations when dependent subclasses are used to categorize the prospectively planned primary analyses of clinical trials. We provide the computations necessary for the case of $S = 2$ subclasses of events. Consider a clinical trial that is designed to have five primary analyses. that have been divided into two subclasses $\{(2)\ (3)\ (4)\}$ and $\{(1)\ (5)\}$. The first subclass has $S_1 = 3$ primary analyses, and the second subclass $S_2 = 2$ primary analyses. Let $D_{m(1)}$ be the minimum of $D_{3|2}$ and $D_{4|2,3}$, which are the two dependency parameters from the first subclass. Let $D_{5|1}$ be the dependency parameter reflecting the relationship between the two primary analyses in the second subclass. Assume that the two subclasses of hypothesis tests are independent of each other.

We continue by denoting ξ_1 as the familywise error level for the first subclass and ξ_2 as the familywise error level for the second subclass. Since the subclasses are independent of each other, we can write

$$\xi = 1 - (1 - \xi_1)(1 - \xi_2),\qquad (6.41)$$

or, more constructively, choose ξ_1 and compute ξ_2 as

$$\xi_2 = 1 - \frac{1 - \xi}{1 - \xi_1}.\qquad (6.42)$$

Once the levels ξ_1 and ξ_2 are chosen, which are the familywise error levels for the two subclasses of primary analyses $\{(2)\ (3)\ (4)\}$ and $\{(1)\ (5)\}$, respectively, we then simply apportion the type I error levels within the two subclasses. For the first subclass made up of the primary analyses (2), (3), and (4) we are required to compute α_2, α_3, and α_4 where $\alpha_2 \geq \alpha_3 \geq \alpha_4$. Then we

(1) Choose $\alpha_2 < \xi_1$.

(2) Compute

$$\alpha_3 = \min\left[\alpha_2,\ \frac{\xi_1 - \alpha_2}{(1 - \alpha_2)(1 - D_{m(1)}^2)}\right].\qquad (6.43)$$

(3) Compute

$$\alpha_4 = \min\left[\alpha_3,\ \frac{[1 - \alpha_2][1 - \alpha_3(1 - D_{m(2)}^2)] - (1 - \xi_1)}{[1 - \alpha_2][1 - \alpha_3(1 - D_{m(2)}^2)][1 - D_{m(2)}^2]}\right].\qquad (6.44)$$

The process is easier for the second dependent subclass consisting of primary analyses (1) and (5), ordered such that $\alpha_1 \geq \alpha_5$.

(1) Choose $\alpha_1 < \xi_2$.

(2) Compute

$$\alpha_5 = \min\left[\alpha_1, \frac{\xi_2 - \alpha_1}{(1-\alpha_1)(1-D_{5|1}^2)}\right] \tag{6.45}$$

and since $\xi_2 = 1 - (1-\xi)/(1-\xi_1)$, we can rewrite the second expression of the minimum function in (6.45) as

$$\frac{\xi_2 - \alpha_1}{(1-\alpha_1)(1-D_{5|1}^2)} = \frac{1 - \dfrac{1-\xi}{1-\xi_1} - \alpha_1}{(1-\alpha_1)(1-D_{5|1}^2)} = \frac{(\xi - \xi_1) - \alpha_1(1-\xi_1)}{(1-\xi_1)(1-\alpha_1)(1-D_{5|1}^2)}. \tag{6.46}$$

6.6.2 Therapy for CHF

As an example of the possible use of dependent subclasses of primary analyses within a clinical trial, consider the circumstance of a clinical trial that is designed to determine the effect of a randomized intervention in CHF. In this study, the investigators will recruit only patients suffering from moderate CHF who meet the requirements of the NYHA classification system for class II or class III heart failure. Every patient recruited for the study will receive the standard level of care for heart failure (life style alteration, diuretics, digitalis, ACE-i therapy, and beta blocker therapy). In addition, patients who are randomized to the active group will receive the new intervention while patients in the control group will receive placebo therapy.

The investigators discussed thoroughly the choice of endpoints. They would like to choose primary analyses that are unambiguously measured and directly interpretable, such as the effect of therapy on the total mortality rate or the effect of therapy on the all-cause hospitalization rate. However, the physicians designing the trial recognize that, despite their best efforts, the number of patients that they will recruit for their clinical trial will be too small to carry out an analysis on these important primary analyses with adequate power. However, the investigators would like to retain some ability to declare that their clinical trial is positive for a finding of important magnitude for these endpoints. These scientists declare that the analyses for the effect of the intervention on the cumulative mortality rate and the effect of the intervention on the cumulative hospitalization rate are primary analyses and allocate type I error level to each of them.[1] Since a smaller sample size is

---

[1] As discussed in Chapter 4, this procedure will allow the investigators to say the study is positive if the p-value at the end of the concordantly executed trial is less than the type I error level allocated to it prospectively. However, since these analyses will be underpowered, the

required for the analyses that directly measure exercise tolerance, the investigators prospectively choose its measure as the primary analysis for the trial. Thus, the investigators settle on four primary analyses for this study (Table 6.5).

Table 6.5. Prospective planned primary analyses.

Exercise Tolerance
The effect of therapy on the 6-minute walking distance
The effect of therapy on the 9-minute treadmill

Clinical Morbidity and Mortality
The effect of therapy on the cumulative total mortality rate
The effect of therapy on the cumulative total hospitalzation rate

---

The four prospectively defined primary analyses for these studies may be considered as two subclasses of endpoints. The first subclass consists of the two primary analyses that focus on the two measures of exercise tolerance (exercise subclass). The second subclass of analyses (clinical subclass) consists of the two primary analyses: (1) the effect of the intervention on the cumulative total mortality rate and (2) the effect of the intervention on the cumulative total hospitalization rate.

The familywise error for this clinical trial is set to the 0.05 level, a level that is to be allocated among the four primary analyses. The investigators begin by acknowledging that, after considering the twin conditions of endpoint coincidence and therapy homogeneity, the two subclasses of primary analyses are independent of each other.[2] The investigators then partition the familywise error rate ξ by allocating $\xi_1 = 0.04$ to the exercise subclass and $\xi_2 = 0.01$ to the clinical subclass. This division was justified because the analyses for the clinical subclass will be underpowered, indicating that a paucity of events is expected for these analyses. This anticipated small number of events will require a substantial saving of lives, or a substantial reduction in the cumulative hospitalization rate to persuade the medical community that the therapy is efficacious for these primary analyses. The joint consideration of large effect size and small p-value would be most persuasive (Table 6.6).

---

absence of a positive finding cannot be interpreted as a null (or no effect) finding but as merely uninformative.

[2] This process was discussed in Chapter 5, Section 5.2.

Table 6.6. Alpha allocation example with four primary endpoints.
Two dependent subclasses: First design scenario.

Primary analyses	Type I error level subclass	Type I error level analysis specific	Dependency parameter
Exercise Subclass 6-minute walk 9-minute treadmill	0.040		
Clinical Subclass Total mortality Total hospitalizations	0.010		

Initial assignment of familywise error levels for each of the two subclasses.

The investigators then proceed by allocating a type I error within each of the two subclasses. If the investigators assume that there is no intra-subclass dependence within each of the two primary analyses subclasses, this is easily accomplished. For example, the investigators allocate a type I error event rate of 0.030 for the effect of the intervention on the 6 minute walk, leaving approximately $0.040 - 0.030 = 0.010$ for the maximum type I error level acceptable for the effect of the intervention on the 9-minute treadmill test. Analogously, the allocation of $\alpha_3 = 0.008$ for the effect of therapy on the cumulative mortality rate leaves a residual of α_4 for the effect of therapy on the effect of the randomly allocated intervention on the cumulative total hospitalization rate (Table 6.7). This is the allocation assuming no intra-dependence subclasses.

However, in this circumstance there will be dependency between the primary analyses within each of the two subclasses. This dependence can be used to conserve type I error within each of the exercises and clinical primary analyses subclasses. The investigators believe that there is strong dependence between each of the two exercise tolerance endpoints. Patients who perform well on the 6-minute walk will also tend to perform above average on the 9-minute treadmill test. Also, the investigators have every reason to suspect that the effect of therapy will be the same on each of these two endpoints; it would be extremely unlikely, and there is no prior evidence to suggest that the randomly allocated intervention would produce a benefit on the 6-minute walk and not on the 9-minute treadmill test. These considerations lead the investigators to settle on a high value of the dependency parameter between these two primary analyses within the exercise-dependent subclass; $D = 0.90$. This value of D can be used to compute the type I error level for the 9-minute treadmill test from expression (6.45).

$$\alpha_2 = \min\left[\alpha_2, \frac{\xi_1 - \alpha_1}{(1-\alpha_1)(1-D^2)}\right],\tag{6.47}$$

with $\xi_1 = 0.04$, $\alpha_1 = 0.030$, this indicates that $\alpha_2 = 0.03$.

Table 6.7. Alpha allocation example with four primary endpoints. Two dependent subclasses: Second design scenario.

Primary analyses	Type I error level subclass	Type I error level analysis specific	Dependency parameter
Exercise Subclass	0.040		
6-minute walk		0.030	
9-minute treadmill		0.010	
Clinical Subclass	0.010		
Total mortality		0.008	
Total hospitalizations		0.002	

Assignment of test specific α levels assuming complete within subclass and between subclass hypothesis test dependence.

A similar analysis is provided for the clinical subclass of primary analyses. In this case, the investigators believe that 75% of patients who die in this clinical trial will be hospitalized, or $c = 0.75$. They expect a high degree of therapy homogeneity in the effect of therapy on those patients who die but are not hospitalized first, or $h = 0.75$. Thus, from (5.39)

$$\begin{aligned} D &= c\left[1-(1-c)(1-h)\right] \\ &= 0.75\left[1-(1-0.75)(1-0.75)\right] \\ &= 0.75[1-(0.25)(0.25)] \\ &= 0.75[0.9375] = 0.7031 = 0.70. \end{aligned}\tag{6.48}$$

This computation leads to the calculation using (6.16) that the test-specific α level α_4 for the evaluation of the effect of the randomly assigned intervention on the cumulative incidence rate of all-cause hospitalizations is 0.004 (Table 6.8).

Table 6.8. Alpha allocation example with four primary endpoints
Two dependent subclasses: Third design scenario.

Primary analyses	Type I error level subclass	Type I error level analysis specific	Dependency parameter
Exercise Subclass	0.040		0.90
6-minute walk		0.030	
9-minute treadmill		0.030	
Clinical Subclass	0.010		0.70
Total mortality		0.008	
Total hospitalizations		0.004	

Assignment of test-specific α levels assuming intrasubclass
dependence and intersubclasss independence.

A comparison of the α allocation between Table 6.7 and 6.8 reveals the increase in the test-specific α levels for the effect of therapy on the 9-minute treadmill evaluation from 0.01 to 0.03. Analogously, there has been an increase in the test-specific α level α_4 for the evaluation of the effect of the randomly allocated intervention on the cumulative incidence rate of total hospitalizations from 0.02 to 0.04. Note that the sum of the type I error rates for the 6-minute walk and 9-minute treadmill exceed the 0.04 α probability for the exercise subclass. The same is the case for the sum of the α error rates for the analysis of the effect of therapy for the clinical endpoints. Because there is dependence between the analyses within the subclass, the test-specific α error rates can be larger than in the case of statistical independence.

6.7 Conclusions

The use of multiple statistical analyses in clinical trials, while providing the disciplined researcher with several opportunities to identify a positive effect of the randomly allocated intervention, also complicates that scientist's work by requiring her to allocate a type I error rate across each of several primary analyses. Since the familywise error level for the entire trial is typically fixed at 0.05, the test-specific α levels for each of a large number of hypothesis tests become small very quickly. In Chapter 4, we discussed the procedures that a researcher might utilize to control the familywise error rate. However, we must acknowledge that even by triaging the analyses, and then allocating α differentially among these primary analyses, the investigator commonly faces the difficulty that prospectively set α levels for some of these primary analyses will be very small.

The recognition that some of these primary analyses will be dependent each other and that this dependence will lead to some type I error level conservation has been the focus of much of the statistical literature devoted to the multiple analyses issue. That body of literature was reviewed in Chapter 5. Clearly, there are several approaches one can take in incorporating dependence between endpoints. However, regardless of the selection the investigators make, the procedure they embed in the clinical trial's analysis plan must be embedded prospectively.

Chapters 5 and 6 have provided what I hope is an intuitive procedure for the clinical investigators as they grapple with the notion of incorporating dependent hypothesis testing in their clinical trial designs. While Chapter 5 focused on the basic notion of statistical dependence between hypothesis testing and provided illustrations of its use in the circumstance of two prospectively specified primary analyses, Chapter 6 concentrated on the use of this dependency tool in more complicated clinical trial designs. Clearly, the more complicated the dependency relationship between subsets of the primary analyses, the more complex the prospective α allocation procedure can be. However the development provided in these two chapters demonstrates the flexibility of the notion of dependency. If there are many different multiple endpoints, the approach used in this chapter is both applicable and straightforward.

An important question is the response of the regulatory community to the notion of incorporating dependency in hypothesis tests. The FDA has shown itself to be open and receptive to this process. A case in point is the study of the use of integrilin as a post cardiac angioplasty therapy [1]. At the advisory committee meeting that first discussed the approval of this product, the Cardiovascular and Renal Drugs Advisory Committee focused not on the use of dependency, but on whether the analysis plan that was prospectively identified was the one that ultimately governed the analyses that the sponsor defended. The sponsor's choice to prospectively embed dependency between hypothesis tests was not the major methodological concern. If the use of dependency (1) is carefully considered, (2) avoids extremes, (3) is prospectively applied, and (4) steers clear of the hyper-dependence issues discussed in Chapter 5, then there will be minimal difficulty with its successful incorporation (using the tool developed in this textbook or others discussed in the statistical literature) into a clinical trial program on the trajectory for regulatory approval.

At this point, we have developed both the nomenclature and the methodological tools that we need to carefully examine the most common settings in which multiple analyses are used in clinical trials. The use of combined endpoints, subgroup analyses, and multiple treatment groups will be the focus of the next six chapters.

Problems

1. Construct a table of joint probabilities for the joint occurrence of type I errors from $K = 3$ independent primary analyses in a prospectively designed clinical trial analogous to Table 5.2 which was constructed for the case of $K = 2$.

2. A clinical trial is prospectively designed with three primary analyses. The familywise error rate is to be conserved at the 0.05 level. Assume that the first two primary analyses are independent of each other, with test-specific type I errors levels $\alpha_1 = 0.025$ and $\alpha_2 = 0.015$. The third primary analysis is dependent

on the first two, and has a test-specific α error level α_3. Compute the range of values for α_3 as $D_{3|1,2}$ increases from 0 to 1.

3. Consider a clinical trial with three prospectively defined primary analyses, with test-specific α levels α_1, α_2, and α_3 respectively, and dependency parameters $D_{2|1}$, and $D_{3|1,2}$. Let $\alpha_2(d)$ be the test-specific type I error that is computed

    as $\alpha_2(d) = \min\left[\alpha_1, \dfrac{\xi - \alpha_1}{(1 - \alpha_1)(1 - D^2)}\right]$. Why must α_2 be less than $\alpha_2(d)$ in order

    for type I error to be distributed across the three primary analyses?

4. Compute the test-specific type I errors rate for α_4 for four prospectively defined primary analyses in a clinical trial for decreasing dependency levels. Assume $\alpha_1 \le \xi$ is given, $D_{3|1,2} = D_{2|1}{}^2$: $D_{4|1,2,3} = D_{3|1,2}{}^2$, where $\alpha_2 = \alpha_2(d)/2$ and $\alpha_3 = \alpha_3(d)/2$ where

    $$\alpha_3(d) = \min\left[\alpha_2, \frac{[1 - \alpha_1][1 - \alpha_2(1 - D^2)] - (1 - \xi)}{[1 - \alpha_1][1 - \alpha_2(1 - D^2)](1 - D^2)}\right].$$

5. Compute the test-specific type I errors rates α_1, α_2, α_3, α_4 for four prospectively defined primary analyses in a clinical trial for increasing dependency levels. $D_{3|1,2} = D_{2|1}{}^{1/2}$: $D_{4|1,2,3} = D_{3|1,2}{}^{1/2}$, where α_2 is defined as in problem 3 and α_3 is defined as in problem 4.

6. Verify formula (6.27) for $K = 3$, 4, and 5.

7. Verify formula (6.28) for $K = 3$, 4, and 5.

8. Show that in expression (6.38), the formula for full dependence reduces to the formula for conservative dependence when $D_{k|1,2,3\ldots,k-1} = D_m$ for $K = 1$ to K when there are K prospectively defined primary endpoints.

9. Why can the second and third expressions in (6.38) be referred to as generalizations of the Bonferroni inequality?

References

1. Transcript of the Federal Food and Drug Administration Cardiovascular–Renal Advisory Committee. February 28, 1997.

Chapter 7

Introduction to Composite Endpoints

This chapter is the first of seven consecutive chapters that applies the multiple analyses methodology that we have developed thus far to specific, complex circumstances that commonly occur within modern clinical trials. Both this and the next chapter focus on the use of the composite or combined endpoint as a primary analysis variable. Composite or combined endpoints are defined as the combination of component (singleton) endpoints, each of which has clinical significance in its own right. In this chapter, the complications involved in the construction of the composite endpoint are discussed, and the issue of homogeneity versus heterogeneity of treatment effect is addressed.

7.1 Introduction

Composite or combined[1] endpoints have been incorporated into the design of many clinical trials over the past 30 years. The use of these complicated endpoints has expanded both in scope and in complexity as investigators have become more accustomed to their features. A well-designed clinical trial that prospectively embeds a composite endpoint into its primary analysis plan is empowered to measure small effects. The use of the combined endpoint improves the resolving ability of the clinical trial, strengthening its capacity to pick out weaker signals of effect from the background noise of sampling error. If larger effect sizes are of interest, then a trial using a composite endpoint can gauge the effect of therapy using a smaller sample size (everything else being equal).

However, the entry of a composite endpoint into a clinical trial introduces that trial to complications in both endpoint construction and endpoint interpretation, complexities that can weaken the trial's ability to reach reliable conclusions. In some circumstances, the combined endpoint can be exceedingly difficult to analyze in a straightforward, comprehensible manner. The components of the endpoint, if not carefully chosen, may produce a conglomerate endpoint that is off balance. The medical community's resultant difficulty in understanding the meaning of this unequilibrated endpoint can cast a shadow over the effect of the clinical trial's intervention. This can reduce what appeared as a stunningly successful demonstration of clinical and statistical efficacy to merely the demonstration of tepid and ultimately irrelevant effectiveness against an endpoint that in the end was seen to be of dubious clinical value.

---

[1] The terms *combined endpoint* and *composite endpoint* are synonymous and will be used interchangeably.

7.2 Definitions and Motivations

While our ultimate focus in this chapter will be on the complications that composite endpoints add to the problem of multiple statistical analyses in clinical trials, we will begin our discussion with an introductory overview of the combined endpoint, assessing its strengths and weaknesses.

A combined or composite endpoint in a clinical trial is a clinically relevant endpoint that is constructed from combinations of other clinically relevant endpoints, termed *component endpoints* or *singleton endpoints*. Two examples of singleton endpoints are (1) the cumulative incidence of total mortality and (2) the cumulative incidence of total hospitalization. A patient experiences a combined endpoint based on these two singleton endpoints if they either die or are hospitalized. If a patient experiences either or both of these component events during the course of the clinical trial, then that patient is considered to have experienced the composite endpoint, commonly referred to total mortality/total hospitalization or total mortality + total hospitalization.

7.3 Notation

We can introduce some elementary notation to further clarify the constitution of the composite endpoint. Consider a composite endpoint that is composed of the two singleton endpoints A and B. Then as stated earlier, the composite endpoint occurs if either the event A or the event B has happened. We can denote this occurrence as $A \cup B$ where $\cup$ is called "union". $A \cup B$ (said as "A union B") denotes the occurrence of either the event A, the event B, or both events. Simply put, $A \cup B$ means that at least A or B has occurred. If A denotes the occurrence of a death during the course of a trial and B denotes the occurrence of a hospitalization during the course of the trial, then $A \cup B$ accurately describes the combined event of at least a death or a hospitalization. Thus, the union event is precisely the combined endpoint.

7.4 Motivations for Combined Endpoints

There are theoretical and practical motivations that guide investigators as they consider the use of a composite endpoint as a primary analysis variable in a clinical trial. Each of these motivations must be considered in turn so that we might gain some insight into how to prospectively construct a functional combined endpoint for such a study.

It is a truism that disease, and certainly chronic disease, manifests itself in different ways. As an example, consider CHF. CHF can produce death; CHF also increases the likelihood of hospitalization, as well as prolonging it. CHF impairs the patient's ability to exercise, and reduces that patient's quality of life. In addition, CHF is associated with chronic effects on measures of cardiac function including but not limited to LVEF, end systolic volume, end diastolic volume, stroke volume, cardiac output, and blood pressure. If the investigator wishes to attempt to measure the effect of an intervention in alleviating the signs and symptoms of CHF, which of these measures should she use?

As we saw in Chapter 4, the investigators who design a clinical trial attempt to choose a measure of disease that the intervention will positively affect. However, considering the many possible signs and symptoms of CHF, this choice can seem to be an impossible one for investigators to make, even after following the analysis triage tactic reviewed in Chapter 4. Alternatively, by building a combined endpoint from several of the signs and symptoms of CHF outlined above, the investigators can simultaneously focus on several manifestations of the disease process. Thus, the use of the combined endpoint can represent an earnest attempt by the investigators to construct a "whole" of the disease's varied effects that may be greater than the "sum" of the combined endpoint's components.

7.4.1 Epidemiologic Considerations

Additionally, epidemiologic assessments of singleton endpoints reveal that the isolated interpretation of a single component endpoint can be misleading. As an example, consider the correct interpretation of a clinical trial that is prospectively designed to examine the effect of an intervention on the occurrence of MIs. There is one prospectively identified primary analysis in this study, and that is the effect of therapy on the cumulative incidence rate of nonfatal MI. The experiment is concordantly executed and, at its conclusion, the study demonstrates both a clinically significant and a statistically significant reduction in the nonfatal MI rate.

In this illustration, the randomly allocated intervention reduced the occurrence of nonfatal heart attacks. However, the intervention may not be as effective as it first appeared. By focusing solely on a nonfatal endpoint, the investigators might miss the possibility that the intervention may have produced a harmful effect on another measure of this same disease—one that was not captured by the primary analysis of the effect of therapy on nonfatal MI. For example, it is possible that the therapy reduced the incidence of nonfatal heart attacks by increasing the incidence of fatal heart attacks (Figure 7.1). That is, even though the number of nonfatal heart attacks was reduced in the active group of the clinical trial, the total number of heart attacks was increased in the active group, and the majority of these events were fatal heart attacks. Because the intervention's influence on mortal events may be hidden if the principle analysis involves the measurement of only a morbidity endpoint, the morbidity endpoint can be combined with the mortality endpoint to provide a more complete depiction of the effect of therapy.

7.4.2 Sample Size Concerns

An additional motivation for the use of the composite endpoint is to insure that there is adequate power for the primary analyses of the study. Combining component endpoints permits their endpoint rates to be accumulated, and this increased event rate can be translated into a reduction in the minimum number of patients required for the clinical trial.

Recall from Appendix E that one of the critical factors included in the sample size formula is the control group endpoint event rate. The larger this rate is, the greater the number of endpoint events that will be accumulated in the study. Thus, if all other assumptions remain constant, we find that the greater the probability of an endpoint, the smaller the number of subjects that will be required to produce an adequate number of those endpoint events. It is this relationship that is taken advantage of in the construction of a composite endpoint.

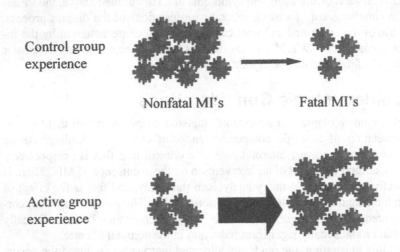

Control group
experience

Nonfatal MI's   Fatal MI's

Active group
experience

Figure 7.1. The active group converts more nonfatal MI's to fatal ones and therefore produces the misleading result of fewer MIs.

Consider an investigator interested in studying the effect of a new therapy on CAD death. His preliminary data suggest that the annual event rate in the control group of the study for the population of patients he is planning to recruit is 0.015. The investigator will be able to follow these patients for 5 years. Thus, the 5 year cumulative incidence rate of CAD death is 0.073.[2] The investigator believes that the randomly allocated intervention will reduce the cumulative event of CAD death by 20%. A computation[3] reveals that the required minimum number of patients required for this clinical trial, assuming 90% power and a two sided type I error probability of 0.05 is 12,132 patients, to be divided equally between the two groups (Table 7.1).

---

[2] If the annual event rate is r, then the cumulative event rate over y years is $1-(1-r)^y$ The reasoning behind this formula is that one first computes the probability of no events in y years as $(1-r)^y$ and then computes the probability of at least one event in y years, which is $1-(1-r)^y$.

[3] The formula for this computation is provided in Appendix D.

Table 7.1. Sample Size computation as a function of the composite endpoint.

Primary analyses	Annual Event rate	Cumulative control group event rate	Efficacy	Alpha (two-tailed)	Power	Sample size
CHD death	0.015	0.073	0.20	0.05	0.90	12132
CHD death + nonfatal MI	0.025	0.119	0.20	0.05	0.90	7092
CHD death + nonfatal MI + unstable angina	0.040	0.185	0.20	0.05	0.90	4260

Sample size decreases for combined event rates with larger annual event rates

    This is a large sample size, and the investigator believes he will be unable to recruit and follow this number of patients for 5 years. However, if this investigator were to combine with CAD death the event of survival and nonfatal MI, then the cumulative event rate of this combined endpoint will include not just CAD death but also the cumulative event rate for the nonfatal MI component. The cumulative annual event rate is 0.025 for this combined analysis, leading to a cumulative 5-year event rate of 0.119 and a sample size of 7092.

    The investigator can take the additional step and add yet another singleton endpoint to this combined endpoint to gain a further reduction in the sample size. If the investigator was to consider patients who survived the study and did not experience a nonfatal MI but did experience unstable angina pectoris during the course of the trial as a third component endpoint, then the annual event rate for this triple composite endpoint of CAD death + nonfatal MI + unstable angina increases to 0.040. The 5-year cumulative incidence rate for this new composite endpoint is 0.185, and the resultant sample size is 4260 patients. By choosing a combined endpoint, the investigator was able to decrease the sample size of the trial from 12,132 to 4,260 solely by adding component endpoints to the composite endpoint. This reduction in the clinical trial's sample size produces a clinical trial requiring fewer resources to execute.

    In the assembly of the composite endpoint, each singleton endpoint contributes an event rate that is included in the event rate of the combined endpoint. Thus with each new component endpoint, the sample size will decrease because the event rate increases.

7.4.3 Improved Resolving Power

Another advantage of the well-considered use of a composite endpoint derives from the increase in the number of patients with events that the trial introduces. In the previous section we saw how the increase in the control group event rate in a clinical trial decreases the sample size required for the study. One other perspective on this multifaceted sample size computation is that the larger event rate provides a more sensitive test of the effectiveness of the therapy.

    As an illustration of this principle, consider an investigator interested in designing a clinical trial to detect the effect of an intervention for the treatment of heart failure. The intervention is relatively safe and is free (e.g., a change in lifestyle). The investigator is interested in demonstrating that the effect of the randomly allocated intervention in patients with heart failure will lead to a 10% to 12% reduction in heart failure clinical consequences. He chooses as the single primary analysis for this trial the effect of therapy on the cumulative incidence rate of CHF mortality. He anticipates being able to randomize no more than 4000 to 5000 patients for this study.

The investigator estimates an 18 month CHF mortality rate will be 15% in the control group. Assuming 80% power and a two sided type I error of 0.05, the original sample size for this research effort reveals that it will take 4066 patients to demonstrate a 20% reduction in the actively treated group. However, the investigator believes that in this population a 10% to 12% reduction is the minimal clinical threshold that is worth detecting. In order to be able to detect this low level of efficacy with any statistical reliability, 11,731 patients must be recruited. However, if the investigator chooses to add to the CHF mortality the clinical event of CHF hospitalization, the number of events experienced in the placebo group will increase. In fact, if the cumulative control group event rate for this new combined endpoint of CHF death/CHF hospitalization is 34%, a sample size of 4094 patients will identify a 12% reduction in events that is due to the therapy. The ability of a sample size of approximately 4100 patients to identify clinically significant but smaller levels of therapy efficacy has been improved with the use of the combined endpoint (Figure 7.2).

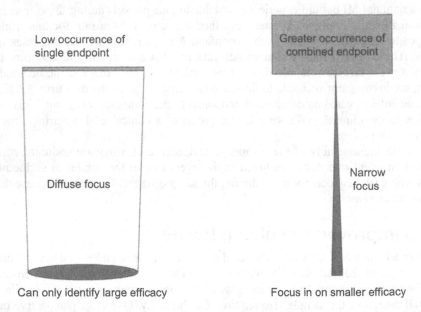

Figure 7.2. The use of a combined endpoint increases the resolving ability of a clinical trial to examine smaller clinically significant effect sizes.

The two advantages of adding a composite endpoint are broadening the measure of the therapy's effect on the disease and decreasing the required sample size or increasing the trial's ability to detect smaller efficacy levels. However, these advantages must be weighed against the problems with incorporating a combined endpoint into a clinical trial.

7.5 Properties of Combined Endpoints

We have just defined a combined endpoint. To appreciate the complications of embedding a composite endpoint into the structure of a clinical trial, we must develop the properties of combined endpoints. These properties can be divided into (1) coherence, (2) endpoint equivalence, and (3) therapy homogeneity.

7.6 Component Endpoint Coherence

There are many manifestations of chronic disease, and as we have pointed out, investigators who wish to study the effect of a therapy on the occurrence of that disease using a combined endpoint must choose the component endpoints from among these signs and symptoms. Some manifestations may measure common clinical and pathophysiologic correlates (e.g., fatal and nonfatal MI); others measure disparities (e.g., intraocular pressure and popliteal nerve conduction velocities in patients with diabetes mellitus). The component endpoints that make up the combined endpoint must be coherent-they should measure the same underlying pathophysiologic process and be consistent with the best understanding of the causes of the disease the investigators wish to study. Consideration of coherence requires an examination of the degree to which different component endpoints may measure related pathology. A balance must be struck between coincidence and separation of the singleton endpoints.

7.7 Coincidence

Since the combined endpoint is "built up" from the contributions of at least two and many times several singleton endpoints, the clinical relevance of the composite endpoint derives from the clinical meaning of its component endpoints from which it was constructed. Each component endpoint must measure not just the same disease process, but the same underlying pathophysiology. When each component endpoint is measuring the progression of the same pathology, then the investigator can be assured that the component endpoint is measuring the process which is best understood to excite the production of the disease's manifestations.

However, the component endpoints should not be so closely related that a patient is likely to experience all of them. These types of component endpoints we will term *coincident endpoints*. If a patient experiences one of two coincident endpoints, they are likely to experience the other. In this situation, there is no real advantage in using the combined endpoint instead of one of its component endpoints. Constructing component endpoints that are too interrelated will make the combined endpoint redundant.

For example, consider a clinical trial will study the effect of a randomly allocated medication in patients with diabetes mellitus. In this trial, patients will undergo a baseline blood sugar evaluation, receive the study medication (active or placebo), and then be followed for 6 months, at which time a second blood sugar evaluation will take place. The investigator could choose as the principle analysis the effect of the intervention on the combined endpoint of reduction in fasting blood glucose + reduction in HbA1c. There is no doubt that these two component endpoints measure the same underlying pathophysiology, i.e., the presence of glucose in the blood. A fasting blood glucose measurement reports the current level of blood sugar, a level that is transient and changes from day to day. The HbA1c level evaluation provides a more stable measure of blood sugar levels over approximately 3 months.

The randomly allocated therapy being evaluated in the trial is likely to reduce each of these measures of plasma glucose over the course of the study. At the conclusion of the study, patients who experience important reductions in their elevated blood sugar are also likely to experience reductions in their HbA1c. Thus, patients who experience one component endpoint are likely to experience the other. The events of reduction in blood sugar and reduction in HbA1c, while measuring the same underlying pathophysiology (abnormalities in carbohydrate metabolism) are measuring "too much of the same thing."

Even though they should measure the same underlying pathophysiology, the component endpoints of a composite endpoint should be different enough that a patient can experience either of the component endpoints, not just both. We might express this formally as follows in the case of a combined endpoint that is constructed from two component endpoints A and B each of which have incidence rates (e.g., total mortality or total hospitalizations). Recall that we defined the composite endpoint as the occurrence of either A, B, or both and denoted that event as the union of component endpoint A and component endpoint B. We wrote the combined endpoint as $A \cup B$.

Since the clinical trial will randomize a fixed number of subjects and follow them for a prespecified period of time, measuring the new occurrence of events, the event rates the trial will measure are incidence rates. We can use the probability of the occurrence of the endpoints in the placebo group as a representation of the placebo group incidence rate. Thus, $P[A \cup B]$ is the incidence rate of the composite endpoint over the course of the trial. From elementary probability, we can write

$$P[A \cup B] = P[A] + P[B] - P[A \cap B], \tag{7.1}$$

where $P[A]$ and $P[B]$ are the component event incidence rates for the singleton endpoints A and B. $P[A \cap B]$ is the incidence of the joint occurrence of the two of the component endpoints A and B. Recall also from elementary probability that

$$P[A \mid B] = \frac{P[A \cap B]}{P[B]}. \tag{7.2}$$

This can be written as $P[A \cap B] = P[A \mid B]P[B]$. Substituting this result into (7.1) reveals

$$P[A \cup B] = P[A] + P[B] - P[A \cap B]$$
$$= P[A] + P[B] - P[A \mid B]P[B] \qquad (7.3)$$
$$= P[A] + P[B](1 - P[A \mid B])$$

This last formulation directly links the probability of the occurrence of the combined endpoint to the probability of each of the component endpoints and the conditional probability of the occurrence of the component endpoint A given component endpoint B has occurred. When the P $[A \mid B] = 0$, the composite endpoint event rate $P[A \cup B]$ reaches its maximum value, i.e., the sum of the incidences rates for component endpoints A and B. What type of events must A and B be in order for the $P[A \mid B] = 0$ and for the cumulative incidence rate $P[A \cup B]$ to reach its maximum value?

7.8 Mutual Exclusivity and Disparate Events

In probability, when we consider the properties of events, a useful observation to make is whether the occurrence of one event excludes the occurrence of another event. We describe such joint events which cannot occur together (or for these purposes, cannot occur in the same patient during the course of the trial) as mutually exclusive events. As an illustration of this property, consider a clinical trial in which patients who have died are categorized by their cause of death. In this example let there be only two possible causes of death; cardiovascular death, or noncardiovascular death. If a patient is judged to have died a cardiovascular death, than that patient cannot have died a noncardiovascular death. We say that the event of dying from a cardiovascular event and the event of dying from a noncardiovascular death are mutually exclusive. The occurrence of one of these events excludes and makes impossible the occurrence of the other event.

When component endpoints A and B are mutually exclusive, then their joint occurrence is impossible and $P[A \cap B] = 0$. Thus, the probability that component endpoint A has occurred, given that endpoint B has occurred is zero (i.e., P $[A \mid B] = 0$). This implies that $P[A \cup B] = P[A] + P[B]$, When events are mutually exclusive the cumulative event of the union of events is simply the sum of the cumulative incidence rate of the composite endpoints. Thus, when the component endpoints cannot occur in the same patient, the largest combined endpoint event rate is attained. Mutual exclusivity of component events directly translates into the smallest sample size for the trial.

It is now easier to think through the problem with coincident component endpoints. If the component endpoints are very coincident, then the conditional probability $P[A \mid B]$ is close to one, and the cumulative event rate for the combined endpoint is only marginally larger than the incidence rate for the component endpoint A. The larger the conditional probability $P[A \mid B]$, the more coincident the component endpoints become. This in turn leads to a lower frequency of occurrence of the combined endpoint (i.e., smaller) $P[A \cup B]$ and a larger sample size for the clinical trial.

7.9 The Problem with Mutual Exclusivity

The prior discussion suggests that the selection of mutually exclusive component endpoints would be advantageous in constructing a combined endpoint. However, the difficulty with the use of mutually exclusive singleton endpoints is that they can measure different characteristics of the same disease that physicians are unaccustomed to linking together. This can produce serious problems in the interpretation of the results. Even though the choice of mutually exclusive component endpoints minimizes the required sample size for an evaluation of the effect of the intervention on the combined endpoint, care should be taken to assure that the component endpoints are not too disparate.

As an example of the problems that disparate component endpoints can produce, consider a clinical trial that will measure the effect of a randomly allocated intervention on the signs and symptoms of diabetes mellitus. The combined endpoint for this trial is blood sugar levels > 300 mg/dl + the occurrence of peripheral neuropathy. This is a difficult composite endpoint to defend. There is no doubt that diabetes mellitus produces both elevations in blood glucose and peripheral neuropathy. However, the two events are not closely linked. Changes in blood sugar can be acute, while the development of peripheral neuropathy is chronic, appearing after many years of exposure to the complex metabolic derangements produced by the disease. It is difficult to make clinical sense out of a combined measure of two manifestations of a disease that themselves are not very clearly linked together pathophysiologically. If the component endpoints become too disparate, it can become very difficult to describe exactly what the combined endpoint is measuring that is of direct clinical relevance. Choosing component endpoints, several of which are likely to occur in the same patient, may not produce the combined endpoint that leads to the smallest sample size but it can make the trial's results much easier to interpret.

The occurrence of multiple component endpoints in the same patient during the course of the trial, however, admits a possible problem with the use of combined endpoints that the trial planners must overcome. Since it is possible that a patient can experience each of the components of a combined endpoint, care must be taken to ensure that the patient is not considered to have reached the combined endpoint multiple times. Consider a clinical trial in which the prospectively defined primary analysis is the effect of therapy on the combined endpoint of total mortality + hospitalization due to CHF. It is possible (perhaps even likely) that a patient who meets the inclusion/exclusion criteria of the study could experience a hospitalization for CHF (perhaps experience multiple distinct hospitalizations for CHF) and then subsequently die. In the analysis of this endpoint, even though the patient has satisfied the criteria for the combined endpoint more than once, that patient can only be counted as having reached this endpoint once.[4] Commonly, the prospective

---

[4] This does not mean that in a randomized clinical trial in which patients are expected to be followed for 5 years, a patient who reaches one nonmortal component of the prospectively defined combined endpoint early in their follow-up should not be followed for the duration of the study. Post-event measurements, which include the occurrence of adverse events and the possible occurrence of secondary endpoints subsequent to the occurrence of the primary

determination is made that the first time the patient reaches the primary endpoint of the study, the patient is considered to have reached the endpoint. In our example, the patient who suffered multiple hospitalizations for CHF and subsequently died during the hospitalization is considered to have reached the primary endpoint upon the first hospitalization.

7.10 Balancing the Separation

Component endpoints in clinical trial are commonly not mutually exclusive; patients can experience combinations of the singleton endpoints which make up the component endpoint. However, the component endpoints of a composite endpoint should be contributory and coherent—they must make sense. Each of the components endpoints should measure the same underlying pathophysiology, but be different enough that they add a dimension to the measurement of the disease process that has not been contributed by any other component endpoint.

As an example of a combined endpoint whose component endpoints reflect a balance of distinct component endpoints, consider the design and results of the Cholesterol and Recurrent Event (CARE) trial [1]. CARE evaluated the effect of the HMG-CoA reductase inhibitor pravastatin on the reduction in morbidity and mortality in patients at risk of developing atherosclerotic disease. The CARE trial recruited 4159 patients with a history of recent MI and with low-density lipoprotein (LDL) cholesterol levels between 115 mg/dl and 174 mg/dl. These patients were randomized to either standard care or standard care plus pravastatin 40 mg once a day. The prospectively chosen primary endpoint that was the only primary analysis of this study was fatal CAD + nonfatal MI. Each of the two component endpoints of this composite endpoint is an important manifestation of the same atherosclerotic cardiovascular disease process. Each singleton endpoint is in its own right an important clinical manifestation of ischemic heart disease.

After randomization, patients were followed for a median duration of time of 5 years. During that time, the investigators worked to ensure that the investigators assigned to determine whether any of the singleton endpoints had been reached were blinded from knowing whether the patient had been assigned active therapy or placebo therapy. In CARE, this also meant that investigators were not to receive information about the patient's plasma lipid levels. Treatment guidelines based on lipid levels were provided by the trial's coordinating center to a matched patient. This matched patient received study medication in addition to mask any additional therapy required by a patient at the same clinical center in the opposite randomized group[5]. From the results of CARE [2] we can assess the degree to which the component endpoints measure the same event (Table 7.2).

---

endpoint are two of many reasons why patients should continue to be followed until the end of the study.

[5] This required tremendous effort in the trial, but insulated the trial from the criticism that it was unblinded de facto.

Table 7.2 Component Endpoint Frequency of Occurrence in CARE

	Number of events	Incidence rate
Fatal CHD	215	0.052
Nonfatal MI	308	0.074
Joint Occurrence	37	0.009

In CARE, there were 215 patients who experienced the fatal CAD component of the primary endpoint. The nonfatal MI component endpoint was observed in 308 patients and 37 patients had both a nonfatal MI and a CAD death.

We can utilize formula (7.2) to compute the probability that a patient has a CAD death given that they experienced a nonfatal MI as 0.009/0.074 = 0.12. If these two component endpoints were coincident, then there would have been many more patients who experienced both a nonfatal MI and a fatal CAD death. In CARE, even though the component endpoints measure the same underlying pathophysiology, these singleton endpoints are not coincident.

Perhaps a useful rule of thumb in determining whether there is sufficient difference in what the component endpoints are measuring is whether the component endpoints require different documentation. Within the clinical trial mechanism, the occurrence of multiple events in the same trial participant often translates into the requirement of different and distinct documentation to confirm the occurrence of each of the singleton endpoints. In the example of a clinical trial for which the composite endpoint is total mortality + hospitalization for CHF, the documentation for the occurrence of total mortality is insufficient to document the occurrence of a hospitalization for CHF. Each of these two component endpoints requires its own standard of documentation. The total mortality singleton endpoint will require information such as a death certificate and perhaps eye witness accounts that describe the circumstances surrounding the patient's death. Documentation of the occurrence of a hospitalization for CHF will at least require a hospital discharge summary. The difference in the type of documentation required by these two endpoints is a reflection of the distinctions between these morbid and mortal events. Thus, although the component endpoints of a combined endpoint should be coherent, i.e., they should be reflections of the same disease process, they require different documentation as a demonstration of their distinctive features.

7.11 Component Endpoint Equivalence

There is no doubt that component endpoints have been very useful in the design and analysis of clinical trials. However, the techniques and tools of analysis of these endpoints can be complex. In some circumstances, the complications induced by the analyses of these complicated endpoints can undermine and even negate any advantage the combined endpoint itself offered.

The component endpoints that make up the composite endpoint are typically of two types. One type is the endpoint measurement that is itself a number e.g., change in blood pressure. Since a patient's blood-pressure change over time can assume any value (within a reasonable range) including fractions, this type of endpoints is defined as a *continuous endpoint*. Other examples of continuous endpoints are changes in LVEF and reductions in HbA1c levels. Other endpoint measures are not continuous. They either occur or they do not occur. The simplest and best example is death—a patient either dies or survives. In this case there is no intermediate value. An endpoint such as death is described as a *dichotomous or (0–1) endpoint*. While death is the clearest example of a dichotomous endpoint, other examples are hospitalization (a patient is either hospitalized or not), or the requirement of chemotherapy.[6]

Analysis tools for component endpoints which are either continuous or dichotomous are well described [3], [4]. However, analysis tools for combinations of these endpoints can be complex, and sometimes may not be generally accepted. Even in the simplest cases, the analysis of the composite endpoint may make some questionable assumptions. As an illustration, consider the circumstance of a clinical trial whose prospectively defined combined endpoint is assembled from two dichotomous component endpoints. The first component endpoint is death and the second component of this composite endpoint is hospitalization. The patient is considered to have met the criteria for the combined endpoint (said to have "reached" the combined endpoint) if they have either died during the course of the trial, or they survived the trial but were hospitalized during the study. In the case of a patient who is hospitalized and then dies during the clinical trial, only the first endpoint is counted. As described earlier, this analytic tool avoids the problem of counting a patient more than once if they have experienced multiple hospitalizations.

While this analysis is useful, it makes the explicit assumption that each of the two components of this combined endpoint is analytically equivalent to the other. Whether a patient meets the hospitalization part of the endpoint or the mortality part of the endpoint doesn't matter as far as the analysis is concerned. But is a hospitalization the same as a death? Is this assumption of equivalence a true reflection of clinical reality? While one might possibly make the argument that a patient who is admitted to a hospital in stage four heart failure is close to death, an investigator would not need to look very far to find someone who disagrees with the assumption that this complicated hospitalization is equivalent to death. Obviously, less sick patients can be hospitalized but survive to lead productive lives, a circumstance that is clearly not the clinical equivalent of death.

A similar debate might be sparked in the consideration of the equivalence assumption for patients who reach the prospectively defined composite endpoint of fatal or nonfatal MI. Since patients who suffer and survive heart attacks can live for years, be involved in gainful employment, participate in community activities, en-

---

[6] Sometimes a continuous endpoint is converted to a dichotomous endpoint prospectively. An example of this type of conversion would be reduction in blood sugar, in which case the endpoint is not the magnitude of the reduction in blood sugar, but whether the blood sugar has been reduced by a prespecified amount, e.g., 25 mg/dl.

joy their families, and even be enrolled in subsequent clinical trials whose entry criteria require a prior MI, is it reasonable to assume that MI and subsequent survival is equivalent to MI with immediate death?

This equivalence can be a troubling assumption and can complicate acceptability of the combined endpoint. Of course, there are alternative algorithms that are available that would provide different "weights" for the occurrence of the various component endpoints of a combined endpoint. For example, one might assume that for the combined endpoint of death + hospitalizations a death is three times as influential as a hospitalization. However, it is very difficult for investigators to reach a consensus on the correct weighting scheme to use, and any selection of weights that the investigators choose that is different from equal weighting for each of the components of the combined endpoint is difficult to defend. Unfortunately, at this point there is no commonly accepted way out of this analytic enigma in clinical trials.

The situation only worsens when continuous and dichotomous component endpoints are combined in the same composite endpoint. How would one construct an analysis tool for the combined endpoint that has two component endpoints: (1) death or (2) reduction by at least ten units in LVEF? Not only is there the equivalence issue, but there is also the fact that, while the exact date of the patient's death is known, the date when the patient first experienced a ten unit reduction in their ejection fraction after they were randomized is not known.[7] Complicated analysis procedures that address this issue have been developed [5]. However, as revealed at conversations held by the Cardiovascular and Renal Drugs Advisory Committee of the FDA, these endpoints can be difficult to understand, and their acceptance by the medical community is guarded at best [6].

7.12 Therapy Homogeneity

As pointed out in the previous section, an important trait of a combined endpoint is that each of its component endpoints should reflect an important clinical manifestation of the disease. However, the purpose of the selection of a combined endpoint is that it not only provides a persuasive depiction of disease morbidity and mortality, but that it also be a useful metric against which the effect of the clinical trial's intervention will be tested. Therefore, from the investigators' point of view, it would be most useful if the composite endpoint is sensitive to the therapy that will be assessed in the clinical study. This situation is most likely to occur if each of the component endpoints that make up the combined endpoint is itself responsive to the therapy to be tested in the clinical trial. The homogeneity of the therapy effect for each of the singleton endpoints permits a fairly straightforward assessment of the prediction of the effect of therapy on the combined endpoint; this is a necessary feature in the traditional sample size computation of the trial[8]. In addition, therapy

---

[7] This could only be known if the patient had an ejection fraction measured each day of the trial.

[8] A brief primer on sample size computations is provided in Appendix D, and an exploration of sample size computations in the presence of heterogeneity of singleton endpoints is provided in Appendix E.

homogeneity helps to avoid interpretative difficulties when the medical community considers the intervention's effect at the conclusion of the study. In addition, as recalled from Chapters 5 and 6, the presence of therapy homogeneity can be exploited in allocating type I error among dependent statistical hypothesis tests.

As an example of a combined endpoint, whose component endpoints reflect consistent therapy homogeneity, we can return to the example of the CARE trial. Recall that CARE evaluated the effect of the HMG-CoA reductase inhibitor pravastatin on the reduction of morbidity and mortality in patients at risk of developing atherosclerotic disease. The primary analysis in CARE was the evaluation of the effect of pravastatin on the cumulative incidence rate of fatal CAD + nonfatal MI. As pointed out earlier in this chapter, each of the two component endpoints of this composite endpoint measures the same pathophysiology; however, the endpoints are distinct enough from each other to capture different manifestations of the same pathology.

For the prospectively defined analysis in CARE, patients were considered to have met the composite endpoint if they either (1) died from coronary artery disease or (2) survived the trial, but during the course of the trial, experienced a nonfatal myocardial infarction[9]. The effect of pravastatin was assessed at the conclusion of the trial (Table 7.3).

Table 7.3. Effect of pravastatin on the combined endpoint in CARE.

Endpoint	Placebo (n = 2078)		Active (n = 2081)		Relative Risk	95% CI	p-value
	n	%	n	%			
Combined endpoint							
Fatal CHD + nonfatal MI	274	13.2	212	10.2	0.76	[0.64 - 0.91]	0.003
Component Endpoints							
Fatal CHD	119	5.7	96	4.6	0.80	[0.61-1.05]	0.1
Nonfatal MI	173	8.3	135	6.5	0.77	[0.61-0.96]	0.02

Pravastatin therapy lowered the mean low-density lipoprotein (LDL) cholesterol level by 32% and maintained average levels of LDL cholesterol of 97 to 98 mg/dl throughout the 5 years of follow-up. During follow-up, the LDL cholesterol level was 28% lower in the pravastatin group than in the placebo group, the total cholesterol level was 20% lower and the high-density lipoprotein (HDL) cholesterol level was 5 % higher.

---

[9] A patient could, of course, suffer both a nonfatal MI and subsequently die from CAD. In the analysis of a composite endpoint which is not continuous (e.g., blood pressure change, that can have a large number of values) but death, (that either occurs or does not, described as dichotomous), the time to the event is taken into account in the analysis. In this circumstance, when a patient experiences each of two dichotomous component endpoints, the patient is not counted twice. Instead, the earliest occurring of the two endpoints is the endpoint that is counted.

CARE was a positive study. The frequency of the composite primary endpoint was 10.2% in the pravastatin group and 13.2% in the placebo group, reflecting a 24% reduction in risk. The use of pravastatin produced a relative risk of 0.76, representing a 24% reduction in the incidence of the combined endpoint of fatal CAD + Nonfatal MI. Note, however, the degree to which pravastatin affected each of the two components of the composite endpoint. Pravastatin produced a relative risk of 0.80 for the fatal CAD component of the primary endpoint, and a 0.77 relative risk for the nonfatal MI component of the endpoint. Not only was the combined endpoint coherent, but it also demonstrated therapy homogeneity.

7.13 Composite Endpoint Measurement Rules

The previous sections of this chapter discussed the considerations that the investigators must give to the details of the composite endpoint's construction. However, there are additional requirements that must be satisfied for the successful incorporation of a composite endpoint into a clinical trial. These additional requisites will now be reviewed.

7.14 Prospective Identification

As pointed out in the earlier chapters of this book, the incorporation of an endpoint into the primary analysis of a clinical trial must follow certain principles. These principles require the prospective identification of the endpoint and the plan for its analysis. The motivations for this rule have been discussed in detail in Chapters 2 to 4. Although that discussion focused on a single endpoint (e.g., total mortality), the guiding concept also applies to the evaluation of the effect of a randomly allocated intervention in a clinical trial on a composite endpoint.

As was the case for the single endpoint, the composite endpoint must be specified in great detail during the design phase of the trial. This description must include how each of the composite endpoint's components will be ascertained. In addition, a committee of investigators is commonly chosen to determine whether a component endpoint has occurred. The procedures put in place to blind or mask these investigators from the identity of the randomly allocated therapy to which the patient was assigned should be elucidated. In addition, the analysis plan for the combined endpoint must also be detailed. Any weighting scheme that will be used in assessing the contribution each component endpoint makes to the combined endpoint must be determined a priori, and should be acceptable to the medical and regulatory community. If there are plans to submit the results of the clinical trial to a regulatory agency, then that agency should be completely and fully informed about the details of both the construction of the combined endpoints and its analysis before the experiment begins.

The requirement of concordant trial execution is critical to the successful implementation of the composite endpoint in a study. Just as it is unacceptable to change the definition of the endpoints used in a study's principle analyses, it is equally crucial to keep the constitution of the clinical trial's combined endpoint fixed. Specifically, the component endpoints of a composite endpoint should be prospectively chosen and locked in. New component endpoints should not be added nor should established components be removed. The same chaotic effects[10] that can weaken and destroy the interpretation of a clinical trial, whose principle analyses involve a single endpoint,can also wreak havoc on the evaluation of a composite endpoint primary analysis.

7.15 Combined Endpoint Ascertainment

The accurate assessment of the component endpoint's interpretation in a clinical trial is both critical and complicated. To understand this new complexity introduced by the use of a composite endpoint, first consider a clinical trial that has the effect of the intervention on the cumulative incidence of CAD death as its sole primary analysis. At the conclusion of the research, the study's investigators must classify the experience of each of the randomized patient's as one of (1) survival, (2) death due to a non-CAD cause, or (3) death due to CAD.

In well-conducted clinical trials, specific documentation is collected to confirm that a patient reported by an investigator to have died is actually dead and, if they are dead, the cause of that death. These confirmatory steps are taken in order to ensure that living patients are not mistakenly assumed to have died. However, the investigators must also collect data confirming that a patient believed to be alive is in fact alive, a check that avoids the opposite mistake of assuming that a dead patient is actually living. While this last step is a straightforward matter for patients who have attended each visit, there is commonly a subset of patients who have missed several of the most recent visits and from whom no information has been collected. It is on these patients that intense activity is exerted to determine if they are either alive (as suspected) or have died.

The situation is much more complicated when a composite endpoint is to be part of the primary analysis of a clinical trial. If, in the above illustration, the investigators chose as a primary endpoint not just CAD death, but CAD death + nonfatal MI, the investigators have an additional inspection to complete. Not only must they assure themselves of the vital status of each patient; they must also determine whether an MI has occurred in all patients. Of course, specific documentation will be collected from patients who volunteer the information that they have suffered an MI. However not every patient who experiences a heart attack reports the event to the investigators.[11] Occasionally, in some patients, the MI may have produced no symptoms at all (silent MIs). Mistakenly assuming that these patients who have experienced an MI were infarct free would lead to an inaccurate count of the number of patients who had this event.

The provision of assurance that patients who did not report a MI in fact did not experience an MI can be an expensive task. Investigators, after determining that a patient has survived the trial, must also ask that surviving patient if they suffered a heart attack during the course of the study that the patient did not previously re-

---

[10] These effects are described in Chapter 2.

[11] For example, the MI and associated hospitalization might have occurred while the patient was on vacation and the patient was out of contact with the clinical trial's investigator.

port.[12] The determination of the occurrence of silent MIs can be especially problematic. Although many of these silent events can be identified by requiring every patient to undergo annual electrocardiograms, obtaining and interpreting these evaluations is expensive. Also, if a silent MI is found to have occurred, its exact date can be impossible to determine.

As a final complication, consider the task awaiting investigators who have prospectively chosen the combined endpoint of CAD death/nonfatal MI/unstable angina pectoris. The evaluation of the unstable angina component, whose occurrence is commonly unrecognized and unreported, can add an overwhelming logistical burden onto the clinical trial apparatus. However, the study's investigators must complete this onerous task. Recall that, in the analysis of the composite endpoint, the occurrence of unstable angina is just as critical as the occurrence of the other two components of the combined endpoint. If each of the component endpoints is important, then each must be measured with the same high standard of accuracy and precision. Clearly, the greater the number of component endpoints in the study, the more work the investigators must complete in order to assure both themselves, the medical community, and the regulatory community that they have an accurate count of the number of endpoints which have taken place during the course of the study. This is one additional problem of embedding a complicated composite endpoint into a clinical trial that has limited financial and logistical resources.

7.16 Conclusions

The implementation of composite endpoints in clinical trials holds both great promise and great danger. A carefully constructed combined endpoint can helpfully broaden the definition of a clinical endpoint when the disease being studied has different clinical consequences. This expansion commonly increases the incidence of the endpoint and this property can be used to either reduce the sample size of the trial or, if a larger sample size is maintained to increase the sensitivity of the experiment to detect moderate levels of therapy effectiveness. However, if the combined endpoint is too broad it can become uninterpretable and ultimately meaningless to the medical and regulatory communities. Thus, the combined endpoint should be both broad and simultaneously retain its interpretability. We have termed this property coherence. Additionally, there should be some experiential evidence or at least theoretical motivation justifying the expectation that the therapy to be studied in the trial will have the same effect on each of the component endpoints of the combined endpoint. This we have termed the homogeneity of therapy effect.

In the next chapter, we will review some examples of the use of composite endpoints in clinical trials and describe how the number of confirmatory evaluations, that derive both from an evaluation of the effect of therapy for the composite endpoint and its components, may be expanded.

---

[12] As we stated earlier in this chapter, the time to the first component event experienced is the critical measure used in the analysis of the effect of the intervention on the composite endpoint, thus MI ascertainment is also important for patients who died during the course of the study.

Problems

1. Briefly describe the advantages that the use of composite endpoints bring to a clinical trial? What are the problems that these complicated endpoints introduce to the trial's execution and interpretation?
2. Why or why not should the singleton endpoints of prospectively defined primary endpoints be mutually exclusive?
3. What is the epidemiologic difficulty with an endpoint that captures only nonfatal clinical events?
4. Can you explain, without using mathematics, why the sample size of a clinical trial decreases when the primary endpoint event rate on which the sample size is based increases?
5. In a clinical trial designed to measure the effect of an anti-inflammatory drug on reducing the sequela of atherosclerotic cardiovascular disease, comment on the utility of the combined endpoint of fatal CAD death/automobile accidents. What would be the advantage of such an endpoint? What would be its interpretative disadvantages?
6. Discuss the weakness of the proposed combined endpoint of coronary artery bypass surgery/hospitalization from the perspective of coincident singleton endpoints. What does the coronary artery bypass surgery component add to the combined endpoint? Would you expect the probability of hospitalization given the patient is to have coronary artery bypass surgery to be close to one or close to zero?
7. How does the notion of homogeneity of therapy effect among the singleton endpoints of a composite endpoint affect that combined endpoint's interpretability?
8. Describe the impression that is introduced into the assessment of the impact of a randomly allocated therapy on a combined endpoint when different levels of quality assurance are implemented for the different singleton endpoints.

References

1. Pfeffer, M.A., Sacks. F.M., Moyé, L.A. et. al for the Cholesterol and Recurrent Events Clinical Trial Investigators (1995). Cholesterol and Recurrent Events (Cholesterol and recurrent events clinical trial) trial: A secondary prevention trial for normolipidemic patients. *American Journal of Cardiology*.76:98C–106C.
2. Sacks, F.M., Pfeffer, M.A., Moyé, L.A., Rouleau, J.L., Rutherford, J.D., Cole, T.G., Brown, L., Warnica, J.W., Arnold, J.M.O., Wun, C.C., Davis, B.R., Braunwald, E., for the Cholesterol and Recurrent Event Trial Investigators (1996). The effect of pravastatin on coronary events after myocardial infarction

in patients with average cholesterol levels. *New England Journal of Medicine*. **335**:1001–1009.

3. Meinert, C.L. (1986). *Clinical Trials Design, Conduct, and Analysis*, New York. Oxford University Press.

4. Piantadosi, S. (1997), *Clinical Trials: A Methodologic Perspective*. New York. John Wiley.

5. Moyé, L.A., Davis, B.R., Hawkins, C.M. (1992). Analysis of a clinical trial involving a combined mortality and adherence dependent interval censored endpoint. *Statistics in Medicine* **11**:1705–1717.

6 . Transcript of the Cardiovascular and Renal Drugs Advisory Committee to the FDA Captopril. February 16, 1993.

Chapter 8

Multiple Analyses and Composite Endpoints

In this chapter, we continue our discussion of the combined endpoint in clinical trials. Examples of the use of combined endpoints are provided, and illustrations of both exemplary and somewhat questionable incorporations of these complex entities within clinical trials are provided. Finally, we focus on the uses of the two tools; (1) unequal allocation of type I error and (2) measures of dependency between statistical hypothesis tests in the analysis of combined endpoints. When these devices are prospectively implemented within a clinical trial, the concordant execution of that trial permits confirmatory assessments of the effect of a randomly allocated intervention on both the combined endpoint and each of its component endpoints.

8.1 Examples of Composite Endpoint Use

As we saw in the last chapter, the decision to incorporate a combined endpoint into a clinical trial can be difficult. Its inclusion into a study expands the measurement of the disease process that the randomly allocated therapy was designed to improve. This broadened measure decreases the sample size of the trial and thereby reduces the administrative and logistical burden of the study's execution. Alternatively, use of a composite endpoint can enable the clinical trial to identify treatment effect sizes that may be modest but clinically significant. These smaller effect sizes may be too small to identify (with appropriate concern for type I and type II error rates) in a clinical trial in which a single endpoint was used as the primary analysis of the study, but can be successfully resolved through the use of a composite endpoint.

However, these complex composite endpoints that are constructed from other endpoints bring their own share of new difficulties. As with single endpoints, combined endpoints must be prospectively defined in extensive detail, and the clinical trial that tests the effect of the intervention on the composite endpoint must be concordantly executed. The successfully implemented combined endpoint must be broad enough to measure different aspects of the disease's manifestations, but should avoid a conglomeration of clinically disparate signs or symptoms of the disease process. There should be a knowledge base that supports the assumption that the randomly allocated therapy will be equally effective for each of the component endpoints. Finally, the use of a combined endpoint in a clinical trial requires that each of the combined endpoint's component endpoints must be measured with equally high precision.

The following represent three examples of the incorporation of a combined endpoint into a clinical trial.

8.2 Lipid Research Clinics

One of the earliest examples of the prospective incorporation of a combined endpoint into a clinical trial was the Lipid Research Clinic (LRC) experience [1]. The LRC study was prospectively designed as a randomized, controlled clinical trial that focused on the benefits and costs of controlling serum cholesterol levels in patients at risk of developing CAD.

As originally conceived, LRC was designed to evaluate the ability of the cholesterol-reducing agent, cholestyramine, to reduce the number of mortal events. Men between 35 and 60 years of age with total cholesterol levels greater than 265 mg/dl would be randomized to receive either diet alone or diet plus cholestyramine for the management of their lipid levels. The initial design of this trial concentrated on the ability of cholestyramine to reduce the cumulative incidence rate of fatal CAD. However, the sample size requirement for this trial exceeded the number of patients that were available [2]. The investigators therefore chose to evaluate the effect of therapy on a combined endpoint; the cumulative incidence rate of the CAD death + nonfatal MI. This prospectively chosen analysis was the primary analysis for the study. The primary results of this study were reported as positive [3] (Table 7.4).[1]

It is interesting to note the large number of events the nonfatal MI component contributes to the combined endpoint; there are more than four times as many patients with nonfatal MIs as there are patients who died a CAD death. We can examine the degree of coincidence between the two singleton endpoints by (see Table 7.4) computing the conditional probability of a CAD death given that a nonfatal MI has occurred. Let A be the component event of a fatal CAD death and B be the event of a nonfatal MI. From Table 7.4, there were 158 + 38 - 187 = 9 patients who had both a nonfatal MI and a CAD event (joint events) in the placebo group and 130 + 30 - 155 = 5 joint events that were observed to have occurred in the active group.

We have the information that we need to compute the probability of a CAD death given that a patient suffered a nonfatal MI. We first compute the probability of the joint occurrence (i.e., the occurrence of both events in the same patient) of a fatal MI or a CAD death from Table 4 as

$$P[A \cap B] = \frac{9+5}{1900+1906} = 0.0037.$$

Again, using data from Table 7.4, we can compute the probability of a nonfatal MI is

$$\frac{158+130}{1900+1906} = 0.076.$$

---

[1] The interpretation of the LRC trial was not without controversy. See Moyé [2], p. 132–133.

These are the preliminary calculations that we need to compute the conditional probability of a fatal CAD death given the occurrence of a fatal MI as

$$P[A \mid B] = \frac{P[A \cap B]}{P[B]} = \frac{0.0037}{0.076} = 0.049.$$

Patients who had a nonfatal MI in LRC were not very likely to have a CAD death.

As reported by the LRC, the effect of cholestyramine therapy produced a 24% reduction for the fatal component and 19% reduction in the nonfatal component, representing a reasonable degree of therapy effect homogeneity.

Table 8.1. Component Endpoint Frequency of Occurrence in The Lipid Research Clinic Study

N	Placebo 1900		Active 1906	
	Events	Rate	Events	Rate
CHD death	38	0.020	30	0.016
Nonfatal MI	158	0.083	130	0.068
Combined	187	0.098	155	0.081

LRC demonstrates fine prospective implementation of a combined endpoint in a clinical trial. The two singleton endpoints of CAD death and nonfatal MI were different manifestations of the same pathophysiology. The combined endpoint increased the placebo group event rate considerably above that of the component endpoint CAD death by (1) taking advantage of the relatively high event rate for the nonfatal MI component and (2) producing a low conditional probability of a CAD death given the occurrence of a nonfatal MI. Thus, the sample size of the trial based on the combined endpoint was considerably smaller than that for the component endpoints. Finally, the therapy effect was homogeneous across the two endpoints. The use of the composite endpoint carefully expanded the measure of atherosclerotic disease from the original design, decreased the sample size of the trial, and maintained therapy effect homogeneity.

8.3 UKPDS

An example of a clinical trial with a more complicated combined endpoint is the United Kingdom Prospective Diabetes Study (UKPDS). This was a multicenter, prospective, randomized, intervention trial of 5102 patients with newly diagnosed type 2 (non-insulin-dependent) diabetes mellitus from 23 centers in England, Northern Ireland, and Scotland. The UKPDS investigators have published 57 manuscripts describing various features of this study's design, execution, and analysis. However, we will concentrate here on the construction, alteration, and interpretation of the combined endpoint of this trial.

This study was designed to evaluate the impact of improved blood glucose control on the complications of diabetes mellitus with particular emphasis placed on reductions in morbidity and mortality [4]. Patients who had newly diagnosed type II diabetes mellitus were randomized to either diet for control of their hyperglycemia (control group), or to insulin and a sulfonylurea therapy (active group). The investigators believed that the pharmacologic therapy employed in the active group would reduce blood glucose to near normal levels. Thus, the UKPDS was putting to the test the theory that reduction of blood sugar to near normal levels would reduce the incidence of long-term complications of diabetes mellitus. This important concept in the treatment of diabetes remained unanswered after the controversial conclusions of the University Group Diabetes Program (UGDP) which found that there was no clinical benefit from the use of insulin or sulfonylurea/metformin therapy in patients with type II diabetes, and that tolbutamide was associated with an increase in cardiovascular mortality [5].

The protocol for this trial was written in 1976. Recruitment took place from 1977 to 1991. The study ended in 1997 at a cost of £23 million.

The endpoint that the UKPDS investigators chose was quite complex (Table 7.5). Diabetes mellitus increases the cumulative total mortality rate. It has been associated with an increase in the rate of MIs (both fatal and nonfatal), and strokes (fatal and nonfatal). In addition, diabetes mellitus increases the cumulative incidence rate of renal failure, amputations, and blindness. The UKDPS investigators were interested in testing the effect of reductions in blood sugar to near normal levels on the cumulative incidence rate of each of these major complications. However, many of these complications take years to develop, especially in a population that consists of newly diagnosed diabetic patients.

Even though the UKPDS investigators planned to follow the randomized cohort for many years [6], they suspected that this duration of follow-up would not be long enough to accrue enough events for any of the component endpoints to justify the use of that component endpoint as a primary analysis of the study. Therefore, in order to increase the number of events, the UKPDS investigators prospectively combined many of the component endpoints, reflecting all of the major consequences of diabetes mellitus into a supercombined endpoint. The combined endpoint had fatal and nonfatal components that reflected the longterm cardiovascular, renal, peripheral vascular, and ophthalmologic sequela of diabetes mellitus (Table 8.2).

Table 8.2. Prospectively chosen combined endpoint in UKPDS.
fatal and nonfatal complications of diabetes mellitus

Fatal Endpoints: Diabetes Related Deaths
        Cardiac death
        Stroke death
        Renal death
        Hyperglycemic/hypoglycemic death
        Sudden death

Nonfatal Endpoints
        Nonfatal MI
        Angina pectoris
        Major stroke
        Minor limb complications
        Blindness in one eye
        Renal failure

When the UKPDS was started in 1977, the investigators believed that the improved blood glucose control might reduce the incidence of diabetes-related complications by 40% [7]. The original sample size computation revealed that 3600 patients were required in order to detect this large an effect with 81% power and a two sided type I error rate of 0.01. This was, at the time, the single largest clinical trial that examined the effect of "tight control" of blood glucose on the long-term consequences of diabetes. According to the investigators "If intensive therapy for 11 years is found to be either neutral or disadvantageous in effect, we would conclude that the potential degree of benefit may not be worth the effort of intensive therapy including the increased risk of hypoglycemia" [6, p. 443].

However, midway through the trial a change was made. In 1987, an interim review of the data revealed that is was very unlikely that a 40% reduction in the cumulative incidence of the endpoints would be seen. The investigators were now interested in detecting at least a 20% reduction in the incidence of the combined endpoint, for which they had adequate power [4, Table 6]. Later, as the trial progressed, the investigators determined that a 15% reduction in the occurrence of the composite endpoints was more realistic. An additional sample size computation revealed that the randomization of 3867 patients would provide adequate power (81% power) to measure the effect of intensive therapy on the cumulative incidence rate of the composite endpoint.

The results of UKPDS were reported in 1998 [7] (Table 8.3). This trial demonstrated a 12% reduction in the cumulative incidence rate of any diabetes-related complication (95% CI 1% to 21%; $p = 0.029$). At first glance, these results are statistically significant, although there are major interpretative problems due to the discordant trial execution. We cannot help but notice that the demonstration of a 12% reduction in any complication of type II diabetes mellitus falls far short of the initial prospective determination of a 40% efficacy and, in fact, is even

Table 8.3.   Results of United Kingdom Prospective Diabetes Study (UKPDS)

	Active rx. (n = 2729)	Conv. rx. (n = 1138)	P-value	Rel. risk	95% CI*
Composite endpoints	963	238	0.029	0.88	[0.79 – 0.99]
Fatal endpoints	285	129	0.340	0.90	[0.73 – 1.11]
Fatal MI	207	90	0.630	0.94	[0.68 – 1.30]
Stroke deaths	43	15	0.600	1.17	[0.54 – 2.54]
Renal deaths	8	2	0.530	1.83	[0.21 – 12.49]
Glucose related**	1	1	0.523	0.420***	[0.03 – 6.66]
Sudden death	24	18	0.047	0.54	[0.24 – 1.21]
Death from PVD****	2	3	0.120	0.26	[0.03 – 2.77]
Nonfatal endpoints					
Nonfatal MI	197	101	0.067	0.79	[0.58 – 1.09]
Angina pectoris	177	72	0.910	1.02	[0.71 – 1.46]
Major stroke	114	44	0.720	1.07	[0.68 – 1.69]
Amputation	27	18	0.990	0.81	[0.28 – 1.33]
Blindness	78	38	0.390	0.84	[0.51 – 1.40]
Renal failure	16	9	0.450	0.76	[0.53 – 1.08]
Photocoagulation*****	207	117	0.003	0.71	[0.53 – 0.96]

*Confidence Interval
**Hypoglycemic or hyperglycemic death.
*** p- value and confidence interval were computed by the author from data.
presented in the manuscript.
****Peripheral vascular disease.
****Retinal photocoagulation (not prospectively stated).

less than the 20% efficacy level and the 15% efficacy levels that were the newly stated design parameters of UKPDS in the middle of this study.

Although the results of the United Kingdom Prospective Diabetes Study are controversial, our focus here will be on the construction of its combined endpoint. The assembly of this structure was complex, since it included aspects of cardiovascular disease (cardiac death, stroke, angina pectoris), renal disease (renal death and renal failure), peripheral vascular disease (amputation), death due to the extreme and unpredictable post-randomization fluctuations in blood sugar (hypoglycemic/hyperglycemic death), and ophthalmologic findings (blindness in one eye). This is a very diverse endpoint examining the effects of diabetes on multiple organ structures. However, in all fairness to the investigators, they hoped to demonstrate that an active aggressive plan to maintain blood sugar levels as close as possible to normal would have a uniformly beneficial effect on each of these endpoints. Thus, while this composite endpoint may seem very broad, it measures exactly those manifestations of diabetes mellitus that the UKPDS investigations believed would be affected by therapy.

However, it was not only the efficacy of the design parameter that was allowed to change during the course of the trial; the constitution of the composite endpoint appears to have altered as well. The UKPDS design manuscript [4] that listed the components of the combined endpoint did not mention that retinal photocoagulation would be part of the UKPDS endpoint. However, at the conclusion of the study, we find that retinal coagulation was included as part of the combined endpoint.

The inclusion of this new endpoint introduces a new complexity into the UKPDS result analysis. Unlike other component endpoints of death, or amputation, which can be directly interpreted by the medical community, the assessment of the effect of intensive therapy on photocoagulation can be problematic. Its occurrence is based on visits to physicians and eye doctors and referrals. While these effects would be expected to be nonpreferentially distributed across the two treatment groups, this distribution does not dismiss the concern for the addition of the photocoagulation endpoint. As we have pointed out in Chapter 2, changing clinical trial design parameters (e.g., efficacy measures and endpoints) after the trial has been initiated, introduces complexities that can make the results of that trial uninterpretable. What is to be gained by adding a photocoagulation measure to the UKPDS combined endpoint when the investigators already had a straightforward, easily interpreted measure of ophthalmologic disease in UKPDS—blindness?

The addition of the photocoagulation endpoint to the composite endpoint of UKDPS is all the more remarkable because this component endpoint makes up $(207+117)/(963+438) = 23\%$ of all the component endpoints used in the combined endpoint. This non-prospectively defined, singleton endpoint contributes over 20% of the total number of endpoint events that compose the composite endpoint of the UKPDS. In a very real sense, photocoagulation dominates the other component endpoints. Unfortunately, this most prevalent component of the combined endpoint is also its least persuasive.

Equally remarkable is the observation that, of all the component endpoints in the UKPDS combined endpoint, only retinal photocoagulation is even nominally statistically significant. Each of the other component endpoints is consistent with no effect of intensive therapy. In fact, it is the finding for the effect of therapy on the photocoagulation component that produces the statistical significance of the composite endpoint. These observations do not increase our confidence in the findings of the UKPDS.

8.4 HOPE

The final illustration of a clinical trial that integrated a composite endpoint into its primary analyses is the Heart Outcomes Prevention Evaluation (HOPE). By the mid 1990s, ACE-i therapy had demonstrated its effectiveness as an important treatment not just for systemic hypertension but also for the treatment of CHF. The clinical trials SOLVD [8], [9] and Survival and Left Ventricular Enlargement (SAVE)

[10] demonstrated that the administration of ACE-i therapy could reduce morbidity and prolong survival in patients who have left ventricular dysfunction and CHF. However, there was interest in testing the effectiveness of ACE-i inhibitor therapy in reducing morbidity and mortality caused by ischemic cardiovascular disease.

The HOPE trial was designed to test the effectiveness of the ACE-i therapy (ramipril and vitamin E) in reducing morbidity and mortality in patients who were at risk of developing ischemic cardiovascular disease [11]. HOPE was a randomized, prospective, double-blind clinical trial. Patients who were recruited for this study were required to have either (1) evidence of cardiovascular disease (coronary artery disease, peripheral vascular disease, or a prior stroke), or (2) the presence of risk factors for the development of ischemic cardiovascular disease (diabetes mellitus plus at least one of the following: hypertension, cigarette smoking, hyperlipidemia, or microalbuminuria). Patients were to be randomized to either (1) placebo therapy (2) vitamin E alone (3) ramipril alone, or (4) vitamin E + ramipril. This experimental design provided the investigators the flexibility that they needed to evaluate the effect of each of the two active compounds alone or in combination.[2]

The primary analysis for the effect of ACE-i therapy in HOPE was the effect of ramipril on the composite endpoint of cardiovascular death + nonfatal MI + nonfatal stroke. The investigators believed that a clinically important and biologically plausible risk reduction would be 15% to 20% [11, p. 133]. For this they would need to recruit over 9000 patients and follow them for 3.5 years. However, it was also prospectively stated that the Data and Safety Monitoring Board was empowered to increase the duration of follow-up, which it chose to do, prolonging the follow-up period to 5 years.[3]

The results of HOPE were remarkable [12]. Ramipril produced a 22% reduction in the relative risk of the combined endpoint. In addition, the effect of therapy was homogeneous across each of the component endpoints from which the composite endpoint was constructed (Table 8.4). This uniformity of response to treatment demonstrated that ramipril's effect was not just on one component of the composite endpoint, but instead, ramipril had a beneficial effect on each of the singleton measures of cardiovascular disease. Regardless of the prospectively defined manifestation of cardiovascular disease, ACE-i therapy reduced its cumulative incidence. This is a very clear and very powerful message.

---

[2] This style of design, where two separate treatments are provided individually and in combination with different patients in a completely randomized way is commonly referred to as a *factorial design*.

[3] Making a decision based on data demonstrating the effectiveness of the therapy opens the door to the possibility that the data from this preliminary examination of the trial's results determined the interim decision to continue follow-up, a process that is at the heart of random research (Chapter 2). The HOPE investigators have assured the scientific community that this decision to prolong the study was made in the absence of knowledge about the interim results of the trial.

Table 8.4. Primary analyses of the HOPE trial.

Endpoint	Placebo rx. (n = 4652)		Active rx. (n = 4645)		Rel risk	95% CI*	p- value
	n	%	n	%			
Combined endpoint							
MI**, stroke, or CV*** death	826	17.8	651	14	0.78	[0.70 – 0.86]	<0.001
Component endpoints							
CV death	377	8.1	282	6.1	0.74	[0.64 – 0.87]	<0.001
MI	570	12.3	459	9.9	0.80	[0.70 – 0.90]	<0.001
Stroke	236	4.9	156	3.4	0.68	[0.56 – 0.84]	<0.001

*Confidence interval.
**MI.
***Cardiovascular.

The investigators designed HOPE to identify an effect of ramipril on the combined endpoint with a low type I error probability. Thus, given that ramipril was so effective, it comes as no surprise that the effect of the therapy produces a small p-value ($p < 0.001$) for the composite endpoint. What is surprising is that the effect of ramipril resulted in large effect sizes and small p-values for not just the combined endpoints, but for the effect of therapy on each of the component endpoints as well. For the singleton endpoints (1) death from a cardiovascular cause, (2) nonfatal MI, and (3) stroke, the relative risks associated with therapy revealed at least a 20% reduction and the p-values are each < 0.001. Since one of the primary motivations for using a combined endpoint is to identify a clinically significant treatment effect when the event rates for the component endpoints will not yield statistical hypothesis tests of adequate power, one might wonder why the investigators did not choose the effect of therapy on a singleton endpoint (such as the cumulative incidence rate of cardiovascular death) as HOPE's principle analysis. Although there might be several reasons, one of them is that the trial was initially designed to have a 3.5 year follow-up. In that duration of time, a smaller number of events would occur in the trial, most likely producing an underpowered environment for the hypothesis tests to evaluate the effect of therapy for each of the component endpoints. It is possible that if the data were truncated at 3 years, the findings for the component endpoints might not be so strong, By increasing the duration of follow-up to 5 years, the additional observation period produced more events. Given the effectiveness of ACE-i therapy, this increased number of events decreased the standard error of the relative risk estimate and decreased the p-value.

8.5 Principles of Combined Endpoint Use

Combined endpoints are useful and effective tools to evaluate the effect of therapy in a clinical trial when the evaluation of the effect of therapy on the occurrence of that event will be underpowered. The FDA has accepted the use of combined endpoints in clinical trials as a useful tool in the development of a clinical trial program to evaluate the effect of an intervention. However, the implementation of these composite endpoints can be complicated. We have thus far established the following principles for the use of combined endpoints:

Principle 1.   The endpoint must be clinically relevant to the medical and regulatory communities. *(principle of clinical relevance.)*

Principle 2.   Both the combined endpoint and each of its component endpoints must be prospectively specified in detail *(principle of prospective deployment).*

Principle 3.   Each component of the combined endpoint must be carefully chosen to add coherence to the composite endpoint. The component endpoint that is under consideration must not be so similar to other components so that it adds nothing new to the mixture of singleton endpoints that will make up the combined endpoint, yet it should not be so dissimilar that it provides a measure which is customarily not clinically linked to the other component endpoints *(principle of coherence).*

Principle 4.   The component endpoints that constitute the combined endpoint are commonly given the same weight in the statistical analysis of the clinical trial. Therefore, each of the component endpoints must be measured with the same scrupulous attention to detail. For each component endpoint, it is important to provide documentation not just that the endpoint occurred, but it is equally important to confirm the absence of the component endpoint *(principle of precision).*

Principle 5.   The analysis of the effect of therapy on the composite endpoint should be accompanied by a tabulation of the effect of the therapy for each of the component endpoints, allowing the reader to determine if there has been any domination of the combined endpoint by any one of its components, or if the findings of the effect of therapy for component endpoints are not consistent *(principle of full disclosure).*

Careful attention to detail is required to incorporate a composite endpoint into a clinical trial's primary analyses in accordance with these four enunciated principles. Although following these principles can simplify the interpretation of the combined endpoint, assembling a combined endpoint based on them does not guarantee that the familywise error rate ξ will be conserved. We will now turn our attention to this matter, which is at the heart of the multiple analysis issue that affects the interpretation of composite endpoints in clinical trials. To guide our work, we will make the assumption that the investigators approve of and accept each of these four principles described above for the incorporation of the combined endpoint into their clinical trial.

8.6 α Allocation and Combined Endpoints

In this section, we provide useful guidelines for the use of composite endpoints in clinical trials, and then turn our attention to the allocation of type I error rates for the statistical hypothesis tests that evaluate the effect of therapy on these complicated endpoints.

8.6.1 Familywise Error Control Procedures

In our development of the use of composite endpoints in clinical trials, the concern for the familywise error probability now becomes a dominating issue. This issue was central to the correct interpretation of the effect of a randomly allocated intervention on a single endpoint in the clinical trial. In that circumstance, ethical concern focused on the possibility of misleading the medical community and the population at large about a promising beneficial therapy effect that was merely a spurious finding that appeared in the research sample just through the play of chance. We developed the concept of the familywise error rate, or the probability that at least one of the primary analyses that suggested a beneficial effect of therapy in a clinical trial was false (due to sampling error), and saw that the rate of this error increased with the number of statistical hypothesis tests that was executed.

Our approach in coming to grips with this issue has incorporated (1) recognition and acknowledgment of the investigators' desire to use a single data base to address many scientific questions, and (2) the ethical requirement that we must control the familywise error probability below a bound that is acceptable to the medical community. In order to balance the acknowledgment of the motivation and the requirement of the error rate, investigators should (1) triage analyses into the categories of primary analyses, secondary analyses, and exploratory analyses and (2) allocate a type I error rate prospectively to each of the primary analyses. Procedures were provided so that the computation of error rates could be completed in either the setting of hypothesis testing independence[4] or dependence.[5] These same procedures will be utilized here to allocate a type I error rate for primary analyses which include combined endpoints.

8.6.2 Multiple Analyses and Composite Endpoint Distress

While the composite endpoint, as we have defined it in the previous chapter is considered and analyzed as though it was a single endpoint, its common and appropriate usage imbues it with features that must be addressed within a multiple analysis paradigm. This is because the composite endpoint is made up of component endpoints that in and of themselves have special and particular meaning to the

---

[4] Chapter 4.
[5] Chapters 5 and 6.

medical community. In fact, commonly, it is the singleton endpoint's low cumulative event rate and not its medical relevance that preclude it from consideration as the endpoint for a primary analysis of a clinical trial. It is therefore no surprise that interest continues in the medical and regulatory communities for an examination of the effect of therapy on the singleton endpoints that constitute the composite endpoint (principle of full disclosure).

In addition, there are circumstances that can bedevil the interpretation of a clinical trial. These situations can be obviated by the formal incorporation of multiple analysis procedures. Consider a clinical trial that intends to evaluate the effect of a new therapy on patients with nonischemic cardiomyopathy. Patients who are severely ill and debilitated from this condition are recruited for this trial, and then randomized to receive either standard therapy plus placebo (control group) or standard therapy plus the new treatment (active group).

The trial designers plan on only one primary analysis; the effect of therapy on the occurrence of the composite endpoint of all-cause mortality + all-cause hospitalization. The anticipated cumulative incidence rate for this composite endpoint in the control group is 35% and the investigators are interested in demonstrating a 20% reduction in this rate attributable to the therapy. Assuming a two-sided type I error level of 0.05 and 90% power, the sample size goal for this study is 1842 patients, a goal that is achieved. The investigators report the results of the trial at its conclusion (Table 8.5).

In this trial, the effect of the therapy on the prospectively specified primary endpoint of death + hospitalization is small. The relative risk is clinically insignificant, and the p-value of 0.09 is greater than the 0.05 threshold set in the design phase of the trial. However, the evaluation of the effect of therapy on the total mortality component of the composite endpoint provides a striking finding. The relative risk for the effect of therapy on the cumulative mortality rate is quite small, and the associated p-value of 0.03 is difficult to ignore. Should this study be considered positive based on the finding for the total mortality component endpoint?

Table 8.5. Results of ischemic cardiomyopathy trial.

Analyses	Prespecified type I error level	P-value at trial's conclusion	Relative risk
Death + hospitalization	0.05	0.09	0.91
Total hospitalization	Not specified	0.15	0.99
Total mortality	Not specified	0.03	0.60

The rules that we have provided thus far say the answer to this question should be no. The total mortality analysis had not been prespecified; we are giving the total mortality analysis attention not because we prospectively said we would, but because the result is intriguing. However, counterarguments state that the investigators are obligated to report the total mortality analysis as they comply with the full disclosure principle for composite endpoint use in clinical trials. Shouldn't these results that they are required to report be considered? In addition, there is clearly some dependence between the findings for the total mortality analysis and that of the combined endpoint, since the total mortality endpoint is a component of the composite endpoint. This dependency should lead to some α error level conservation which is not reflected in Table 7.8.

This ambiguous set of circumstances could be avoided if the combinations of trial design precaution and innovation, used to develop multiple hypothesis testing strategies for a singleton endpoint, could be applied in the combined endpoint analysis setting. It is appropriate for the investigators, who recognize that they must provide a complete endpoint assessment, to give consideration to the possibility of not just reporting the results for the component endpoints, but to actually draw confirmatory conclusions from these singleton endpoint analyses as well. This requires that the discussions of Chapters 2 to 6 be considered for the prospective identification of primary analyses among the evaluations for (1) the combined endpoint and (2) the component endpoints. This will be the focus of the remainder of this chapter.

8.7 Example 1: Design for a Heart Failure Trial

Consider the example of investigators who are interested in determining the effect of therapy to reduce morbidity and mortality in patients with CHF. In this study, patients will be followed for 18 months. Specifically, the investigators for the study are interested in demonstrating the effectiveness of the randomly allocated medication on the reduction in (1) the rate of hospitalization for CHF and (2) the cumulative incidence rate of total mortality. The investigators' attention is focused on an evaluation of the effect of therapy on a combined endpoint (death + hospitalization), but the trial scientists would also like to be able to make a confirmatory statement about the effect of the therapy on the two singleton endpoints (total mortality and total hospitalization) as well. These investigators anticipate that the event rate for total hospitalizations will be 30% over the course of the trial and that the cumulative event rate for total mortality will be 15%, producing a 40% cumulative event rate for the combined endpoint. With an expectation that patients randomized to the treatment group will experience a 20% reduction in the occurrence of hospitalizations, and a 25% reduction in total mortality,[6] the investigators proceed with the first sample size computation[7] (Table 8.6).

---

[6] The investigators actually anticipated that the randomly allocated medication would produce a 25% reduction in events; however, the medication quite likely would produce hospitalizations in some patients immediately after randomization. Recognition of this finding leads to a reduction in the efficacy of the compound for both the total hospitalization singleton endpoint and the combined endpoint from 25% to 20%.

[7] Sample size computations are discussed in Appendix D.

Table 8.6. Alpha allocation example for composite endpoint: First design scenario.

Primary analyses	Cumulative control group event rate	Efficacy	Alpha (two-tailed)	Power	Sample size
Death + hospitalization	0.40	0.20	0.050	0.90	1503
Total hospitalization	0.30	0.20	0.050	0.90	2291
Total mortality	0.15	0.25	0.050	0.90	3397

For this initial sample size computation, there is no attempt to control the familywise error probability and the power level is initially chosen as 90% for each of the three analyses. The required sample size for examination of the effect of therapy for the composite endpoint is substantially less than for the analysis of the therapy's effect on either of the singleton endpoints because of the composite endpoint's larger event rate. The largest possible event rate for this combined endpoint event is 0.45, which is the sum of the two events rates for total hospitalization and total mortality. However, since there are patients who will be hospitalized and subsequently die, the cumulative event rate for the composite endpoint is less than the sum of the rates for the singleton endpoints[8]. This state of affairs does not provide the maximum cumulative composite endpoint event rate for the study. However, the fact that patient in this study are both hospitalized and die suggests that the disease process affects the occurrence of each of these. This increases our confidence that the combined endpoint is capturing different although not completely independent manifestations of the same disease process, i.e., that the prospectively chosen composite endpoint is a coherent one.

Table 8.6 provides sample sizes only for the single type I error rate of 0.05. The investigators take the next step of adjusting the type I error rates for each of the three primary analyses to conserve the familywise error rate (Table 8.7).

---

[8] In Section 7.3.1, we pointed out that the lower the probability of the occurrence of a singleton event given the occurrence of another singleton event, the greater the composite endpoint event rate will be. From Table 7.8, we can compute the conditional probability of a death given that the patient is hospitalized. If A is the event of hospitalization and B is the event of death, then we can first compute $0.40 = P[A \cup B] = P[A] + P[B] - P[A \cap B]$. Since we know that $P[A]=0.15$ and $P[B]=0.30$, then we can find $P[A \cap B] = 0.30 + 0.15 - 0.40 = 0.05$. The probability of a death given hospitalization has occurred is then $P[B \mid A] = P[A \cap B]/P[A] = 0.05/0.30 = 0.167$.

Table 8.7. Alpha allocation example for composite endpoint: Second design scenario.

Primary analyses	Cumulative control group event rate	Efficacy	Alpha (two-tailed)	Power	Sample size
Death + hospitalization	0.40	0.20	0.025	0.90	1775
Total hospitalization	0.30	0.20	0.010	0.90	3244
Total mortality	0.15	0.25	0.015	0.90	4460

Of course, the sample sizes for each of the three analyses have increased now that the test-specific α error rates have been reduced. However, the clear relationship between the composite endpoint and the component endpoints from which it is constructed makes it quite reasonable to expect that there will be dependency among these endpoints' hypothesis tests. This recognition allows the investigators to apply the notation and tools of Chapters 5 and 6 to recompute the test-specific type I error rates.

Specifically, in this setting, there are two dependency parameters that the investigators will need to estimate, identified as $D_{2|1}$ (representing the occurrence of a type I error for the effect of therapy for the total hospitalization endpoint given the occurrence of a type I error in the examination of the effect of therapy on the combined endpoint) and $D_{3|1,2}$ (the occurrence of a type I error for the effect of the randomly allocated intervention given that a type I error has occurred on each of the examinations of the effect of therapy on the composite endpoint and total hospitalizations).

Recall that in the consideration of hypothesis test dependency, the two factors that must be considered in estimating $D_{2|1}$ and $D_{3|1,2}$ are (1) coincidence, or the degree to which the combined endpoint and the singleton endpoints occur in the same patient; and (2) homogeneity of therapy effect. However, these two concepts are precisely those ideas that entered into our development of the concept of the composite endpoint, and we may take full advantage of that one-to-one correspondence here. Turning our attention first to the estimation of the value of $D_{2|1}$, recall from Chapter 5 that a useful starting approximation for the value of $D_{2|1}$ is (5.39) and reproduced here.

$$D_{2|1}(e) = c_e \left[1 - (1 - c_e)(1 - h_e) \right].$$

(8.1)

Remember that, in this formulation, $c_e{}^9$ is the coincidence level (between zero and one) that measures the degree to which each of the endpoints occur in the same person and, the quantity h_e measures the homogeneity of therapy effect (again, between zero and one). Examination of the event rates provided in Table 7.9 reveals that the preponderance of events that occur for the composite endpoint of death + hospitalization will be hospitalizations. This observation points to a large value of c, taken here as 0.80.

The investigators anticipate that there will be a high level of homogeneity of therapy effect between the combined endpoint and the total hospitalization singleton endpoint, estimated by $h = 0.90$. They then compute $D_{2|1}$ as

$$D_{2|1}(e) = 0.80\left[1-(1-0.80)(1-0.90)\right] = 0.80[1-(0.20)(0.10)]$$
$$= (0.80)(0.98) = 0.78. \tag{8.2}$$

An analogous computation can now be executed for $D_{3|1,2}$. The coincidence between the occurrence of a death and the occurrence of a composite endpoint and a hospitalization is high, though not as high as the coincidence between the occurrence of a combined endpoint and hospitalization; the investigators estimate $c = 0.65$. However, homogeneity of therapy effect is estimated to very high ($h = 0.90$). Thus, the investigators compute

$$D_{3|1,2}(e) = c_e\left[1-(1-c_e)(1-h_e)\right],$$
$$D_{3|1,2}(e) = 0.65\left[1-(1-0.65)(1-0.90)\right] = 0.65[1-(0.35)(0.10)] \tag{8.3}$$
$$= (0.65)(0.965) = 0.63.$$

The investigators choose to use the familywise error probability of 0.05. Using (5.31) they can compute the upper bound for α_2, the test-specific α error rate for the effect of therapy on the cumulative incidence rate of hospitalization. Furthermore, using the values of α_1, α_2 and $D_{2|1}$ the investigators can compute α_3 from (6.14), the investigators compute the type I error rates for each of the three principle analyses for their clinical trial (Table 8.8). The incorporation of the dependency parameter controls the familywise error rate at the 0.05 level even though the sum of the type I error levels for each of the three hypotheses is above 0.05.

---

[9] We use the subscript e to denote the perspective of dependency between endpoints. In Chapter 11 we will discuss dependency from the perspective of subgroup analysis.

Table 8.8. Alpha allocation example for composite endpoint: Third design scenario.

Primary analyses	Cumulative control group event rate	Efficacy	Alpha (two-tailed)	Power	Sample size
Death + hospitalization	0.40	0.20	0.025	0.90	1775
		$D = 0.78$			
Total hospitalization	0.30	0.20	0.025	0.90	2706
		$D = 0.63$			
Total mortality	0.15	0.25	0.025	0.90	4013

The investigators next choose to reduce the sample sizes further by decreasing the power for the analysis of the effect of therapy on the cumulative incidence of each of the singleton endpoints from 90% to 80%, which is currently the standard minimum power level that divides null analyses from uninformative assessments[10] (Table 8.9).

Table 8.9. Alpha allocation example composite endpoint Fourth design scenario.

Primary analyses	Cumulative control group event rate	Efficacy	Alpha (two-tailed)	Power	Sample size
Death + hospitalization	0.40	0.20	0.025	0.90	1775
		$D = 0.78$			
Total hospitalization	0.30	0.20	0.025	0.80	2072
		$D = 0.63$			
Total mortality	0.15	0.25	0.025	0.80	3073

The result of this exercise is three analyses that demonstrate the medication's effect on total mortality and hospitalization rates. If the investigators can randomize no more than 2072 patients for the study, then there would be two adequately powered confirmatory analyses: (1) the effect of therapy on the composite endpoint of death + hospitalization, and (2) the effect of therapy on the cumulative incidence rate of total hospitalization. The analyses for the medication's efficacy as measured by total mortality could continue to be confirmatory; however, the low power for this evaluation (60% power for the effect of therapy on the total mortality endpoint)

---

[10] Defined in Chapter 4, a null analysis for the effect of a randomly allocated intervention in a clinical trial allows the conclusion that the therapy has no meaningful effect. An uninformative analysis only allows one to say that the effect of therapy cannot meaningfully be evaluated.

means that non-rejection of the null hypothesis is an inconclusive, uninformative result. However, if trial resources permit 3100 patients to be recruited for this study, then one can take advantage of the hypothesis dependency which naturally occurs between the three endpoints to obtain a full confirmatory analysis of the effect of therapy on the cumulative incidence rate of total mortality in this illustration. This action would reduce the required sample size for an adequately powered statistical evaluation of the effect of the randomly allocated intervention for each of the component endpoints.

8.8 Composite Endpoints: Diabetes Mellitus

As a final consideration of the use of composite endpoints in clinical trials, we will return to the evaluation of therapy effectiveness in the treatment of diabetes mellitus. In this hypothetical trial, patients who have been newly diagnosed with this condition will be randomized to specific treatment and followed for many years to evaluate the effect of therapy in reducing the occurrence of long-term consequences of type II diabetes mellitus.

This clinical trial will recruit adult patients who have been recently diagnosed with diabetes mellitus into one of two randomly assigned treatment arms (control therapy versus active therapy). Patients who are randomized to the control group will be placed on a strict diet and exercise program. The weight reduction program consists of (1) weight reduction, (2) reduction and control of total intake of fat, (3) reduction and control of saturated fat intake, and (4) increased intake of fiber. This plan, in concert with a vigorous physical exercise routine, was found to be instrumental in reducing the development of type II diabetes mellitus [13]. In addition, the control group will be subject to the aggressive control of essential hypertension, treatment of dyslipidemic states with lipid reducing agents, and cigarette smoking cessation. Patients who are randomized to active therapy will receive control group therapy plus the addition of agents that will reduce blood sugar levels. The treating physician can choose from the sulfonylurea (either sulfonylurea or placebo), biguanides (or placebo), and/or thiazolindienediones (or placebo).

The trial will be executed in a double-blind fashion with neither randomized patients nor treating physicians learning the identity of the pharmacologic therapy the patient is receiving for the treatment of their diabetes. Patients who are randomized to the control group will receive placebo compounds for the treatment of their blood sugars. To minimize the possibility that a patient's blood sugar will rise to a level that would produce dangerous ketoacidosis, patients will have their HbA1c level measured on a regular and routine basis. Patients whose HbA1c levels rise get too high will be treated with open label therapy to reduce their blood sugar from these dangerous levels. To keep the blind in place, a matching patient in the opposite treatment group whose blood sugar is above the median value for the group to which they are randomized will also receive open label therapy (placebo therapy if the matching patient's blood sugar is not too high).

Diabetes mellitus is a complex disease that affects every major organ system. In order to measure each of these manifestations, the investigators consider creating a composite endpoint that will measure the occurrence of each of the cardiac, cerebrovascular, peripheral vascular, renal, ophthalmologic, and neurological consequences of this disease. Such an endpoint, composed of these different disease manifestations, would produce a relatively large event rate. This large event rate could be used by the investigators to either decrease the sample size of the trial, or to increase the sensitivity of the study by detecting levels of efficacy which are clinically significant but beyond the resolving ability of clinical trials that recruit smaller numbers of subjects. However, this assumes that the therapy will be effective for reducing the occurrence of each of the component endpoints of this hyper composite endpoint. The trial designers feel that such an endpoint would be plagued with interpretative difficulty, especially if there is a heterogeneity of therapy effect across its many component endpoints. Lacking evidence that pharmacologic therapy would be equally effective in reducing cardiovascular clinical endpoints on the one hand, and reducing renal, ophthalmologic, or neurological endpoints on the other, the investigators plot a different strategy; they rely on combined endpoints for the analysis plan, but assemble them differently (Table 8.10).

Table 8.10. Alpha allocation example for diabetes trial: First design scenario.

Primary analyses	Cumulative control group event rate	Efficacy	Alpha (two-tailed)	Power	Sample size
Analysis Set A					
Stroke and coronary artery disease	0.280	0.20	0.050	0.90	2516
Fatal/nonfatal MI	0.210	0.20	0.050	0.90	3642
Fatal/nonfatal stroke	0.100	0.20	0.050	0.90	8595
Analysis Set B					
Other Morbidity/mortality	0.050	0.20	0.050	0.90	18,052
Fatal/nonfatal kidney disease	0.010	0.20	0.050	0.90	93,705
Blindness (one eye)	0.035	0.20	0.050	0.90	26,157
Amputation	0.015	0.20	0.050	0.90	62,183

No attempt has been made at this early stage in the computation to adjust the familywise error rate.

The trial designers are interested in determining the magnitude of the effect of the randomly allocated therapy on the many long-term manifestations of this disease. These scientists decide that the major effort of this research will be to identify the effect of pharmacologic interventions for diabetes mellitus on two sets of outcomes. The first outcome of interest (Analysis Set A) is the composite endpoint of the occurrence of stroke and coronary artery disease. However, this combined endpoint stroke + CAD is itself constructed from two composite endpoints: (1) fatal/nonfatal MI, and (2) fatal/nonfatal stroke. The mechanism by which diabetes mellitus affects the atherosclerotic pathogenesis of these lesions suggests that these two manifestations of diabetes may both be influenced by the effect of therapy. Since a single patient can, but often will not suffer from both a MI and a stroke, the combined endpoint of fatal/nonfatal MI + fatal/nonfatal stroke measures different manifestations of the same disease process. Also they believe that evidence supporting the homogeneity of the therapy effect exists for this evaluation.

As we have seen, the component endpoints of a combined endpoint are in and of themselves of clinical interest; that is clearly the case here. The investigators plan to make a confirmatory statement about each of the combined endpoints: (1) fatal/nonfatal MI and (2) fatal/nonfatal stroke. These two confirmatory statements would be in addition to their confirmatory statement about the effect of therapy on the cumulative incidence of stroke + CAD. This development reveals that, just as the fatal/nonfatal MI endpoint (as well as the fatal/nonfatal stroke endpoint) can serve as a useful combined endpoint, it can serve as a functional component endpoint of a larger and more complex composite endpoint as well.

The second major focus of analysis for this trial is the occurrence of other morbidity and mortality as a consequence of diabetes mellitus (Analysis Set B). This is also a composite endpoint, constructed from a combination of an additional composite endpoint (fatal/nonfatal kidney disease) and the singleton endpoints: (1) blindness (one eye) and (2) amputation. These consequences of diabetes are debilitating; however these particular sequela occur with too low a cumulative incidence rate to have a beneficial effect of therapy identified with adequate power.

As seen from Table 8.10, the sample sizes for this trial vary dramatically. The situation becomes much worse after a first attempt to control the familywise error rate for the trial at 0.05 (Table 8.11) The investigators are demanding many confirmatory analyses from this design and sample sizes indicate the price they may have to pay to achieve their goals. Essentially, type I error is divided between the two analysis sets. Analysis Set A, focusing on an evaluation of the effect of therapy on the occurrence of stroke and CAD will have an α error probability of 0.02. The effect of therapy on other morbidity/mortality measures for diabetes mellitus (Analysis Set B), will have an α error rate of 0.03.

Within Analysis Set A, the entire α error probability is equally distributed across the stroke + CAD endpoint and its two component endpoints (each of which is a combined endpoint). This produces sample sizes from 3790 to 12,947. However, the distribution of type I error rate is carried out differently for Analysis Set B.

Table 8.11. Alpha allocation example for diabetes trial: Second design scenario.

Primary analyses	Cumulative control group event rate	Efficacy	Alpha (two-tailed)	Power	Sample size
Analysis Set A			0.020		
Stroke and coronary artery disease	0.280	0.20	0.007	0.90	3790
Fatal/nonfatal MI	0.210	0.20	0.007	0.90	5485
Fatal/nonfatal stroke	0.100	0.20	0.007	0.90	12,947
Analysis Set B			0.030		
Other morbidity/mortality	0.050	0.20	0.030	0.90	20,468
Fatal/nonfatal kidney disease	0.010	0.20	0.001	0.90	186,424
Blindness (one eye)	0.035	0.20	0.001	0.90	52,040
Amputation	0.015	0.20	0.001	0.90	123,711

Preliminary adjustments in the type I error rates for all of the analyses.

The major focus of the evaluation of the effect of therapy for this analysis set is the combined endpoint (other morbidity/mortality). While the investigators are interested in the identification of the effect of therapy for the component endpoints of this composite endpoint, they recognize that the number of endpoint events will be too small to provide a persuasive argument to the medical and regulatory communities for the effect of therapy at moderate α error rates (0.01 to 0.05), even if the power for Analysis Set B is reduced from 90% to 80% (Table 8.12). The investigators therefore place the overwhelming majority of the α error probability on the combined endpoint (other morbidity/mortality) in Analysis Set B. This action allows the investigators to still claim that the study is positive if the low type I error levels for the effect of therapy on either of fatal/nonfatal kidney disease, blindness, or amputation are not exceeded. If these α error levels are exceeded, the correct interpretation for the effect of therapy on these component endpoints will that the results are uninformative [11].

The investigators now come to grips with the notion of dependency. They decide that (1) there is no demonstrated evidence that suggests that type I errors for the Analysis Set A will influence the likelihood of type I error occurrence for Analysis Set B, and (2) within Analysis Set B, there is no evidence of type I error dependency among the combined endpoints (denoted by other morbidity/mortality) and its component endpoints fatal/nonfatal kidney disease, blindness, or amputation. The notion of dependent subclasses, introduced in Chapter 6 may be brought to bear here. The only dependency they will embed in the analysis is within Analysis Set A.

---

[11] The distinction between uninformative results and null results is defined in Chapter 4.

Table 8.12. Alpha allocation example for diabetes trial: Third design scenario.

Primary analyses	Cumulative control group event rate	Efficacy	Alpha (two-tailed)	Power	Sample size
Analysis Set A			0.020		
Stroke and coronary artery disease	0.280	0.20	0.007	0.90	3790
Fatal/nonfatal MI	0.210	0.20	0.007	0.90	5485
Fatal/nonfatal stroke	0.100	0.20	0.007	0.90	12,947
Analysis Set B			0.030		
Other morbidity/mortality	0.050	0.20	0.030	0.80	15,583
Fatal/nonfatal kidney disease	0.010	0.20	0.001	0.80	152,274
Blindness (one eye)	0.035	0.20	0.001	0.80	42,507
Amputation	0.015	0.20	0.001	0.80	101,049

Reduction in power for Analyses Set B.

Focusing on Analysis Set A, the trial designers recognize that the largest component of the stroke + CAD is its fatal/nonfatal MI component. The investigators also reason that there will be substantial homogeneity of therapy ($h = (1)$ for these endpoints. They therefore compute using (8.1) that $D_{2|1}$ (the dependency parameter reflecting the relationship between the occurrence of a type I error for the stroke + CAD and the fatal/nonfatal MI component endpoint) = 0.75. A similar computation leads to $D_{3|1,2}$ (expressing the relationship between the occurrence of a type I error for the hypothesis test evaluating the effect of therapy for the fatal/nonfatal stroke component and a type I error for the effect of therapy on each of (1) stroke and CAD and (2) fatal/nonfatal MI) = 0.50. The result of this effort provides the sample sizes required for each analysis (Table 8.13).

These computations reveal that with a sample size of 15,583 patients, the investigators will have adequate power to assess the effect of pharmacologic therapy in patients with type II diabetes mellitus for several measures of the long-term consequences associated with this illness. Confirmatory statements will be available for the effect of therapy on stroke and CAD as a combined endpoint as well as for each of its component endpoints. In addition, this trial design permits a confirmatory evaluation of the effect of therapy on other measures of morbidity and mortality produced by diabetes mellitus which are not directly related to the occurrence of cerebrovascular accidents and MIs. Finally, it will be possible to make a confirmatory positive statement about the effect of therapy specifically for each of the endpoints: (1) fatal/nonfatal kidney disease, (2) blindness, and (3) amputations.

Table 8.13. Alpha allocation example for diabetes trial: Fourth design scenario.

Primary analyses	Cumulative control group event rate	Efficacy	Alpha (two -tailed)	Power	Sample Size
Analysis Set A			0.020		
Stroke and Coronary Artery Disease	0.280	0.20	0.012	0.90	3446
		D = 0.75			
Fatal/Nonfatal MI	0.210	0.20	0.012	0.90	4988
		D = 0.50			
Fatal/Nonfatal Stroke	0.100	0.20	0.004	0.90	14255
Analysis Set B			0.030		
Other Morbidity/Mortality	0.050	0.20	0.030	0.80	15583
Fatal/Nonfatal Kidney Disease	0.010	0.20	0.001	0.80	152274
Blindness (one eye)	0.035	0.20	0.001	0.80	42507
Amputation	0.015	0.20	0.001	0.80	101049

Dependency is now embedded for Analyses Set A.

8.9 "Soft" Components

As investigators work to assemble a combined endpoint, they must consider the persuasive ability of the final product. The more persuasive the individual components of the endpoint, the more persuasive the effect of randomly allocated intervention effect on that endpoint will be. However, combined endpoints are commonly constructed from singleton endpoints that are persuasive and others which are not so persuasive.

As an illustration, consider a clinical trial that will randomize patients who are at risk of ischemic cardiovascular disease to either standard therapy plus placebo (control group) or standard therapy plus an active compound. Patients will be followed for 2 years. The investigators believe that they will be able to randomize between 10,000 to 15,000 patients for this clinical trial.

After much discussion, the investigators have settled on a single primary analysis for the effect of therapy on the cumulative incidence rate of a combined endpoint. That composite endpoint has four components: (1) fatal/nonfatal MI, (2) fatal/nonfatal stroke, (3) revascularization, and (4) unstable angina. They have estimated the incidence rates of these four components and have computed initial sample size estimates for the composite endpoint (Table 8.14).

Table 8.14. Alpha allocation example composite endpoint:First design scenario.

Primary analyses	Cumulative control group event rate	Efficacy	Alpha (two-tailed)	Power	Sample size
Composite endpoint	*0.20*	*0.20*	*0.05*	*0.90*	*3867*
Fatal/nonfatal MI	0.04	0.20	0.05	0.90	22,780
Fatal/nonfatal stroke	0.04	0.20	0.05	0.90	22,780
Revascularization	0.08	0.20	0.05	0.90	10,959
Unstable angina	0.06	0.20	0.05	0.90	14,900

The required sample for the composite endpoints is 3867, well within the range of the investigators to recruit subjects. However, an issue that the investigators will need to address, and one they can begin addressing in the design phase of the study is that the combined endpoint's components appear to be divided between endpoints that are the easiest to measure unambiguously (hard endpoints) such as fatal/nonfatal MI and fatal/nonfatal stroke on the one hand, and the softer endpoints of revascularization and unstable angina. These latter two singleton endpoints are subject to either regional practice, changing definitions, or the willingness of a patient to accurately report symptoms. A review of the endpoint event rates in Table 8.14 reveals that these softer endpoints will comprise most of the component endpoints that occur. This may reduce the ability of the trial to convince the medical and regulatory community of the benefit of the therapy.

The findings of the effect of therapy in this trial will be supported if a confirmatory analysis could be executed on the MI and stroke components of the composite endpoint. In order to investigate this possibility, the trial designers create a second composite endpoint constructed from the fatal/nonfatal MI component and the fatal/nonfatal stroke component of the first composite endpoint (Table 8.15) In addition to the inclusion of the hard endpoint composite, there has been a reassignment of the type I error rate during the design phase of this study. The type I error probability for the composite endpoint has been reduced to 0.01, and the hard endpoint composite will be assessed at the trial's conclusion at the 0.04 level. The sample size for this evaluation is 13,390 patients. Although this is well within the investigators ability to recruit patients, this patient's requirement can be reduced by decreasing the power of the hard endpoint composite to 80% (Table 8.16).

The trial will have two principle analyses, each of which will be the effect of therapy on a combined endpoint. The role of the soft endpoints has been effectively reduced to that of prospectively defined secondary endpoints, and the effect of therapy on each of them will be reported in accordance with the expectation of the medical and regulatory communities as outlined in the principle of full disclosure.

Table 8.15. Alpha allocation example composite endpoint: Second design scenario.

Primary analyses	Cumulative control group event rate	Efficacy	Alpha (two-tailed)	Power	Sample size
Composite endpoint	0.20	0.20	0.01	0.90	5476
Hard endpoint composite	0.07	0.20	0.04	0.90	13,390
Fatal/nonfatal MI	0.04	0.20	0.05	0.90	22,780
Fatal/nonfatal stroke	0.04	0.20	0.05	0.90	22,780
Revascularization	0.08	0.20	0.05	0.90	10,959
Unstable angina	0.06	0.20	0.05	0.90	14,900

Table 8.16. Alpha allocation example composite endpoint: Third design scenario.

Primary analyses	Cumulative control group event rate	Efficacy	Alpha (two-tailed)	Power	Sample size
Composite Endpoint	0.20	0.20	0.01	0.90	5476
Hard Endpoint Composite	0.07	0.20	0.04	0.80	10,091
Fatal/Nonfatal MI	0.04	0.20	0.05	0.90	22,780
Fatal/nonfatal stroke	0.04	0.20	0.05	0.90	22,780
Revascularization	0.08	0.20	0.05	0.90	10,959
Unstable angina	0.06	0.20	0.05	0.90	14,900

8.10 Conclusions

The principles of concordant trial design apply equally to the use of combined endpoints in clinical trials. Both the composite endpoints and its components should be identified prospectively and remain unchanged during the course of the clinical trial. The disciplined trial execution will produce interpretable estimates of effect sizes, confidence intervals, and p-values at the study's conclusion.

Finally, although composite endpoints are constructed to be of interest to the medical and regulatory communities, interest remains in the effect of therapy on their component endpoints. The application of the principles of differential α allocation discussed in Chapter 4, and the procedures for allocating type I error during the dependent hypothesis testing in chapters five and six permit the design of clinical trials that can provide confirmatory statements not solely about the effect of therapy on the composite endpoint, but also the therapy effect on several if not each of the composite endpoint's components. These tools can be extended to allow the design of clinical trials whose prospectively defined primary analysis consists of the effect of therapy not just on a composite endpoint, but, in addition, on component endpoints that are themselves composite endpoints. A combination of research discipline and imagination can produce clinical trial designs that are both innovative and conform to the established dictums of prospectively designed research.

Problems

1. What are five useful principles that govern the use of a composite endpoint in a clinical trial?
2. A clinical trial has a composite endpoint composed of two singleton endpoints. If a type I error rate is be prospectively applied to the composite endpoint, must type I error rates be prospectively announced for each of the singleton endpoints? If not, what is the best interpretation of the results of the trial if the effect of therapy on one of the singleton endpoints produces a p-value less than 0.05 but the effect of therapy on the composite endpoint is slightly greater than 0.05.
3. What arguments can be developed to support the notion of using dependent hypothesis testing procedures when there is a prospective desire among the investigators of a clinical trial to carry out hypothesis testing for the composite endpoint and its component endpoints as well?
4. In general, is it easier to support an argument for therapy homogeneity among the singleton endpoints of a composite endpoint than among individual endpoints not combined into a composite endpoint?
5. Consider a clinical trial that will assess the effect of therapy on the component endpoint and each of its two composite endpoints. In the presence of substantial coincidence and homogeneity of therapy, why is there greater type I error conservation when the test-specific α error rate for the composite endpoint hypothesis test is close to 0.05?
6. A clinical trial will test the effect of therapy on each of a composite endpoint and its two singleton endpoints. Can you think of a circumstance in which it may be best to assign the maximum test-specific error rate to one of the singleton endpoints and not the composite endpoint? Can the framework used in chapters seven and eight be applied in this analyses scenario?

References

1. The Lipid Research Clinic Investigators (1979). The Lipid Research Clinics Program: The coronary primary prevention trial; design and implementation. *Journal of Chronic Diseases* **32**:609–631.
2. Moyé, L.A. (2000). *Statistical Reasoning in Medicine: The Intuitive P-value Primer*. New York. Springer. pp. 132–133.

3. The Lipid Research Clinic Investigators. (1984). The Lipid Research Clinics Coronary Primary Prevention trial results. *Journal of the American Medical Association* **251**:351–74.

4. UK Prospective Diabetes Study Group (1991) UK Prospective Diabetes Study (UKPDS) VIII. Study, design, progress and performance. *Diabetologia* **34**:877–890

5. University Group Diabetes Program. (1970). A study of the effects of hypoglycaemic agents on vascular complications on patients with adult–onset diabetes II. Mortality results. *Diabetes* **19** [Suppl 2]:789–830

6. Turner, R.C., Holman, R.R. on behalf of the UK Prospective Diabetes Study Group. (1998). The UK Prospective Diabetes Study. Finnish Medical Society DUOCECIM, *Annals of Medicine* **28**:439–444

7. UKPDS Study Group. (1998). Intensive blood glucose control with sulphonylureas or insulin compared with conventional treatment and risk of complications in patients with type 2 diabetes. *Lancet* **352**: 837–853.

8. SOLVD Investigators. (1991). Effect of enalapril on survival in patients with reduced left ventricular ejection fractions and congestive heart failure. *New England Journal of Medicine* **325**:293–302.

9. SOLVD Investigators (1992). Effects of enalapril on mortality and development of heart failure in aymptomatic patients with reduced left ventricular ejection fractions. *New England Journal of Medicine* **327**:685–691.

10. Pfeffer, M.A., Braunwald, E., Moyé, L.A., Basta, L., Brown, E.J., Cuddy, T.E., Davis, B.R., Geltman, E.M., Goldman, S., Glaker, G.C., Klein, M., Lamas, G.A., Packer, M., Rouleau, J., Rouleau, J.L., Rutherford, J., Wertheimer, J.H., Hawkins, C.M., on behalf of the SAVE Investigators. (1992). Effect of captopril on mortality and morbidity in patients with left ventricular dysfunction after myocardial infarction. Results of the survival and ventricular enlargement trial. *New England Journal of Medicine* **327**:669–677.

11. The HOPE Study Investigators. (1996). The HOPE (Heart Outcomes Prevention Evaluation) Study: The design of a large, simple randomized trial of an angiotensin–converting enzyme inhibitor (ramipril) and vitamin E in patients at high risk of cardiovascular events. *Canadian Journal of Cardiology* **12**:127–137.

12. The Heart Outcomes Prevention Evaluation Study Investigators (2000) Effects of angiotensin–converting enzyme inhibitor, ramipril, on cardiovascular events in high–risk patients. *New England Journal of Medicine* **342**:145–53

13. Tulmilehto, J., Lindström, J., Eriksson, J.G., Valle, T.T., Hämäläinen, H, Ilanne-Parikka P., Keinanen-Kiukaanniemi, S., Laakso, M., Louheranta, A., Rastas, M., Salminen, V., Uusitupa, M. for the Finnish Diabetes Prevention Study Group (2001). Prevention of type 2 diabetes mellitus by changes in lifestyle among subjects with impaired glucose tolerance. *New England Journal of Medicine* **344**:1343–1350.

Chapter 9

Introduction to Subgroup Analyses

This is the first of three chapters that discusses the role and interpretation of subgroup analyses in clinical trials. Subgroup analysis in a clinical trial is the evaluation of the effect of the randomly allocated intervention within only a fraction of the patients in the entire research cohort. This chapter provides some general background on the issue of subgroup evaluation, and discusses some of the interpretative difficulties that occur during the assessment of the effect of therapy within subgroups.

9.1 Introduction

A subgroup analyses in a clinical trial is the evaluation of the effect of the randomly allocated intervention within a fraction of the recruited subjects. The analysis of subgroups is a popular, necessary, and controversial component of the complete evaluation of a controlled clinical trial. Indeed, it is difficult to find a manuscript that reports the results of a clinical trial that does not report findings within selected subgroups.

Subgroup analyses as currently utilized in clinical trials are tantalizing and controversial. There may be no better maxim for guiding the interpretation of subgroup analyses in this setting than "Look, but don't touch," As described in the beginning of Chapter 3, the results from subgroup assessments have traditionally been used to augment the persuasive power of a clinical trial's overall results by demonstrating the uniform effect of the therapy in patients with different demographic and risk factor profiles. This uniformity leads to the development of easily understood and implemented rules to guide the use of therapy[1]. Some clinical trials report these results both in the manuscript announcing the trial's overall results [1], [2], [3], [4] and separately [5], [6], [7]. Such subgroup analyses potentially provide new information about an unanticipated benefit (or hazard) of the clinical trial's randomly allocated intervention.

However useful and provocative these results can be, it is well established that subgroup analyses are often misleading [8], [9], [10], [11]. Assmann et al. [12] has demonstrated how commonly subgroup analyses are misused, while others point out the dangers of accepting subgroup analyses as confirmatory [13]. For example, the amlodipine controversy that was discussed in Chapter 2 [14], [15] was based on a subgroup analysis. Nevertheless, the medical community continues to be tantalized by spectacular subgroup findings from clinical trials. A recent example is the subgroup analysis-based suggestion that medication efficacy is a function of

---

[1] The finding that a particular lipid lowering drug works better in women than in men can complicate the already complex decisions that practitioners must make as the number of available compounds increase.

race; this has appeared in both peer-reviewed journals [16, 17] and the lay press [18].

In this chapter, we will review the definitions, concepts, and limitations of subgroup utilization in clinical trials.

9.2 Definitions and Basic Concepts

While the concept of subgroup analysess is straightforward, the terminology can sometimes be confusing. We will therefore devote some effort to defining and classifying subgroup analyses.

9.2.1 Subgroups Versus Subgroup Strata

A subgroup is the description of patient based characteristic, e.g., gender, that can be subdivided into categories. These different categories are described as strata, one stratum level for each category. For example, if an investigator is interested in creating a gender subgroup, patients are classified according to their sexual characteristics; the resultant gender subgroup consists of two strata—male and female.

The classic subgroup analysis itself is an evaluation of the effect of therapy within each of the subgroup strata. In this example of a gender-based subgroup, the subgroup analysis consists of an evaluation of the effect of therapy for males and an evaluation of the effect of therapy for females. Thus each stratum analysis produces an effect size with its standard error, a confidence interval, and a p-value.

The characteristics that form the basis of these subsets are chosen by the investigators. However, over time, a commonly evaluated set of subgroup evaluations has emerged. Although there are differences from one medical subspecialty to another, the most common of these subgroups are based on demographic criteria e.g., gender, ethnicity, and age. Frequently used sociologic determinants are marital status, education, and acculturation.[2] In addition, there are subgroups that are based on lifestyle choices. Some examples of these are alcohol use, tobacco use, dietary intake, and exercise. Of course findings from medical histories (e.g., history of cancer, history of CHF, history of endocrine disorders) and physical examination (e.g., body mass index or DBP) are among commonly appearing subgroups in clinical trials as well.

The definition of a subgroup can be more complicated than a first glance would suggest. Consider the marriage status subgroup. One might think that this is easy to define. Is the patient married or not? Phrased this way, this suggests that the marriage subgroup should have two strata. However, the choices can be much more complex than this. The patient could be married now, or have been married in the past and is single now. The patient could be separated, divorced, or remarried. These alternative classifications can either be useful, or merely distractions depending on the purpose for which the evaluation will take place. For example, in some research which is not primarily sociologic, these additional classifications may be

---

[2] Acculturation is the degree to which a community composed primarily of immigrants accepts with approval and is involved in the activities of the surrounding society.

unnecessary. However, in other research efforts, the intricate differentiation of marriage history details is very important. Thus, one must know how the subgroup analysis will be used so that the most useful strata membership criteria can be developed. Once each of the subgroup strata have been identified, the clinical trial workers will know what data to collect that will be the most useful.[3]

9.3 Interpretation Difficulties

The illustrations of the previous sections have demonstrated that there are many possible ways to subgroup patients. However, we must keep in mind that, in a collection of subgroup analyses, it is the same patients who are being stratified in different ways. This observation can complicate the interpretation of a subgroup evaluation.

For example, consider a randomized, controlled clinical trial which is in its analysis phase. At this time, all of its patients are classified by gender, grouping patients into male and female sub-cohorts. Once the stratum membership assignment is finished, the effect of the randomly allocated intervention is assessed in each of the two gender strata. It is seen that the effect of therapy appears to depend on gender, with males experiencing a different effect than females.

When completed, these same patients are then reaggregated based not on gender, but on age. Subjects are placed into one of the following three age strata: (1) less than 40 years of age, (2) between 40 and 60 years of age, and (3) greater than 60 years of age. When the subgroup analysis is carried out for the age strata, it appears that the effect of therapy is the same in each of the age groups.

The results from these two subgroup analyses essentially demonstrate that the same patients when characterized one way (by gender) provide a different result than when characterized another way (by age). Was it really gender that modified the effect of therapy or was it the chance collection of patients that made it appear that gender was an influence? Since we can expect that the effect of treatment within a subgroup stratum depends on the patients within that stratum, then the value of the subgroup analysis must be tightly linked to the ability to demonstrate that it is the stratum characteristic that is producing the interesting effect and not just the random aggregation and reaggregation of patients.

9.4 Random Subgroups

Investigators work to identify subgroup classifications that are meaningful. When examination of the therapy effect within a subgroup appears, it is only natural for the investigator to believe the rationale for the choice of the subgroup was justified. Furthermore, the scientist may think that the stratum specific therapy effect is due to some effect-mediation ability produced by the subgroup trait. However, the very fact that patients are classified and divided can induce a subgroup effect.

Consider the following simple experiment. A courtroom chosen at random has a capacity of seating 60 observers. These 60 seats are divided by a central aisle, with 30 seats on each of the left-hand and right-hand side of the courtroom. Sixty

---

[3] Another subgroup that has grown in complexity is that for race/ethnicity.

people seat themselves as they choose, distributing themselves in an unrestricted manner among the seats on each side of the courtroom. When all are seated, we measure the height of each person, finding that the average height is exactly 67 inches. Does that mean that the average height of those seated on the left-hand side of the courtroom will be 67 inches? No. The average height of those seated on the left-hand side of the courtroom will be either less than 67 inches or greater than 67 inches, but it will not be exactly 67 inches (because the average is based on only thirty of the sixty people). If the average height on the left-hand side of the court-room is less than 67 inches, then those seated on the right-hand side will have an average height greater than 67 inches[4]. Is it fair to conclude that those who sit on the right- hand side of the courtroom are in general taller than those who sit on the left-hand side?

The simple, random aggregation and subaggregation of the observations has induced a subgroup effect that is based only on the play of chance. This random subgroup effect appears in all subgroup analyses, and we will have to integrate it into our interpretation of any subgroup effect that we see. Some interesting findings of random subgroup analyses are available [19]. These occurrences help to justify the admonition that the best descriptor of the effect in a subgroup is the finding that is observed in the overall cohort.

As an illustration, consider the result of a hypothetical clinical trial in which the investigators report that the randomly allocated intervention produced a 20% reduction in the prospectively defined endpoint of total mortality. The initial reaction to the demonstration of a beneficial effect of therapy in a well-designed, well executed clinical trial is naturally to assume that the effect of therapy is ho-mogenous. Our first response is to therefore believe that all collections of patients in the active group were beneficiaries of this 20% benefit, and that the beneficial effect of therapy provides protection is broadly distributed (Figure 9.1)

Figure 9.1. Homogenous therapy effect when viewed from in a population.

---

[4]If the average height of all in the courtroom is 67 inches, and the average height on the left side is less than 67 inches, then the average height on the right hand side must be greater than 67 inches

        This treatment effect uniformity may in fact be the truth in the population
at large. However, the examination of the same therapy effect within different subgroups of the clinical trial sample reveals a mosaic of treatment effect magnitudes
(Figure 9.2).

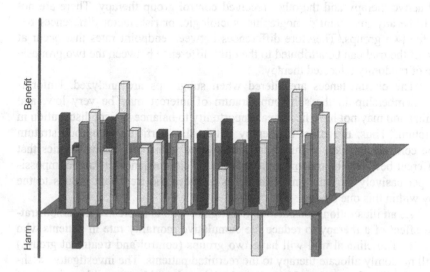

**Figure 9.2. Population homogenous treatment effects when viewed from a
sample. Each bar is the effect of the therapy in a different subgroup.**

        At first glance, it appears that the uniform mortality benefit has been re-
placed by a much more heterogeneous response. However, in reality, the 20%
benefit has been well disguised by the presence of background clutter that is produced by sampling error. The uniform 20% reduction in the total mortality effect is
still there; the population from which the research sample was derived still experienced a 20% reduction in mortality. However, when that uniform effect is viewed
through the prism of a small sample, the uniform effect is distorted. The subgroups
appear to define different levels of responses. However, all that is happening is that
the random selection mechanism causes individuals, whose responses are similar, to
cluster together by chance alone. It is this random variability that produces the differences seen in subgroups that are commonly described as a subgroup effect.

9.5 Stratified Randomization

Another difficulty in the interpretation of subgroup analyses is that the patient classification process can undo one of the most important features of a clinical trial—
the ability to attribute differences in endpoints observed at the end of the study to
the randomly allocated intervention. The absence of this key feature complicates
the interpretation of the subgroup analysis.

        Consider a clinical trial that has a control group and a treatment group.
Recall from Chapter 1 that the random allocation of therapy plays a pivotal role in

clarifying the analysis of the trial's results. It accomplished this by requiring that each patient that is recruited by the trial will have their therapy assigned based on factors other than any of that patient's traits. Frequently, this means that each patient has the same probability of receiving the active intervention as the next patient.[5] This feature distributes patients between the control and active group in such a way that the only difference between the two groups is that one group received active therapy and the other received control group therapy. There are not likely to be any important demographic, sociologic, or risk factor differences between the two groups. Therefore differences between endpoint rates that occur at the end of the trial can be attributed to the only difference between the two groups— the use of randomly allocated therapy.

The circumstances are altered when subgroups are analyzed. Unfortunately, membership in the subgroup stratum of interest may be very low, and randomization may not have had a real opportunity to balance patient distribution in this stratum.[6] Thus, the effect of therapy within that particular subgroup stratum may be confounded, i.e., confused and intertwined with other characteristics that are different between the treatment groups. In this circumstance, it can be impossible to persuasively attribute any differences between the treatment groups to the therapy within this one stratum.

As an illustration, consider an investigator who is interested in demonstrating the effect of a therapy to reduce the cumulative mortality rate in patients who have CHF. The clinical trial will have two groups (control and treatment groups) and will randomly allocate therapy to the recruited patients. The investigator, wishing to generalize the results of her clinical trial to the widest possible universe of patients with CHF, randomizes patients regardless of their NYHA class.[7] Patients must have heart failure, but admission to the clinical trial does not depend on the patient's degree of heart failure.

In addition, this investigator is also interested in examining the effect of therapy in patients with similar levels of heart failure. This investigator plans to carry out an NYHA subgroup analysis at the trial's end, evaluating the effect of the drug in each of the four strata, with a special emphasis on the effect of therapy in patients with the most severe heart failure (NYHA class IV). She therefore assigns each patient an NHYA class score when they are randomly allocated to their blinded therapy assignment at the beginning of the study.

---

[5] Adaptations of this procedure are carried out to ensure that if 100 patients are randomized to a clinical trial with a control arm and a single intervention arm, 50 are randomized to each group. Also, randomized block procedures, which ensure that close to an equal number of patients are recruited in each arm of the clinical trial, modify the probability of therapy assignment slightly. However, even in this case, therapy is not assigned based on a patient's characteristic.

[6] The importance of prospectively declared scientific questions will be addressed later in these discussions.

[7] The NHYA nomenclature groups patients with heart failure into one of four classes based on the severity of their symptoms. There are four classes, and patients with the worst symptomatology are grouped into the higher classes. Class I patients are subjects whose heart failure does not produce limitations in the patient's lifestyle, and patients who are classified into NYHA class IV are subjects whose heart failure symptoms occur at rest.

The investigator recruits 3500 patients for her study. However, upon completion of recruitment, she sees that, as might be expected, very few patients with NYHA class IV heart failure were randomized (Table 9.1).

Table 9.1 Recruiment of CHF patients into NYHA* strata by treatment group.

NYHA class	Therapy group		
	Control	Active	Total
I	450	450	900
II	625	625	1250
III	628	622	1250
IV	60	40	100

*New York Heart Association.

These results portend the difficulty this investigator will have as she attempts to interpret her subgroup analysis. There are far fewer patients in the NYHA class IV category than in the other three groups of patients. The number of patients classified as NYHA class IV actually represent the denominators for the cumulative mortality rate computations within this stratum. These small numbers will produce relatively coarse estimates of the cumulative mortality event rate. Although this problem may be counterbalanced somewhat by the relatively high death rate among these very ill class IV patients, the estimates of the cumulative mortality rate will remain fairly imprecise due to the small number of patients in this subgroup stratum.

An additional problem is that, with only 100 patients in the NYHA class IV stratum, it is unlikely that all patient characteristics will be equally allocated across the two treatment groups. It can be fascinating to observe how quickly the random allocation of therapy provides an equal distribution of patients across treatment groups. However, the large number of demographic, sociologic, risk factor and baseline medical history/physical examination variables makes it difficult to expect that randomly allocating therapy among 100 patients will balance each of these potential influences.[8] Thus, setting the imprecision of the cumulative mortality rate estimates aside for the moment, there will be difficulties in attributing any difference in the mortality rates between the control and active groups to the therapy since many other factors will be different between these patients.

The failure here was that there were not enough patients recruited into the NYHA IV stratum for the random allocation of therapy to become effective. With

---

[8] Although regression analysis may assist in taking these imbalances into account, the number of independent variables that can be placed into a regression model with only 100 observations (at most 12 variables) is very small compared to the large number of characteristics whose influence should be balanced.

more patients, the randomization mechanism would have produced a fair balance of patient characteristics across the two treatment groups. Of course, knowledgeable investigators anticipate the distribution of patients across the subgroup and the resultant small number of patients within some of the subgroup's strata. What these investigators will sometimes do is to actually force the random allocation therapy to work. That is, they adjust the randomization algorithm so that there are an equal number of patients allocated to each of the control and active groups of the trial within the subgroup stratum. This randomization within the strata, or *stratified randomization* ensures that even though there is a small number of patients within the stratum, the allocation of therapy will be more effectively balanced. While not compensating for the imprecise mortality rate estimates stemming from the small number of patients recruited into the stratum, this adaptation does substantially improve the balance of baseline characteristics between the treatment groups, strengthening the ability to ascribe differences in the mortality rate to the randomly allocated therapy.

9.6 Proper Versus Improper Subgroups

A critical preliminary task that clearly must be completed before a subgroup analysis proceeds is the classification of each patient into a subgroup stratum. This is the process by which the subgroup membership for each patient in the study is determined. Although membership determination may appear to be a trivial task, there are circumstances in which this classification is problematic. These concerns revolve around the timing of the subgroup membership determination.

There are two important possibilities for determination of the timing of subgroup membership. The first is the classification of patients into the correct subgroup stratum when the patients are randomized. The second choice is to classify patients into subgroup strata at some time during the execution of the trial. While each has advantages, the determination of subgroup membership at the beginning of the study is preferred.

Determining subgroup membership at the beginning of the trial requires that, not only must the subgroup be defined at the beginning of the study, but also subgroup strata membership should be defined prospectively as well. This is a straightforward procedure to apply to the gender subgroup with its two strata. However, for other subgroups of clinical interest, the process can be complex. As an illustration, consider the design of a clinical trial that will assess the ability of an antihypertensive therapy that has already been established as an effective blood pressure reducing agent to reduce the cumulative incidence rate of strokes in patients with systolic hypertension. Patients will be recruited and randomized to either control therapy or control therapy plus the antihypertensive medication (active group) and followed for a prespecified time.

In addition to the evaluation of the effect of therapy on the cumulative stroke incidence rate, the investigators are interested in examining the degree to which the therapy's influence on the stroke rate is related to SBP (SBP). In order to carry this out effectively, the trial designers will need to determine subgroup membership for each patient, i.e., they must fix the number of strata the SBP subgroup will contain and then decide exactly what SBPs should be contained in each stratum. Before the execution of the study, they decide on two strata: (1) SBP ≤ 140 mg Hg and (2) SBP > 140 mmHg.

Patients who are recruited into this study have their blood pressure measured at baseline and are then placed into one and only one of these strata. If the investigators are concerned about the possibility of confounding the effect of treatment with other baseline variables within any of the two SPB strata, they can determine each patient's treatment group based on a stratified randomization procedure. This is easily accomplished, since the baseline SBP is in hand at the time the therapy allocation is carried out. The product of all of these considerations and actions is the basis of a clear depiction of whether the effect of the blood pressure medication on the cumulative incidence of stroke is related to the baseline SBP (Figure 9.3).[9]

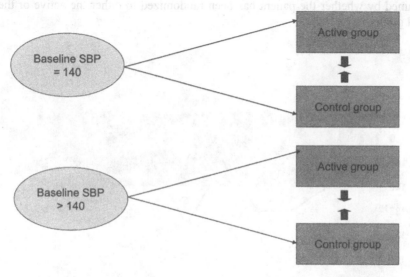

Figure 9.3. Proper subgroup definition provides relatively unconfounded effect of therapy within each subgroup stratum.

However, this is not the only way that the investigators could choose to examine the influence of SBP on the effect of therapy to reduce the cumulative stroke incidence rate. As an alternative, the investigators can prospectively decide to classify patients into one of the two subgroup strata based on each patient's last SBP measurement (which occurs either just before a stroke if the patient experiences this endpoint or is the patient's last blood pressure measurement if they complete the study without experiencing a stroke).

This evaluation is much different, for two reasons. A patient's blood pressure is likely to fluctuate as the patient's measurement is influenced by events that

---

[9] Type I and type II error considerations will have to be factored into the analysis, a procedure that will be discussed later in this chapter.

occur over the course of the trial. Since membership in the SBP subgroup stratum is based on follow-up blood pressure, then as the SBP of the patient changes over time, so too can strata membership (Figure 9.4). Thus, the spurious effect induced by the random aggregation of patients just by chance alone, (discussed earlier in this chapter) will be compounded by random subgroup membership as patients change their SBP during the course of the trial.

Second, and perhaps more importantly, it will be difficult to sort out the effect of SBP on the randomly allocated therapy's influence on the cumulative stroke incidence rate, since therapy has already influenced the SBP. As an example, for patients in the active group, the last SBP is obtained after the patient has in general had substantial and prolonged exposure to the therapy. Since the medication is already known to reduce SBP, subgroup strata membership will to a great degree be determined by whether the patient has been randomized to either the active or the control group.

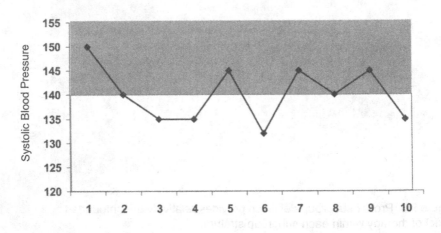

Figure 9.4. As the patient's SBP changes over time, the patient moves back and forth from one SBP stratum (<= 140 mm Hg) to the other (140 mm Hg).

To see this more clearly, we go through the following thought process. Patients assigned to the control group will not receive the active medication and are therefore not very likely to see an important decrease in their blood pressure.[10]

---

[10] Patients in the placebo group may see a slight reduction in SBP for two reasons. The first is that they may go on to active therapy without the study knowing it (e.g., visiting their private physician and that doctor chooses to put them on a blood-pressure-reducing medication). The second reason is regression to the mean. This simply means that a patient who usually had SBPs < 140 before they were enrolled into the clinical trial had an SBP

These patients are more likely to have higher SBPs during the course of the trial, and therefore reside in the greater than then 140 mm Hg subgroup stratum. On the other hand, patients who are randomized to the active group and take their medication will have a greater reduction in their SBP. Since subgroup stratum membership is based on the last SBP, patients who receive active therapy will be more likely to populate this lower SBP subgroup stratum.

Therefore, there will be a predictably large imbalance in the allocation of therapy in each of these groups. The lower subgroup stratum is more likely to be populated by patients randomized to the active group, and the upper subgroup stratum will have a preponderance of patients from the control group. The ability to evaluate the effect of therapy within each of these subgroup stratum will be impaired (Figure 9.5).

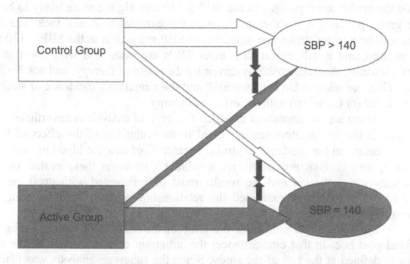

Figure 9.5. The improper definition of subgroups leads to an imbalance in the use of therapy within each stratum, making the within stratum effect of therapy assessment problematic.

In our first example in this section, we acknowledged that there were many factors that influence baseline SBP. Race, gender, family history, prior treatment are but a few of them. However, the randomly assigned intervention did not influence baseline SBP. It is the absence of any relationship between the randomly allocated therapy and the baseline SBP that allows a clear examination of the effect of SBP on the relationship between the intervention and stroke. A subgroup whose strata membership criteria are based on baseline characteristics of the patient is called a *proper subgroup* [20]. Improper subgroups are those whose strata membership can only be determined after the patient has been randomized. Membership

greater than 140 at the time they were enrolled in the study, then "regressed to" their normal SBP values for the duration of the trial.

based on follow-up data is influenced by the randomly allocated therapy and the interpretation is complicated.

The issue becomes even more paradoxical if the investigators wish to evaluate the relationship between SBP and stroke rate (as opposed to the effect of therapy on the stroke rate). When the subgroup definition is proper, allocation of therapy is balanced within each of the two subgroup strata; each of the subgroup strata will contain approximately equal numbers of patients assigned to the active and control groups. The effect of therapy is the same in each of the two subgroup strata, regardless of whether the therapy reduces the stroke rate or not. Thus, the relationship between SBP and the cumulative stroke rate can be clearly observed without having to factor in the effect of the therapy.[11]

However, when the SBP subgroup is improperly defined, patients in the control group are more likely to be in the SBP > 140 mm Hg subgroup stratum, while the predominant patients in the SBP ≤ 140 mm Hg are more likely to be active group patients. If the therapy reduces the cumulative stroke incidence rate, there will be a lower stroke rate in the lower SBP strata than in the SBP > 140 mm Hg stratum, and it will appear that lower SBPs are associated with lower stroke rates. However, this relationship is driven by the effect of therapy, and not the SBP level. Thus the relationship between SBP and the cumulative incidence of stroke is confounded (or bound up) with the effect of therapy.

There are circumstances in which this type of analysis is nevertheless carried out. If the investigators are interested in an evaluation of the effect of lower blood pressure on the incidence of stroke, regardless of how the blood pressure was lowered, then analysis procedures are available.[12] However these evaluations are exceedingly complicated and the results must be interpreted with great caution. Similar evaluations have examined the relationship between lipid lowering and atherosclerotic morbidity and mortality [21], [22], [23].

Finally, we will hold aside the issue of the analysis of a proper subgroup defined post hoc. In that circumstance, the subgroup criteria using baseline variables is defined at the end of the study. Since the subgroup analysis was planned after the data were examined, the analysis is data driven and only exploratory.

9.7 "Intention-to-Treat" Versus "As Treated"

Consider a clinical trial in which patients are randomized to receive an intervention to reduce the total mortality rate from chronic cirrhosis of the liver. At the inception of the study, patients are randomized to receive either control group therapy or the intervention. At the conclusion of the study, the investigators will compare the cumulative mortality rates of patients in each of the two treatment groups. However, at the end of the study, how will the investigators decide what patients should be considered active group patients and which patients should be counted as in the control group? The commonly used approach is to assign treatment group member-

---

[11] We are setting aside the possibility that the therapy may be effective in one subgroup strata, but not another until a later chapter.

[12] Cox hazard analysis with time dependent covariates has been one useful tool in this regard.

ship simply as the group to which the patient was randomized. This is the "intention to treat" principle.

The "intention-to-treat" principle of analysis is the standard analysis procedure for the evaluation of clinical trial results. Undoubtedly, this analysis tends to be a conservative one, since not every patient is treated as they were "intended." For example, some patients randomized to the active group may not take their medication. These patients, although randomized to the active group, will have the control group experience and produce endpoints at rates similar to that of the control group. However, they would be included in the active group since they were randomized to and "intended to be treated" like active group patients. The inclusion of these patients in the active group for analysis purposes tends to make the active group experience look more like the control group experience, increasing the overall active group event rate.[13]

Similarly, patients who are randomized to the control group may nevertheless be exposed to active group medication (e.g., from their personal physician who is not an investigator in the study). These patients will experience event rates similar to the rates of the active group, but since they are considered as part of the control group, the inclusion of these patients will produce an event rate for the control group that is closer to that of the active group. Thus the control group rate will approach that of the active group, while the cumulative event rate in the active group will be closer to that of the control group (described in the previous paragraph). This effect of these combined rate alterations reduces the magnitude of the treatment effect, thereby diminishing the power of the clinical trial.[14]

An alternative analysis to the "intent to treat" principle is one that analyzes the endpoint results using an "as-treated" analysis. In this case, although patients are still randomized to receive either placebo or active therapy, they are classified for analysis purposes based on whether they actually took their medication or not. Since this is determined after the patient was randomized to the medication, and the effect (both perceived beneficial effects, and adverse effects) of the medication may determine whether the patient takes the medication, the "as-treated" evaluation is a confounded analysis. A clearly detailed examination of this issue is available [24].

9.8 Example 1: Diabetes Mellitus in SAVE

As an illustration of a subgroup analysis, consider the Survival and Ventricular Enlargement (SAVE) clinical trial [25]. SAVE was designed to test the effect of the ACE-i therapy captopril on preventing morbidity and mortality in patients with left ventricular dysfunction. This trial recruited 2231 patients, randomizing them to

---

[13] There are occasional complications in an "intention-to-treat" analysis. In some cases, a patient is tested and randomized, but then, subsequent to the randomization the test result reveals that the patient is not eligible for the trial for a prospectively stated reason. In this case, there was no "intent" to randomize this patient when the test result was known, and the patient is removed from the study.

[14] The effect of the magnitude of the treatment effect on the power of a study for fixed sample size is discussed in Appendix D.

receive either standard medical therapy plus placebo treatment or standard medical therapy plus captopril. Patients were followed for an average of 3 years.

SAVE was a positive trial, demonstrating that captopril therapy produced a 19% reduction in the total mortality rate [26]. However, there was interest in the effect of therapy in patients with diabetes mellitus. The primary motivation for this interest began with the recognition that diabetes mellitus is a risk factor for serious morbidity and that the presence of diabetes mellitus increases the likelihood of death in patients with left ventricular dysfunction. Thus the effect of captopril was assessed on the cumulative total mortality rate of patients with diabetes mellitus. The presence of diabetes mellitus was determined by medical history at the time the patient was randomized in the trial (i.e., at baseline). In the diabetes mellitus subgroup, there are two strata: (1) patients with diabetes mellitus and (2) patients without diabetes mellitus. The actual subgroup analysis is the effect of therapy on each of these strata [27] (Table 9.2).

Table 9.2. Effect of captopril in diabetic subgroup in SAVE.

	Control inc. rate*	Active inc.rate	Relative risk	Confidence interval LB†	UB‡	P- value
Total cohort (n = 2231)	0.246	0.204	19	3	32	0.019
Nondiabetic (n = 1739)	0.222	0.181	20	2	35	0.036
Diabetic (n = 492)	0.328	0.292	12	-21	36	0.385

* Incidence rate † lower bound ‡ upper bound.

From Table 9.2 we learn several facts about the presence of diabetes in the SAVE cohort and the effect of therapy within the subgroup strata. Of the 2231 patients randomized to SAVE, 492 or 492/2231= 22% were diabetic. Also we can observe that the cumulative total mortality rate among diabetic patients (32.8%) was greater than for nondiabetic subjects (22.2%) in the trial, reflecting the anticipated increased mortality rate among patients with diabetes mellitus.

However, Table 9.2 suggests several other observations. In SAVE, captopril therapy reduced the total mortality rate by 20% ($p = 0.036$). However, in the diabetic stratum, captopril reduced the cumulative mortality effect by only 12% ($p = 0.385$). A first examination of these results suggests that captopril is effective in non-diabetic patients, but that its effects are just like placebo therapy in patients with diabetes mellitus. Is this an appropriate conclusion?

As we answer this question, there are several methodologic issues we must address. Clearly, the effect of captopril in nondiabetic patients was greater than its effect in diabetic patients in the 2231 patients recruited to SAVE. However, our focus is on the more important issue of what this means for the captopril effect in the larger population of patients from which SAVE's research sample was selected. Is it appropriate to generalize these results?

First, recall from the previous section that just the random reclassification of patients will induce differences in subgroup strata findings by chance alone. Even if there was no difference in the effect of captopril between diabetic and non-diabetic patients, we might expect to see a "subgroup effect" just through the random aggregation of patients in the two subgroup strata.

Second, the number of patients in the two strata is quite different, with there being many more non-diabetic patients then diabetic patients. The effect size for the non-diabetic patient stratum (20%) is very close to that of the overall cohort (19%). One would imagine that if there were 2200 nondiabetic patients, the relative risk (and p-value) of the effect of captopril in the nondiabetic cohort would even more closely match the findings in the total cohort. The reverse would be anticipated for the subgroup strata made up of a smaller number of patients. The results in the smaller cohort will demonstrate wider variability (as demonstrated here by the extremely wide confidence interval for the effect of therapy in the diabetic stratum), and therefore less reliability[15].

Finally, we have said nothing about how this analysis of the diabetic subgroup fits into the a priori analysis plan in SAVE. The absence of a prospective analysis plan for this subgroup makes us less trustful of the estimators of effect size, confidence intervals, and p-values. They are useful for exploratory and not confirmatory purposes.

Consideration of each of these points in turn weakens the persuasive power of this diabetes subgroup analysis. The best conclusion that we can draw from this subgroup evaluation is that the combination of the random play of chance, differences in stratum sizes, and estimator untrustworthiness (produced by the lack of a prospective plan of analysis) produced the differences in the findings in the subgroup strata. If we believe that the SAVE sample is representative of the population at large with left ventricular dysfunction, then the effect of captopril in the overall diabetic and nondiabetic patients in the population is the same as that in the total cohort of SAVE patients. This may be a difficult conclusion to accept based on the wide disparity in the treatment effect seen for the two subgroup strata within SAVE, but is the most accurate conclusion that can be applied to the millions of patients with heart failure who were not recruited into SAVE.

9.9 Subgroup Result Depiction

As discussed earlier in this chapter the evaluation of the effect of therapy within subgroups in clinical trials is a common expectation of the medical and regulatory community. However, the display and description of these expected analyses can be complicated and the task of providing an accurate portrayal of these complex results, within a manuscript that appears in the peer-reviewed journals with severe

---

[15] Another way to say this is that there is inadequate power for the evaluation of the effect of therapy in the diabetic stratum.

word limits, can be challenging. As an alternative to the tabular presentation of subgroup analyses results, an innovative way to show the results of subgroup analyses was developed by Sir Richard Peto. These adaptations, colloquially described as "Petograms," depict the results of the findings for individual subgroup strata within a clinical trial.

As an example, consider the results of the Cholesterol and Recurrent Events (CARE) clinical trial. This clinical trial was carried out to evaluate the effect of the HMG-Co reductase inhibitor pravastatin on atherosclerotic disease morbidity and mortality. CARE recruited 4159 patients with a recent, previous MI, and randomized them to receive standard care (control therapy) or standard care + pravastatin (active therapy). The primary endpoint for this study was fatal CHD + nonfatal MI. The effect of therapy within several subgroup strata was assessed using the post hoc endpoint fatal CAD + nonfatal MI + revascularization.[16]

The results of several of the subgroup analyses are displayed in Figure 9.6. The x-axis depicts the risk reduction for the expanded endpoint in CARE (a positive risk reduction indicates benefit). The y-axis has no quantitative meaning, but simply serves as a convenient dimension in which we can "stack" the subgroup strata one on top of the other.

Each subgroup strata produces an analysis of the effect of therapy on the expanded endpoint in CARE. Each analysis consists of a ball or diamond with a line running through it. The ball is the location of the effect size (a diamond is used to show the effect of therapy in the entire cohort). The size of the ball is proportional to the number of patients in the subgroup stratum, and the location and length of the line going through the ball reflects the confidence interval. Thus, one can quickly and easily gain a sense of the effect size, the precision of the effect size (as portrayed by the width of the confidence interval), and the number of patients in which the analysis was carried out.

There is no inclusion of the p-value in this evaluation. This is not a serious omission if we keep in mind that the majority of subgroup analyses are exploratory. The absence of both a prospective analysis plan and alpha allocation renders the p-values worthless.

In the next chapter we discuss the problems that subgroup analyses have produced for the medical and regulatory communities.

---

[16] Because of the small number of primary endpoint events in the study, the subgroup strata of interest would have contained too few events to provide a precise estimate of the effect of therapy within each of the subgroups of interest. It was therefore decided to use an expanded endpoint that included patients who survived the study, did not have a heart attack during the course of the trial, but did undergo coronary revascularization. An alternative approach to this exploratory evaluation will be provided in Chapter 11.

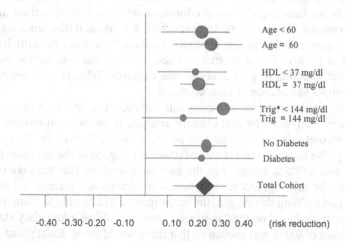

Figure 9.6. "Petogram" of subgroup analyses in CARE as measured by risk reduction.

Problems

1. What are the interpretative problems associated with subgroup analyses?
2. Why do subgroup analyses remain in demand by the medical and regulatory communities?
3. How does an aggregation effect all but guarantee that therapy effect heterogeneity will emerge in the subgroup analysis of a clinical trial.
4. A company has carried out a small clinical trial to learn about the effect of a new medication on the frequency and severity of headaches. In a relatively small, phase II study , the sponsor, using a non-prospective, exploratory analysis, determined that the medication was beneficial in men and not in women. They then conducted a follow-up, phase III study in women only, and, through another nonprospectively specified analysis, determined that the medication produced a benefit in women who believed that their headaches were non-stress related. How would you respond to their argument that they have identified a therapy that is beneficial only in women with non-stress related headaches?
5. A sponsor is interested in testing for the effect of an intervention that has a substantial side-effect profile that will produce a large number of patients who will discontinue therapy and withdraw from the active group. However, if the patients choose to stay on their active therapy, the sponsor believes that the patients will see a modest benefit that can be accrued to the therapy. The company therefore designs the clinical trial for which the primary analysis will be an "as-treated analysis," assigning patients who were originally randomized

to the therapy group based not on randomization, but on whether they could stay on the medication. The intention-to-treat analysis will be carried out, but will be considered a secondary analysis, with a nominal 0.05 α error expenditure. The sponsor believes this approach protects them from the criticism that the study is positive based on an as-treated analysis that was carried out only because the intention to treat analysis was negative. What is your response to the company's solicitation of your opinion?

6. A group of investigators wish to carry out a clinical trial in which there will be two primary analyses. The first primary analysis is an intention-to-treat analysis. The second primary analysis will be an "as-treated" analysis. To conserve the familywise error, an α error rate of 0.045 is assigned to the intention to treat analysis, and 0.005 is assigned to the as-treated analysis (for the sake of conservatism, the investigators do not embed a dependency parameter into their analysis plans). With this design, the investigators will be able to claim that the study is positive based on the "as-treated" analysis. When asked, they state that the threshold of 0.005 was chosen so that there would be no doubt about the effect of the therapy in the "as-treated" analysis. Comment on the advisability of this approach.

References

1. Pfeffer, M.A., Braunwald, E., Moyé, L.A. et al. (1992). Effect of captopril on mortality and morbidity in patients with left ventricular dysfunction after myocardial infarction–results of the Survival and Ventricular Enlargement Trial. *New England Journal of Medicine* **327**:669–677.

2. Sacks F.M. Pfeffer M.A., Moyé, L.A. (1996). The effect of pravastatin on coronary events after myocardial infarction in patients with average cholesterol levels. *New England Journal of Medicine* **335**:1001–1009.

3 The SHEP Cooperative Research Group (1991) Prevention of stroke by antihypertensive drug therapy in older persons with isolated systolic hypertension: final results of the systolic hypertension in the elderly program (SHEP). *Journal of the American Medical Association* **265**:3255–3264

4. The Long-Term Intervention with Pravastatin in Ischaemic Disease (LIPID) Study Group. (1998). Prevention of cardiovascular events and death with pravastatin in patients with CAD and a broad range of initial cholesterol levels. *New England Journal of Medicine* **339**:1349–1357.

5. Moyé, L.A., Pfeffer, M.A., Wun, C.C., et. al (1994). Uniformity of captopril benefit in the post infarction population: Subgroup analysis in SAVE. *European Heart Journal.***15**: Supplement B:2–8.

6. Lewis, S.J., Moyé, L.A., Sacks, F.M., et. al (1998). Effect of pravastatin on cardiovascular events in older patients with myocardial infarction and cholesterol levels in the average range. Results of the Cholesterol and Recurrent Events (CARE) trial. *Annals of Internal Medicine* **129**:681–689.

7. Lewis, S.J., Sacks, F.M., Mitchell, J.S., et. al (1998). Effect of pravastatin on cardiovascular events in women after myocardial infarction: the cholesterol and recurrent events (CARE) trial. *Journal of the American College of Cardiology* **32**:140–146.

8. Peto, R., Collins, R., Gray, R. (1995). Large-cale randomized evidence: Large, simple trials and overviews of trials. *Journal of Clinical Epidemiology* **48**:23–40.

9. MRFIT Investigators. (1982). Multiple risk factor intervention trial *Journal of the American Medical Association* **248**:1465–77.

10. ISIS-1 Collaborative Group (1986) Randomized trial of intravenous atenolol among 16027 cases of suspected actue myocardial infarction–ISIS-1. *Lancet* **ii**;57–66.

11. Lee, K.L., McNeer, F., Starmer, C.F., Harris, P.J., Rosari, R.A. (1980). Clinical judgment and statistics. Lessons from a simulated randomized trial in coronary artery disease. *Circulation* **61**:508–515.

12. Assmann, S., Pocock, S., Enos, L., Kasten, L. (2000), Subgroup analysis and other (mis)uses) of baseline data in clinical trials. *Lancet* **355**:1064–69

13. Bulpitt, C. (1988). Subgroup Analysis. *Lancet*: 31–34 .

14. Packer, M., O'Connor, C.M., Ghali, J.K., et al. for the Prospective Randomized Amlodipine Survival Evaluation Study Group. (1996). Effect of amlodipine on morbidity and mortality in severe chronic heart failure. *New England Journal of Medicine* **335**:1107–14.

15. Packer, M. Presentation of the results of the Prospective Randomized Amlodipine Survival Evaluation-2 Trial (PRAISE–2) at the American College of Cardiology Scientific Sessions, Anaheim, CA, March 15, 2000.

16. Exner, D.V., Dreis, D.L., Domanski, M.J., Cohn, J.N. (2001), Lesser response to angiotensin–converting enzyme inhibitor therapy in black as compared to white patients with left ventricular dysfunction. *New England Journal of Medicine* **334**:1351–7

17.. Yancy, C.W., Fowler, M.B., Colucci, W.S., Gilber, E.M., Brsitow, M.R., Cohn, J.N., Luka, M.A., Young, S.T., Packer, M. for the US Carvedilol Heart Failure Study Group. 2001.Race and response to adrenergic blockade with carvedilol in patients with chronic heart failure. *New England Journal of Medicine* **334**:1358–65.

18. Stolberg S.G. Should a pill be colorblind? *New York Times*. Week in Review. May 13, 2001.p 1.

19. Moyé, L. (2000) *Statistical Reasoning in Medicine: The Intuitive P-Value Primer*. New York. Springer.

20. Yusuf, S., Wittes, J., Probstfield J, Tyroler H.A. (1991).Analysis and interpretation of treatment effects in subgroups of patients in randomized clinical trials. *Journal of the American Medical Association* **266**:93–8.

21. Pedersen, T.R., Olsson, A.G., Faergeman, O., Kjekshus, J., Wedel, H., Berg, K., Wilhelmensen, L., Haghfelt, T., Thorgeirsson, G., Pyòrälä, K., Miettinen, T., Christophersen. B.G., Tobert, J.A., Musliner, T.A., Cook, T.J. for the Scandinavian Simvastatin Survival Study Group. (1998). Lipoprotein changes and

reduction in the incidence of major CAD events in the scandinavian simvastatin survival study (4S). *Circulation* **97**:1453–1460.

22. West of Scotland Coronary Prevention Study Group. (1996). Infleunce of pravastatin and plasma lipids on clinical events in the West of Scotland Coronary Prevention Study (WOSCOPS). *Circulation* **97**:1440–1445.

23. Sacks, F.M., Moyé, L.A., Davis, B.R., Cole, T.B., Rouleau, J.L., Nash, D. Pfeffer, M.A., Braunwald, E. (1998). Relationship between plama LDL concentrations during treatment with pravastatin and recurrent coronary events in the Cholesterol and Recurrent Events trial. *Circulation* **97**:1446–1452.

24. Peduzzi, P.,Wittes, J., Deter, K., Holford, T. Analysis as-randomized and the problem of non-adherence; an example from the veterans affairs randomized trial of coronary artery bypass surgery. (1993). *Statistics in Medicine* **12**:1185–1195.

25. Moyé, L.A. for the SAVE Cooperative Group. (1991). Rationale and design of a trial to assess patient survival and ventricular enlargement after myocardial infarction. *American Journal of Cardiology* **68**:70D–79D.

26. Pfeffer, M.A., Braunwald, E., Moyé, L.A. et al. (1992) Effect of Captopril on mortality and morbidity in patients with left ventricular dysfunction after myocardial infarction–results of the Survival and Ventricular Enlargement Trial. *New England Journal of Medicine* **327**:669–677.

27. The Long–Term Intervention with Pravastatin in Ischaemic Disease (LIPID) Study Group. (1998). Prevention of cardiovascular events and death with pravastatin in patients with CAD and a broad range of initial cholesterol levels. *New England Journal of Medicine* **339**:1349–1357.

Chapter 10
Subgroups II: Effect Domination and Controversy

This second of three consecutive chapters that discusses subgroup analyses covers the rules that govern subgroup analyses interpretation. A distinction is drawn between a subgroup analysis that compares the effect of a randomly allocated intervention in a clinical trial across subgroup strata on the one hand, and the analysis which only seeks to confirm the efficacy of therapy within a single subgroup stratum on the other. Finally three controversial uses of subgroup analyses are provided.

10.1 Effect Domination Principle

We have stated in the previous chapter that, in the absence of confirmatory subgroup evaluations, the best estimate of the effect of randomly allocated therapy within a subgroup strata is the effect of that therapy on the overall cohort. We will call this the principle of *effect domination*— the effect of therapy averaged over all randomized patients dominates the effect seen in the individual subgroup strata.

The effect domination principle was the basis of our decision to overturn the results of several of the subgroup evaluations that were provided in the previous chapter. Although there are many clinical trials designed to provide confirmatory evaluations of their primary analyses, there are far fewer confirmatory evaluations that occur in the assessments of subgroups. Therefore, the effect domination principle is much more frequently required in the interpretation of the results of clinical trials.

Since subgroup analyses have and will, in all likelihood, continue to engender the interest of the medical community, it is logical to ask why there aren't more confirmatory analyses involving subgroup evaluations. This is an especially interesting question since there are clear circumstances in which subgroup evaluations can produce confirmatory results of the therapy effect within (or across) subgroup strata. When executed, these confirmatory results stand on their own, separate and apart from the result of the effect of therapy in the overall cohort. The criteria for these evaluations were clearly characterized by Yusuf et al. [1] and are coincident with our development of confirmatory analyses in this text.

The first of these criteria for the development of confirmatory analyses in clinical trials is that the subgroup analysis must be prospectively designed and proper. This structure is required so that (1) the therapy effect size estimators that the subgroup analysis produces are trustworthy; and (2) that the effect of therapy to be evaluated in a subgroup is not confounded by (i.e., bound up with) post-randomization events as discussed in the previous chapter. In general, there has been no difficulty with meeting this requirement of confirmatory subgroup analyses. Many clinical trials make statements in their protocols describing the plans of investigators to evaluate the effect of therapy within their subgroups of interest. These subgroups are, by and large, proper subgroups, e.g., demographic traits, or the presence of risk characteristics at baseline.

However, the final requirement for a confirmatory subgroup analysis is the prospective allocation of type I and type II error rates. This last criterion has proved to be especially vexing because of the severe sample size constraints this places on subgroup analyses. As we have pointed out earlier, the allocation of type I error rates for confirmatory testing must be such that the FWER, ξ, is conserved. This requires that statistical testing at the level of subgroup analyses will be governed by test-specific α error rates that are generally less than 0.05.

The difficulty of executing subgroup analyses in the presence of FWER control and adequate statistical power is not difficult to understand. In fact, resources are generally strained to the breaking point for the analysis of the effect of therapy in the overall cohort. This overall analysis is typically carried out with the minimum acceptable power (80%) because of either financial constraints or patient recruitment difficulties. By definition, subgroup analyses (and certainly within-stratum subgroup analyses) will involve a smaller number of patients; it is a daunting task to prospectively allocate type I and type II error rates at acceptable levels in a smaller number of patients, although the methodology for the accurate computation of sample size is available [2]. Thus, the growth of the use of subgroups as confirmatory tools has, to some extent, been stunted by the difficulty of constructing a prospective clinical trial with an embedded, prospectively defined proper subgroup for which tight statistical control is provided for type I and type II statistical errors.

10.2 Assessment of Subgroup Effects

The evaluation of subgroup effects in clinical trials focuses on the effect of the randomly allocated therapy on the subgroup of interest. However this assessment can be carried out in two complementary manners. The first is the determination of a differential effect of therapy across subgroup strata. The second is the evaluation of the effect of therapy within a single subgroup stratum. Each approach, when prospectively planned and concordantly executed, can supplement the information provided by the evaluation of the main effect of a clinical trial.

10.2.1 Effect Modification and Interaction Analyses

We commonly think of the effect of the randomly allocated intervention in a clinical trial as an effect across the entire research cohort. The determination that the magnitude of the effect depends upon the subgroup stratum can be provocative, valuable, and the basis of a new indication for the use of the therapy. The examination of a dataset for this effect, while complicated, has become a routine part of the evaluation of the randomly allocated therapy's influence in a clinical trial. The finding of both clinical and statistical significance for this analysis suggests that the effect of therapy is different for one subgroup stratum than for another.

This type of subgroup effect is commonly referred to as a *treatment by subgroup* interaction; a notable product of this analysis is the *p*-value for interaction. Typically, the analysis result is described as identifying how the subgroup strata interacts with the therapy to alter the occurrence of the endpoint, and the evaluation is called an *interaction analysis*. Alternatively, this approach is described as *effect modification*, i.e., it examines the degree to which the subgroup stratum modifies the effect of treatment on the endpoint of interest. Either descriptor is well accepted and serves as an appropriate characterization of the process and interpretation when the analysis is prospectively defined and executed according to its protocol.

Statistically significant effect modification analyses in clinical trials are not common, primarily because the analyses are underpowered. We should not be surprised that this is the case, since the subgroup analyses involve an evaluation of an effect difference between smaller subsets of patients within the research cohort. Everything else being equal, the smaller sample sizes reduce the statistical power of the hypothesis tests. Therefore the occurrence of a statistically significant effect size can be particularly noteworthy.

An example of such a finding occurred in the Cholesterol and Recurrent Events (CARE) clinical trial described in the previous chapter. In that study, an exploratory examination of the effect of the HMG-CoA reductase inhibitor pravastatin was assessed in the gender subgroup. The relevant analysis was the effect of pravastatin on the cumulative incidence rate of the post hoc composite endpoint of CAD death + nonfatal MI + coronary revascularization [7]. There were 4159 patients recruited in the CARE study; of these, 576 (13.8%) were women and 3,583 (86.2%) were men. During the course of the trial the effect of the randomly allocated intervention pravastatin on lipids appeared to be the same in women and men, producing equivalent reductions in total cholesterol (20% in women, 19% in men), low density lipid (LDL) cholesterol (28% in women, 28% in men), and triglycerides (13% in women, and 14% in men). There were equivalent elevations in high-density lipoprotein (HDL) cholesterol (4% in women, 5% in men).

However, the subgroup analysis revealed an apparent difference in the effect of pravastatin therapy on the expanded endpoint in men and women (Table 10.1). Men in CARE experienced a relative risk of 0.761 on pravastatin therapy, while women who were randomly chosen to receive pravastatin therapy experienced a 0.545 relative risk. The *p*-value that assesses the difference in the effect for men and women was 0.05. Within CARE, the effect of therapy appeared to be modified by gender; women being the greater beneficiary of this effect than men. However, the post hoc nature of the analysis provides only hypothesis generating status to these results.

Table 10.1. Interaction effect in CARE for expanded endpoint*
gender modification of therapy effect

Gender strata	Rel. risk	Interaction p-value
Males	0.761	
Females	0.545	
		0.050

*CHD disease death + nonfatal MI + coronary revascularization.

10.2.2 Within-Stratum Effects

The comparison of the effect of therapy across subgroup strata can be a very powerful elucidation of the randomly allocated therapy's effect heterogeneity. However, the interpretation of this analysis can be problematic, since it is often underpowered. In a competitive environment in which only cost effective clinical trials are funded, it is difficult to gather sufficient financial resources to design and execute a clinical trial, one of whose primary missions is to examine a treatment by subgroup strata interaction.

In addition, the evaluation of a subgroup mediated effect modification may not directly address the question the investigators have raised about the subgroup. This is because the investigators' interest may not be in the entire subgroup, but only in selected subgroup strata. Specifically, the investigators may not ask whether the effect of therapy is the same across subgroups, but instead ask whether there is an explicit effect of the intervention in the prospectively defined subgroup stratum of interest. This is a different question than the question which is best answered by an interaction analysis.

Under what circumstances will the investigator be interested in a therapy effect in only one subgroup stratum? One situation would be if the stratum is composed of patients who have a very different prognosis from that of other patients. While investigators may be most interested in the effect of a new intervention on breast cancer, they may be particularly interested in the effect of the therapy in patients with an advanced stage of the disease. This interest does not require the investigators to ask whether the effect of therapy in patients with less advanced breast cancer is different from that of patients with advanced breast cancer; they wish to know only whether the therapy has been shown to have explicit efficacy in patients with advanced breast cancer.

Similarly, a new therapy for the treatment of CHF may hold promise for reducing mortality in all patients with CHF, but the investigator is motivated to demonstrate the effect of this therapy in patients with CHF whose etiology is non-ischemic. She is not interested in comparing or contrasting the efficacy of the intervention between ischemic versus nonischemic etiologies of CHF. She is instead focused on two questions: (1) Is the therapy effective in the entire cohort and (2) Is the therapy effective in the subcohort with CHF-nonischemic etiology?

Is it possible that the therapy could be effective in the entire cohort but not the sub cohort of interest? Yes. Consider the possibility that the therapy in fact is effective for patients with CHF-ischemic etiology but ineffective for patients with a nonischemic etiology for their CHF. Let the research sample primarily contain patients with CHF-ischemic etiology with only a small number of patients who have a nonischemic etiology for their heart failure. Since the research sample mostly contains patients who will respond to the therapy, the result of the concordantly executed clinical trial will be positive (barring an effect that is driven by sampling error). The investigator will then argue that, since the trial is positive, this positive finding will apply to the CHF-nonischemic subgroup as well. Essentially, the conclusion about the nonischemic subcohort is based primarily on the findings of patients who are not in that subcohort at all. This is the consequence of the effect domination principle, in which the findings in the overall cohort devolve on each of the subgroup strata. In this example, the principle produces the wrong conclusion; nevertheless, it is the best conclusion available in the absence of a confirmatory subgroup analysis. In order to avoid this possibility, the investigator is interested in reaching a confirmatory conclusion.

As another illustration of a circumstance in which prospectively specified, stratum-specific subgroup analyses can make an important contribution, consider the situation in which the adverse event profile of a therapy that is being studied in a controlled clinical trial is known to be different between women and men. As an illustration, consider a cholesterol-reducing drug that produces breast cancer in women. In this circumstance, the risk-benefit profile of this drug is different for women than it is for men. Since women will be exposed to a greater risk with this therapy, it is reasonable to require investigators to produce a statistically valid demonstration of efficacy in women. The investigators are not disinterested in an effect in men—but the relatively low risk of the drug in men allows the investigators to be satisfied with deducing the effect of the therapy in men from the effect of therapy in the overall cohort. It is the greater adverse event risk in women that requires an explicit demonstration of efficacy in them.

Perhaps the most useful product of this dialogue is that there are different questions that can be asked of subgroups. Some of these questions can be addressed by a heterogeneity of effect evaluation and an interaction analysis, but there are others which are addressed by the direct demonstration of efficacy in a single subgroup stratum. We will return to this issue in the next chapter.

10.3 Problematic Subgroup Analyses

At this point, it is clear that subgroup analyses (much like multiple statistical analyses) in clinical trials are both prevalent and unreliable. Retrospectively considered, sometimes only casually planned, the conclusions concerning subgroup analysis, while descriptive of the findings in the sample, often do not reveal the truth about the relationship in the larger population. Recent discussions in the literature concerning the wide variation in results by clinical center in the BHAT trial [3], [4], [5] are an illustration of the difficulty in interpreting subgroup assessments. Indeed, the literature [6], [7], [8], [9], [10] recommends that, as currently incorporated in clinical trials, subgroup analyses interpretations are exploratory; they can suggest, but do not confirm, a modification of the randomly allocated therapy's effect in the population at large.

We will next review three current and provocative subgroup analyses in clinical trials. In each case, the controversial nature of the clinical question was allowed to overturn the correct use of subgroup methodology.

10.4 The MERIT Trial

Carvedilol[1] was not the only beta-blocker that was investigated for its effects in patients with CHF. The evaluation of other medications in this same class accelerated in the 1990s, and researchers identified metoprolol CR/XL as a promising compound whose initial results justified a full-scale clinical trial.[2]

The Metoprolol CR/XL Randomized Intervention Trial in CHF (MERIT-HF) was designed to evaluate the effect of metoprolol XL in patients with decreased LVEF and symptoms of heart failure. The protocol of this study was published [11], providing details of it's a priori planned analysis. MERIT-HF was a prospectively designed, randomized, clinical trial. Patients with NYHA class II–IV heart failure of at least 3 months duration and LVEFs ≤ 40% were recruited from both the USA and Europe. Subjects who met all inclusion and exclusion criteria were placed on optimal medical therapy for their CHF. This therapy included the use of diuretics, and ACE-i therapy.) If the ACE-i could not be tolerated, hydralazine or an angiotensin II receptor antagonist was substituted. Patients were then randomly selected to receive either metoprolol CR/XL or placebo therapy. This random allocation was prospectively planned so that the effect of therapy would be balanced for the analyses of the following subgroups; investigational site, age, sex, ethnic origin, cause of heart failure, previous acute MI, (and in patients with previous MI, the time since the last MI), diabetes mellitus, ejection fraction and NYHA functional class. The target dose of the therapy was 200 mg daily. Follow-up visits were required every 3 months.

The investigators in MERIT-HF had prospectively planned two primary analyses and differentially allocated the type I error rate between them. The first primary analysis was the effect of metoprolol on the total mortality rate; the test-specific α error rate for this evaluation was 0.04. A prospectively specified α error of 0.01 was chosen to evaluate the effect of therapy on the combined endpoint of total mortality + total hospitalizations.

Although the protocol stated that the effect of therapy on total mortality would be assessed in the prospectively defined subgroups listed above, no attempt was made to control the type I error allocation for these assessments. Thus, these

---

[1] Discussed in Chapter 1.

[2] The author was a paid consultant for the sponsor during the evaluation of the FDA's interpretation of the MERIT-HF clinical trial.

subgroup evaluations were to be secondary analyses, providing only supportive evidence for the two primary analyses. The sample size goal was 3200 patients (1600 subjects per group), and the trial was monitored by an independent DSMB.

The results of the study were published in 1999 [12]. The MERIT-HF investigators enrolled 3991 patients from 313 clinical sites in 13 European countries and the United States. In the metoprolol CR/XL group, 145 patients died (7.2%); 217 patient died in the placebo group (11.0%). This produced a relative risk = 0.66, and a 95% confidence interval 0.53-0.81. The p-value for this finding was $p <$ 0.001. These results led the DSMB to stop the trial prematurely based on prospectively defined stopping criteria.[3]

Additional findings in MERIT-HF added strength to the hypothesis that metoprolol CR/XL produced a beneficial effect on total mortality. Cardiovascular mortality, sudden death, and death from worsening heart failure were all reduced in the active group. Subgroup analysis [12, Figure 5] revealed the beneficial effect of metoprolol CR/XL on total mortality was homogeneous within each of the prospectively identified subgroup analyses. Editorial comments appearing in the literature [13], while acknowledging that beta-blocker therapy was reported to be associated with a diminished quality of life within the first few weeks of therapy, affirmed that MERIT-HF provided overwhelming evidence of benefit of β-blocker therapy in heart failure. By the definitions adopted in this text, MERIT-HF was a positive trial.

The Metoprolol for CHF New Drug Application (NDA) was submitted by the sponsor to the FDA for review after the conclusion of the MERIT-HF study. The sponsor requested that metoprolol CR/XL be approved for use as a medication that reduced total mortality for patients with CHF. Both the overall results and the subgroup findings of the MERIT-HF trial were reproduced by the FDA's review team. However, during their review of the NDA, the FDA executed an additional analysis that had been neither prospectively planned nor carried out by the MERIT-HF investigators. (Table 10.2).

Table 10.2. Effect of metoprolol CR-XL by country.

Country	Relative risk	95% CI Lower bound	95% CI Upper bound
USA	1.05	0.71	1.56
All others	0.55	0.43	0.70

Interaction p-value = 0.003

---

[3] A description of early termination procedures in clinical trials is provided in Chapter 1.

The FDA created a new subgroup with two strata: (1) patients randomized in the United States, and (2) patients randomized from other countries. The within-strata analyses revealed that metoprolol was less effective in reducing total mortality in the United States than it was in other countries.

The sponsor was informed of the results of this analysis and expressed concerns about attempts to draw conclusions from this evaluation. In response to the Sponsor's concern, the FDA reviewer stated that the United States patient population analysis was carried out mainly to check the internal consistency of the overall trial result. The FDA did not require that there be a statistically significant reduction in the total mortality rate in the United States patients, but insisted that it is at least necessary for the United States mortality outcome not to contradict the mortality findings in the overall cohort. The review also stated that

> ...if the mortality endpoint is the most important among all endpoints, the US sub-population should be the most important subgroup in a multinational trial because the goal of the NDA submission is to gain approval for marketing in the drug in the US. The efficacy outcome in this population must be evaluated carefully as part of the evaluation of totality of the evidence and possible extrapolation of the efficacy evidence from foreign population to US population.[4]

There was no prospective statement about this concern by the FDA during the initial development of the MERIT-HF protocol. Nevertheless, this concern was echoed by other voices within the agency, e.g.,

> Because of demographic differences or differences in concomitant care, a treatment might be beneficial overall but neutral or detrimental in some subpopulations. In particular, even though studies in United States patients were not required for approval, evidence that a treatment is non-beneficial in United States patients (or even in some identifiable subpopulation among United States patients) must not be ignored. The observed mortality among United States patients receiving metoprolol was 105% of that seen in those receiving placebo.

> How should this finding be interpreted? The finding of adverse United States mortality effects could of course be attributable to chance, but it could alternatively be a genuine finding, the result of US-European differences in demographics or concomitant therapy".[5]

On this basis, the FDA did not provide the new indication for total mortality that the sponsor requested.

The analysis that produced this controversy is clearly post hoc and cannot be confirmatory. It is equally clear that the FDA was well aware of the numerous

---

[4] *Statistical Review and Evaluation* (Amendment I), NDA 19,962. May 30, 2000.
[5] Internal FDA memo, May 16, 2000.

problems created by relying on post hoc analyses in general, and on non-prospectively defined subgroup analyses in particular. Certainly, these argument would have been effectively wielded against the sponsor if the results of MERIT-HF were null, but the sponsor was to argue that metoprolol CR/XL should be approved on the basis of a beneficial finding in an unplanned analysis of United States patients.

The sponsor argued in vain that this post hoc, underpowered comparison of the U.S. subgroup against all of the other countries combined was neither logical nor a valid comparison. The non-US countries did not represent a homogenous group regarding social, economic, or standard of care characteristics. The Sponsor also pointed out that there was no evidence that beta-blocker therapy interacted with any of these characteristics. Other analysis findings cast doubt on the excess mortality finding in the US. An examination of the additional endpoints in the MERIT-HF study failed to provide any support for the suggested lower effect on total mortality in the United States subgroup. In fact, the results for the composite endpoint of total mortality and all-cause hospitalizations, as well as the results for sudden death, in the United States subgroup support the overall study findings of compelling benefit in the treatment of heart failure. Nevertheless, the FDA remain unmoved. After much additional discussion, Metoprolol extended release formulation was approved for the treatment of CHF, but was not given a total mortality indication.

10.5 Ethnicity and ACE-i therapy

A current issue in cardiology is the possibility that the treatment of CHF might be tailored to the race of the individual. An exploration of this concept has produced a collection of analyses which have appeared in the peer-reviewed literature.

One of the first evaluations of this issue was a retrospective examination of two clinical trials in heart failure [14]. This analysis reviewed and contrasted the experience of African-American and Caucasian patients with CHF, demonstrating differences in CHF etiology, neurohumoral stimulation, and response to pharmacological agents in these patient groups with CHF. The evaluations were based on the comparisons between 180 African-American male patients and 450 Caucasian male patients in V-HeFT 1 and a second comparison of 215 African-American and 574 Caucasian male patients in V-HeFT II.

An assessment of demographic characteristics revealed that African-Americans had a lower incidence of CHD, a higher incidence of previously diagnosed hypertension, and a greater cardiothoracic ratio than Caucasians. Neurohumoral differences included lower plasma norepinephrine levels in African-Americans and reduced plasma renin activity in African-Americans with a history of hypertension. The authors also identified a trend toward lower mortality of African-American patients being treated with hydralazine plus isosorbide dinitrate, while Caucasian patients who were treated with the ACE-i had a reduced cumulative mortality rate. These findings suggested that there might be a biologic mechanism underlying racial differences in the response to therapy. However, the investigators clearly stated that these evaluations were post hoc, analyses that required confirmation in well-controlled, clinical trials.

To continue the investigation of this interesting concept, the SOLVD investigators provided an analysis of this issue from two clinical trials. The SOLVD clinical trials evaluated the effect of the ACE-i enalapril on the occurrence of morbidity and mortality in patients with left ventricular dysfunction [15] and in patients with frank CHF [16]. These two pivotal clinical trials were among those that led to the recommendation that all patients with CHF be treated with ACE-i therapy as tolerated. The post hoc examination of these SOLVD studies for the influence of race, demonstrated that African-American patients with a history of CHF had a worse outcome then Caucasian patients, with African-American patients being more likely to die from any cause, and 37 % more likely to die from any cause or be hospitalized for heat failure [17].

The investigators now wished to compare the effect of enalapril in African-Americans to that of Caucasians using a *post hoc* analysis structure. In these two studies 800 participants classified themselves as African-American, and 5719 patients were Caucasian. However, there was the problem of attribution of effect, i.e., any differences in event rates between the races might not be ascribed to race, but instead attributed to other differences between these patients. In an attempt to minimize this problem, African-American and Caucasian patients were matched according to which of the two SOLVD trials they were randomized. They were also matched on the basis of baseline LVEF, therapy group, gender and age. As many as 4 Caucasian patients were matched to one African-American patient. However, despite these attempts to match patients, African-American patients were younger and less well educated than Caucasian patients.

The investigators found that event rates were higher among African-American patients than Caucasian patients (12.2 deaths per 100 person years versus 9.7 deaths per 100 person years). The effect of enalapril did not reduce deaths from any cause in either African-American or Caucasian patients. However, while enalapril reduced the hospitalization rate for CHF for Caucasian patients, its use had no effect on the reduction of the hospitalization rate in African-American patients. The authors concluded that enalapril therapy is associated with a significant reduction in the risk of hospitalization for heart failure in Caucasian patients with left ventricular dysfunction but that enalapril produced no significant alteration in this outcome among similar African-American patients.

Yancy et al. examined the effect of race on the response of patients to carvedilol in patients with chronic CHF [17]. The effect of carvedilol therapy on patients with CHF was identified in the United States Carvedilol program[6] In this trial, there were 217 African-American patients and 877 non-African-American patients. As anticipated, the African-American patients were less likely to have CAD and more likely to have hypertension then non-African-American participants. Also, as anticipated, African-American patients had a higher mortality rate than non-African-American patients (8.9% versus 7.5%) and also a greater hospitalization rate (31.5% versus 25.3 %).

The investigators reported that carvedilol lowered the risk of death from any cause by 68% in non-African-Americans and by 56% in African-Americans. In

---

[6] This collection of clinical trials was discussed in Chapter 2.

addition carvedilol reduced the risk of death from any cause or hospitalization by 49% in non-African-American and 43% in African-Americans, and reduced the risk of progression of heart failure by 51% in non-African-American and 54% in African-Americans. None of the statistical comparisons of these rates between African-Americans reached nominal significance.

Taken at face value, these results appear to suggest that African-American patients who suffer from CHF might be better treated with the beta blocker carvedilol than with the ACE-i enalapril. This concept has engendered discussion in the medical literature. In his review of these results, Swartz [18] clearly enunciates the difficulties in the identification of race and the attendant problems of tailoring therapy based on a demographic characteristic which is currently so imprecisely determined. Wood [19] stated that racial differences in the response to drugs not only have practical importance for each of the choice of and dose of drugs but should also alert physicians to the important underlying genetic determinants of the drug response.

However, before we delve into these more enticing issues, we must first ask a more fundamental question. Are these analyses statistically reliable? Do they provide a clear and accurate depiction of the effect of each of enalapril and carvedilol on African-American patients? CHF, whose lethality is race-independent, is particularly acute and tragic in African-American patients with its earlier onset and more rapid production of morbidity and mortality. The suggestion that CHF therapy can be used differently in African-American patients than in Caucasian patients suggests that the need to optimize therapy for CHF should adumbrate treatment practices that are based on the assumption that patients should be treated the same regardless of race, since people, despite differences in skin color, are more alike than they are different.

Do the data in these two evaluations support overturning this well established principle of non-race-based treatment? Without the confirmatory hypothesis testing procedures in place for subgroup evaluations, the best interpretative guide in this matter is that of Yusuf [20], i.e., the most reliable estimate of the effect of a therapy within a subgroup strata in the effect of therapy in the overall cohort. Is there any reason for us to negate this natural conclusion in either of the two foregoing analyses? In the case of the race–therapy assessment from SOLVD, the racial statistical evaluation was entirely post hoc. No prospective plan guided the combination of the two SOLVD studies, nor was there an a priori plan in place to determine how this assessment should take place. This is specifically not the environment in which to draw confirmatory conclusions about the effect of therapy in African-American patients. Thus, we must void the SOLVD racial subgroup analyses and replace them by the findings of the overall SOLVD results.

We may never know why African-American patients taking enalapril in SOLVD did not experience a reduction in their hospitalization rate, (just like we will in all likelihood never know why hypertensive men with baseline ECG abnormalities did worse on antihypertensive therapy in the classic MRFIT study [20]—a finding which threatened to reverse the treatment of hypertension in the early 1980's [19]). These are the spurious outcomes that occur from unplanned subgroup analyses. However, the task is to identify the most reliable therapy for the millions of African-American patients with CHF who were not recruited into SOLVD. The clearest, time tested, most accurate answer SOLVD offers is its overall finding of enalapril benefit, identified in the analysis of the entire cohort.

Turning now to the study involving carvedilol, we see that, as was the case with SOLVD, the assessment of a race mediated therapy effect in the United States Carvedilol program as presented by Yancy et al. was a post hoc analysis. In addition, that study did not produce the effect of carvedilol (stratified by race) on the prospectively defined endpoints of the United States Carvedilol program but instead used substituted endpoints. This is again not a research plan that permits us to draw confirmatory conclusions. Thus, invoking the best interpretative methodology for subgroup analyses in clinical trials leads us to apply the effect of carvedilol on all patients in the United States Carvedilol program to the subset stratum of African-American patients, i.e., that there is no race mediated effect of therapy in the United States Carvedilol program. This is precisely what Yancy's result reveals. In fact, in each of the reported evaluations carried out by Yancy et al., carvedilol had the same effect in African-Americans as it did in non-African-Americans.

The effect of carvedilol in African-Americans is the same as the effect in the entire cohort. However, we must now ask what that overall effect was. In SOLVD the primary analysis of the effect of enalapril on the entire cohort was prospectively written into the protocol and its results were easy to interpret. However, major criticism has been leveled at the US Carvedilol program[7]. Thus, to identify the effect of carvedilol in African-American patients with CHF, use of correct methodologic principles requires us to apply the findings of carvedilol seen in the overall cohort. However, that effect cannot be identified because of the US Carvedilol's program weak analytic methodology.

The medical community's attraction to subgroup analysis is in direct proportion to the healthcare provider's need to treat special subgroup strata that are at unusual risk. Unfortunately, the reliability of the traditional subgroup analyses in clinical trials does not increase with this acutely felt need in the medical community, rendering it particularly vulnerable to misleading subgroup evaluations. Therefore we must be particularly disciplined in the rigorous application of methodologic standards in controversial settings.

10.6 The NETT Study

As a final example of a controversial use of subgroup results, we consider the findings of the National Emphysema Treatment Trial (NETT) Research Group [21]. The treatment of emphysema has been problematic. Lung-volume-reduction surgery (LVRS), or the process by which 20 to 35 % of the emphysematous lung is removed is a controversial tool in the treatment of this chronic disease. The surgery mortality rate is from 4 to 17 %, but commonly, lung function, exercise capacity, and the quality of life can improve in the overwhelming majority of patients who have completed the surgery. NETT is a federally funded clinical trial to assess the effect of LVRS when compared to conventional medical therapy.

---

[7] See the discussion in Chapter 2 on the US Carvedilol program.

The purpose of this study was to compare the survival rates and exercise capacity of patients who receive LVRS to those patients who receive medical therapy. However, an additional goal of NETT was to identify selection criteria for LVRS. The NETT investigators were prospectively interested in carrying out subgroup analyses for the purpose of identifying subgroup strata that either particularly benefit from or do worse as a result of LVRS surgery.

The DSMB for this study was charged with monitoring the safety of the patients who were recruited and followed in the NETT. However, they had one additional, prospectively proscribed role; to periodically review subgroups of patients who may benefit from or be harmed by the procedure. These subgroups were prospectively defined based on age, forced expiratory volume at 1 second (FEV1), arterial CO_2, residual lung volume, as well as carbon monoxide diffusing capacity, maximal work capacity, quality of life, race or ethnic group, and sex. Subgroup data were reviewed every 3 months.

Recruitment began in 1998 and 3.5 years later, 1022 patients had been randomized to either LVRS or medical therapy in 17 clinical centers. There were no deaths in the first 30 days after randomization in the medical group, while the 30 day mortality rate postsurgery was 16%. When the analysis focused on survivors, patients recruited to the surgery group sustained an increase in exercise capacity. However, statistically significant subgroup findings were observed for each of two subgroups (Table 10.3).

Table 10.3. Subgroup analysis in NETT trial.

Subgroup	Surgical therapy deaths (patients)	Medical therapy deaths (patients)	Risk ratio	p-value
FEV1 = 20%* + homogeneous emphysema	23 (46)	5 (48)	5.96 (2.2 – 20.1)	<0.001**
FEV1 = 20% and DLCO < 20%*	22 (44)	8 (43)	2.98 (1.3 – 7.7)	0.001**

* Percents are of the predicted value.
** Computed by the author.

For each of these high-risk subgroups (FEV1 ≤ 20% of predicted plus homogeneous emphysema, and FEV1 ≤ 20% of predicted and DLCO < 20% of predicted), surgery was associated with an elevated risk of mortality. The NETT investigators concluded that they had identified groups of patients who were at high-risk for fatal consequences of LVRS and that these findings have clear importance for the selection of patients for this procedure. They advocated caution in the use of this procedure in these patients who were likely to derive little benefit from it.

The interpretation of these subgroup findings is somewhat more complex than in previous examples, primarily because in the case of NETT, the subgroup evaluations were prospectively stated and provided in detail before the trial was carried out. In fact, one of the principle aims of this clinical trial was to identify the effect of therapy in high-risk subgroups. Deliberative consideration went into the review of subgroup definitions during the design phase of the trial, and the DSMB was prospectively charged with the interim monitoring of the subgroup findings. Thus, the subgroup analyses in NETT are protected from the charge that they were the product of data-based, random research. The estimates of mortality rates, relative risks, and their associated confidence intervals are accurate depictions of the relative effects of surgical versus medical surgery in these patients with chronic disease.

While the prospective choice of these analyses allows us to accept these estimators as trustworthy, we then must ask the question about the conservation of the familywise error probability. If there were no a priori statements about the magnitude of the type I error rates, ordinarily we would conclude that accepting the findings of the NETT investigators would inflate the type I error beyond any reasonable upper bound. However, the small p-values for each of these estimates allays any fears about α error rate inflation. Thus the NETT subgroup analyses are proper and meet with currently accepted methodology, and their findings should be accepted as confirmatory.

10.7 The Difficulties Continue

This chapter demonstrates some of the contemporary difficulties that subgroup analyses create. Yet another force that exerts traction on both investigators and regulators for subgroup interpretation is the lay press. Consider, as an example, an editorial appearing in the Wall Street Journal that purported to have identified an unnecessary obstruction put in place by the FDA slow rapid drug approval [22].

The editorial reported that, in the search to identify vaccines that would be active against cancer, investigators believed that they had identified a substance that would be active against prostate cancer. In a placebo-controlled clinical trial, the active medication was randomly allocated to patients who had late-stage prostatic cancer. At the end of the study, the final analysis that included all of the randomized patients was of reduced statistical significance. However, in those patients with Gleason scores (measures of the degree to which the tumor spreads), of seven or less, the medication was seen to be effective. The FDA appropriately chose not to grant approval of the compound based on this post hoc analysis. The regulatory agency instead required that a new study that would prospectively target patients with lower Gleason scores should be commissioned and completed. The editorial criticized this decision, and asked "why not allow companies to cull the relevant data from existing studies when a certain subgroup is clearly of help?"

Unfortunately, these calls for directed action that are based on misdirected and misleading subgroup analysis are not harmless. The genuine, heartfelt desire to come to the aid of ailing people must be tempered with disciplined research strategy and execution. In the absence of this strength, the research effort produces interventions that have been shown many times not to help our patients in need, but to harm them.

Problems

1. Describe the role of the effect domination principle in the interpretation of subgroup analyses in clinical trials.
2. Recall from Chapter 4 that the role of a prospectively planned secondary analysis in clinical trials is solely supportive. With this as a background, and considering the implications of the effect domination principle, under what circumstances can a subgroup analysis be used as a secondary analysis in a clinical trial?
3. Provide several reasons why confirmatory subgroup analyses are not seen more frequently in clinical trials.
4. What is the common difficulty that confronts investigators who wish to prospectively allocate type I and type II error rates at acceptably low levels for subgroup analyses in clinical trials?
5. How are subgroups used to measure a modification of effect in a clinical trial?
6. What is the difference between the use of subgroup analyses to evaluate the presence of an effect modification and the use of subgroups to identify a stratum specific effect in a clinical trial?

References

1. Yusuf, S, Wittes J., Probstfield, J., Tyroler, H.A. (1991). Analysis and interpretation of treatment effects in subgroups of patients in randomized clinical trials. *Journal of the American Medical Associatio* **266**:93–8.
2. Peterson, B., George, S.L. (1993). Sample size requirements and length of study for testing interaction in a 1 x *k* factorial design when time-to-failure is the outcome. *Controlled Clinical Trials* **14**:511–522.
3. Horwitz, R.I., Singer, B., Makuch, R.W., Viscoli, C.M. (1996). Can treatment that is helpful on average be harmful to some patients? A study of the conflicting information needs of clinical inquiry and drug regulation. *Journal of Clinical Epidemiology* **49**:395–400.
4. Altman, D.G. (1998). Within trial variation—A false trial? *Journal of Clinical Epidemiology* **51**:301–303.
5. Feinstein, A.R. (1998). The problem of cogent subgroups: A clinicostatistical tragedy. *Journal of Clinical Epidemiology* **51**:297–299.
6. Lee, K.L., McNeer, F., Starmer, C.F., Harris, P.J., Rosari, R.A. (1980). Clinical judgment and statistics. Lessons from a simulated randomized trial in coronary artery disease. *Circulation* **61**:508–15.
7. Simon, R. (1982). Patient subsets and variation in therapeutic efficacy. *British Journal of Clinical Pharmacology* **14**:473–482.
8. Pocock, S.J. (1983). *Clinical Trials; A Practical Approach*; Chichester. John Wiley & Sons. p213–215.

9. Friedman, L., Furberg, C., and DeMets, D. (1996). *Fundamentals of Clinical Trials* 3rd ed. New York. Springer.

10. Meinert, C.L. (1986). *Clinical Trials Design, Conduct, and Analysis.* New York: Oxford University Press.

11. The International Steering Committee on behalf of the MERIT-HF Study Group (1997). Rationale, design, and organization of the metoprolol CR/XL randomized trial in heart failure (MERIT–HF). *American Journal of Cardiology* **80**:54–58.

12. MERIT-F Study Group. (1999). Effect of metoprolol cr/xl in chronic heart failure. Metoprolol cr/xl randomized intervention trial in congestive heart failure (MERIT-HF) *Lancet* **353**:2001–2007.

13. Califf, R.M., O'Connor, C.M. (2000). β–blocker therapy for heart failure; the evidence is in, now the work begins. *Journal of the American Medical Association* **283**:1335–1336.

14. Carson, P., Ziesche, S., Johnson, G., Cohn, J.N. (1999). Racial differences in response to therapy for heart failure; analysis of the vasodilator–heart failure trials. *Journal of Cardiac Failure* **5**:357–382.

15. The SOLVD Investigators. Effect of enalapril on mortality and the development of heart filure in aymptomatic patients with reduced left ventricular ejection fraction. *New England Journal of Medicine.* **327**:685–91. [Erratum, *New England Journal of Medicine* **327**:1768.

16. The SOLVD Investigators. (1991). Effect of enalapril on survival in patients with reduced left ventricular ejection fraction and congestive heart failure. *New England Journal of Medicine* **325**:293–302.

17. Dries, D.L., Exner, D.V., Gersh, B.J., Cooper, H.A., Carson, P.E., Domanski, M.J.(1999). Racial differences in the outcome of left ventricular dysfunction. *New England Journal of Medicine* **340**:609–616.

18. Swartz, R.S. (2001). Racial profiling in medical research. *New England Journal of Medicine* **344**:1392–1393.

19. Wood, A.J. (2001). Racial differences in the response to drugs – pointers to genetic differences. *New England Journal of Medicine* **344**.1393–1395

20. MRFIT Investigators. (1982). Multiple risk factor intervention trial *Journal of the American Medical Association* **248**:1465–1477.

21. National Emphysema Treatment Trial Research Group (2001) Patients at high-risk of death after lung–volume–reduction surgery. *New England Journal of Medicine* **345**:1075–1083.

22. Editorial: Now for the real cancer vaccines. *The Wall Street Journa.* November 26, 2002.

Chapter 11

Subgroups III: Confirmatory Analyses

In this last chapter on subgroup analyses, procedures are described that allow subgroup evaluations to be viewed as confirmatory analyses. While we have clearly delineated the investigators' responsibility to prospectively design the analyses for a clinical trial, we now expand that role to encompass a detailed evaluation of the analysis of the effect of therapy within the subgroup strata of interest. The investigator is empowered to make determinations of (1) endpoints, (2) endpoint event rates, (3) efficacy levels, and (4) the precision of the endpoint measurement for the analysis of the effect of therapy within the subgroup stratum of interest. These determinations should be made with the same careful attention to detail required for the analysis of the effect of therapy in the entire cohort.

11.1 Introduction

Some of the most intriguing analyses in clinical trials have been the evaluation of the effect of therapy within subgroups. Unfortunately, many of these analyses have been misleading. For the reasons that have been delineated in Chapters 9 and 10, the typical subgroup analyses in clinical trials are best interpreted as exploratory, and the most accurate estimate of the effect of therapy within a subgroup is the effect of therapy in the overall cohort.

The twin requirements of (1) the detailed, prospective delineation of subgroup membership criteria, and (2) the protection of type I and type II error levels together increases the challenge of carrying out a confirmatory subgroup analyses within a clinical trial. We will develop confirmatory subgroup evaluations in which the focus of the investigators is on the prospective identification of an effect of therapy within a single subgroup stratum, as opposed to the interaction examination. The methodology proposed for evaluating the effect of the study intervention within a subgroup stratum is not a strategy which would supplant interaction testing. It addresses instead a different question—Is there an explicit effect of the intervention in the prospectively defined subgroup stratum of interest?

As we have seen, not all important subgroup evaluations need to be of the interactive type.[1] The subgroup evaluation controversy in MERIT was focused solely on the presence or absence of an effect of the therapy within the U.S. population stratum. As an additional illustration, recall that the National Emphysema Treatment Trial (NETT) investigators were interested in identifying individual subgroup strata that were at particular risk for adverse outcomes following surgery.

---

[1] Effect modification, or interaction subgroup analyses are discussed in Chapter 10, Section 10.2.1.

While each of two subgroup evaluations might be assessed indirectly in an interactive analysis, there is no methodological impediment to their direct examination.

As an additional example, it is not uncommon for an investigator to have a specific, prospective interest in a subcohort that is sicker than that of the overall cohort. These patients with greater morbidity often require multiple concomitant medications. Ill patients are hospitalized more frequently, and have a greater death rate. The explicit demonstration of efficacy in this sicker subcohort could make among the most dramatic differences in these ill patients' prognoses. Thus, while there is certainly an interest in the effect of therapy in the overall cohort, the explicit demonstration of efficacy in this sicker subcohort is also of great prospective importance to the investigator. In this circumstance, the scientific question is not whether there is a greater effect of therapy in the sicker fraction of patients than in the rest of the research cohort—that is a question that requires an interaction evaluation. The question here is much simpler. Does the therapy work in the sicker subgroup stratum?

11.2 Focus on Stratum-Specific Effects

Why isn't the principle of effect domination articulated in Chapter 10 sufficient for the interpretation of a therapy's effect within a subgroup stratum? This principle that the effect of a therapy in a subgroup is best measured by the effect of that therapy in the entire clinical trial cohort is very useful, but must be viewed in the end as a limited statement, the limit being imposed by the inability to make a confirmatory statement about the therapy's effect within the subgroup. The medical community is comfortable which specific, detailed, and reliable data about a treatment effect within a subgroup. It is less certain of the interpretation of a subgroup that must first be translated down from the overall cohort efficacy to the subgroup of interest.

A particular example of the importance of the direct demonstration of efficacy within a subgroup stratum, is the issue of a therapy effect in extremely low or extremely high strata levels. The medical and regulatory communities commonly have an interest in the effect of therapy at these stratum extremes in their desire to construct (and understand) treatment guidelines. For example, consider the clinical question raised in 1996 as the result of four clinical trials that considered the reduction in patients' low-density lipoprotein (LDL) cholesterol [1], [2], [21], [22]. In each of these trials, patients were admitted to the study with a wide range of LDL cholesterol levels. The central question addressed by each of these studies was the effect of therapy on the reduction of clinical events. However, an issue that was also of interest was whether there was a lower range of cholesterol levels within (or below) which there was no beneficial effect of therapy. Each of the trials carried out a subgroup analysis, and the attention of the medical community focused on the response of patients in the lower stratum of LDL cholesterol. Although the community was in general satisfied with the application of the effect domination principle in this example (i.e., that modern lipid reduction strategies would save lives of patients with "average" LDL cholesterol levels), it nevertheless retained a particular interest in the findings within this subcohort with the lowest LDL cholesterol measures. A confirmatory analysis within the stratum of low baseline LDL cholesterol levels would have provided important information in this regard.

11.3 Confirmatory Analyses Requisites

The tasks outlined here will be more than merely prospectively identifying the subgroup stratum in which our interest resides and then "trust to luck" that the investigators will identify a therapeutic effect. To the contrary, targeting this subgroup stratum will require the investigators to give careful consideration to each of the design parameters of the subgroup analysis. We will outline the construction of confirmatory subgroup analyses along the lines of Moyé and Deswal [2]. Specifically, the trial designers must deliberate on the choice of the endpoint, the stratum specific control group event rate for that endpoint, a defensible efficacy, and the type I and type II errors rates. In addition, the notion of dependent hypothesis testing will be incorporated in this development.

The central idea here is that the investigator should design the subgroup analysis with the same attention to detail that is required for the design of the analysis of the effect of the randomly allocated intervention in the entire research cohort. The result will be a confirmatory evaluation of the effect of the randomly allocated intervention of the clinical trial in both the entire cohort and within a pretargeted subgroup stratum that conserves the familywise error probability ξ. Put another way, two confirmatory analysis plans will be deployed at the beginning of the clinical trial. The first is the plan for the evaluation of the effect of therapy in the entire cohort of the controlled clinical trial. The second is the confirmatory plan for the evaluation of the intervention within the subgroup stratum. Each plan is predicated on its own defensible assumptions for statistical error rate, endpoint choice, endpoint event rate, and intervention efficacy.

As we did for Chapters 4–8, in this development we will assume that a randomized, controlled clinical trial, to study an intervention's effectiveness, is the vehicle in which the subgroup will be analyzed. We will also assume that the subgroup stratum in which efficacy is to be examined has been announced prospectively and that the subgroup is a proper subgroup. We will, in addition, assume that the prospectively planned clinical trial is executed concordantly (i.e., the experiment is executed according to its protocol). Thus, in this environment, the estimates the trial provides of the effectiveness of the intervention are trustworthy and need only have appropriately low levels of type I and type II error, in order to produce a confirmatory evaluation of the intervention's effect in the subgroup.

11.4 Incorporating Subgroup Dependency

Just as we recognized that the execution of prospectively defined analyses for a combined endpoint and its component endpoints was a research environment in which dependency between statistical hypothesis tests was very likely, we can easily see that this same concept of dependency can be applied to a collection of well-designed hypothesis tests carried out in both an entire cohort of patients as well as in a subgroup of them.

Recall from Chapter 5 that we developed two characteristics of dependent statistical hypothesis testing; coincidence and homogeneity of therapy effect. The degree to which each of these are present determines the magnitude of the dependence between the hypothesis tests. In fact, a relationship was expressed between the dependency parameter D, the coincidence c and homogeneity of therapy h reproduced here.

$$D = c\left[1 - (1-c)(1-h)\right] \tag{11.1}$$

where c is the coincidence level $0 \le c \le 1$ and h, $0 \le h \le 1$ measures the therapy homogeneity. Here, $h = 1$ denotes perfect therapy homogeneity, i.e., the therapy has the same effect on each of the analyses.

Recall that in Chapter 7 we described coincidence as a characteristic between endpoints. Specifically, it was defined as the degree to which the combined endpoint and a component endpoint occurred in the same person. For our evaluation in the paradigm of subgroup evaluations, coincidence will be a property of the subgroup stratum, i.e., we will define coincidence as the degree to which the same patient appears in each analysis. More precisely, coincidence will be the proportion of patients in the entire cohort that are included in the subgroup stratum of interest.

The following illustrations motivate this definition. Consider a clinical trial that randomly allocates an intervention or placebo therapy to 1100 patients. After a prespecified period of time, the investigators will measure the effect of the therapy on one endpoint, the total mortality rate. The investigators prospectively plan to evaluate the randomly allocated therapy on the cumulative incidence of total mortality using two analyses: (1) the entire cohort and (2) patients ≥ 60 years of age. Assume for the moment that the effect of therapy in the overall cohort is the same as the effect of therapy in patients who are 60 years old and older. If 1050 of these 1100 patients are at least 60 years of age, there is an overwhelming overlap between the two prospectively designed statistical analyses that is entirely due to the fact that the great majority of the patients who are included in the analysis of the entire cohort are included in the age subgroup stratum analysis. Recall that our notion of dependency was based on the commission of a type I error. If a type I error occurs in the analysis for the effect of therapy in the overall cohort of 1100 patients, then it is extremely likely to occur in the analysis of 1050 of the same patients. The level of dependence between the statistical analysis of the effect of therapy in the entire cohort and the analysis of the effect of therapy in the subgroup strata is very high in this case. The smaller the proportion of patients who are at least 60 years of age, the greater the difference in the set of patients analyzed in the entire cohort and the patients analyzed in the overall cohort and, consequently, the lower the dependence between the hypothesis tests. We will refer to c_s as the coincidence property of subgroups.

Similarly, h_s will reflect the degree to which the effect of therapy in the subgroup (or collection of subgroups) is the same as the effect of therapy in the overall cohort. Thus, we may rewrite (11.1) as

$$D_s = c_s\left[1 - (1-c_s)(1-h_s)\right] \tag{11.2}$$

and apply all of the developments of Chapters 5 and 6 and Appendix E to the conservation of the familywise error probability ξ in the context of subgroup analyses. It is useful to examine the relationship between the dependency parameter and both the coincidence parameter c_s and the homogeneity parameter h_s (Figure 11.2)

For a fixed value of the homogeneity of therapy estimate h_s, the dependency parameter increases with increasing coincidence. Also, larger values of the therapy homogeneity parameter are associated with greater hypothesis test dependency.

11.4.1 Therapy Homogeneity in Subgroup Evaluations

The value of h_s must be selected with special care in subgroup analyses. Selecting $h_s = 1$ is equivalent to an assumption that the effect of therapy will be the same in the subcohort and the entire cohort. Since the purpose of the evaluation of the effect of therapy in the subcohort is to obtain a separate assessment of the therapy's effect, it would be incorrect to embed a presumed answer to this question within the dependence parameter. However, to choose a value of $h_s = 0$ is equally inappropriate, since the subcohort findings are included in the overall cohort; this observation alone will produce some homogeneity of therapy effect. A reasonable choice in this circumstance is simply to let $h_s = c_s$.

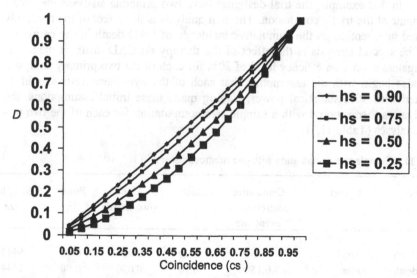

Figure 11.1. Dependency parameter as a function of coincidence (*cs*) and therapy homogeneity (*hs*) in subgroup analyses.

Thus, the homogeneity of therapy effect is governed by the degree to which the subcohort and the entire cohort contain the same patients. In this circumstance

$$
\begin{aligned}
D_s &= c_s \left[1 - (1 - c_s)(1 - h_s) \right] \\
&= c_s \left[1 - (1 - c_s)(1 - c_s) \right] \\
&= c_s \left[1 - (1 - c_s)^2 \right] \\
&= c_s^2 \left[2 - c_s \right]
\end{aligned}
\tag{11.3}
$$

where c_s is the fraction of the overall cohort that is included in the subgroup stratum of interest.

As a very simple example of this concept, consider the design of a placebo controlled clinical trial in which patients with ischemic cardiovascular disease are recruited and then randomly selected to receive either a new antiplatelet agent or placebo therapy to reduce the incidence of CAD death. The investigators have the resources available to recruit 7000 patients for this study. They plan to use 2 years to recruit this cohort and then to follow the last patient who is recruited for 4 years. The investigators have prospectively chosen one endpoint—CAD death. The inclusion and exclusion criteria of this trial are such that the investigators anticipate that the 4 year cumulative incidence rate of CAD death is 15%.

In this example, the trial designers have two principle analyses they wish to compute at the trial's conclusion. The first analysis is the effect of the randomly allocated intervention on the cumulative incidence of CAD death in the entire cohort. The second analysis is the effect of the therapy on CAD death in men. The investigators choose an efficacy level of 20% for each of the two primary analyses. They also begin with the assumption that each of the hypothesis tests should be executed with 90% statistical power. Having made these initial assumptions, the investigators then proceed with a sample size computation for each of the two primary analyses (Table 11.1).

Table 11.1. Sample size computation with one subgroup: Scenario 1.

Primary analyses	Cohort	Cumulative control group event rate	Efficacy	Alpha (two-tailed)	Power	Sample size
CHD death	Total	0.150	0.20	0.050	0.90	5444
CHD death	Men	0.150	0.20	0.050	0.90	5444

With no difference in the design parameters for each analysis, of course, the sample size computations for each of the primary analyses will be the same. Even though the total sample size for the trial is 5444, much less than the maximum of 7000 patients available for the study, the fact that ξ is not conserved in Table 11.1 precludes the researchers from selecting the sample size produced in this table as the goal sample size of the trial.

The investigators then proceed to apportion the α error probability. This increases the sample size requirements since the type I error rates for each of the two hypothesis test are each less than 0.05 (Table 11.2).

Table 11.2. Sample size computation with one subgroup: Scenario 2.

Primary analyses	Cohort	Cumulative control group event rate	Efficacy	Alpha (two-tailed)	Power	Sample size
CHD death	Total	0.150	0.20	0.030	0.90	6172
CHD death	Men	0.150	0.20	0.020	0.90	6744

The investigators now incorporate the notion of dependency into the design of these analyses. They first estimate that 85% of the total number of patients recruited for this study will be men ($c_s = 0.85$). A simple computation based on $D_s = c_s^2 [2 - c_s]$ reveals $D_s = 0.83$. The investigators next prospectively set the FWER ξ = 0.05, and the test-specific α error rate for the hypothesis test on the entire cohort as $\alpha_1 = 0.03$. From the formula introduced in Chapter 5 for the computation of α_2, the test-specific α error probability for the subcohort of men, given ξ and α_1.

$$\alpha_2 = \min \left[\alpha_1, \frac{\xi - \alpha_1}{(1 - \alpha_1)(1 - D^2)} \right]. \tag{11.4}$$

they compute $\alpha_2 = 0.03$ and next recompute the sample sizes based on these considerations (Table 11.3).

Table 11.3. Sample size computation with one subgroup: Scenario 3.

Primary analyses	Cohort	Cumulative control group event rate	Efficacy	Alpha (two-tailed)	Power	Sample size
CHD death	Total	0.150	0.20	0.030	0.92	6622
		D= 0.83				
CHD death	Men	0.150	0.20	0.030	0.85	5326

Note also that the investigators reduced the power of the analysis involving only men from 90% to 85%. For the analysis of the effect of therapy in the male subcohort, 5326 men are required. Since 85% of the recruited sample will be men, the total sample size of the study will be 6172/0.85 = 6266 patients, a number that does not exceed the 7000 maximum number of participants.

The investigators of this trial are now in a position to carry out a confirmatory analysis of the effect of the randomly allocated intervention in each of the total cohort and the male subcohort. This was produced through the incorporation of a conservative estimate of the level of dependence between the two statistical hypotheses, in addition to the differential allocation of the type I error probability.

11.5 Subgroup Stratum-Specific Endpoints

The procedure outlined in the previous section permitted a confirmatory evaluation of the effect of therapy within a subgroup stratum. This goal was achieved solely on the manipulation of the statistical criteria of the two prospectively defined hypothesis tests. Although these adjustments during the design phase of the trial are legitimate and represent devices that we will use repeatedly, they are not the only tools at our disposal. We will now turn to an examination of the clinical assumptions under which a statistical hypothesis test is evaluated, with particular focus on how they might be controlled to achieve confirmatory hypothesis tests within a subcohort.

Heretofore, we have carefully examined the role of endpoints in clinical trials. In Chapter 3, we discussed the logistical reasons as well as the epidemiologic rationale for their incorporation within a single clinical trial. In Chapter 4, the methodology for assessing the effect of therapy based on their occurrence was developed. However, a relatively unexplored aspect of the inclusion of multiple endpoint evaluations in clinical trials is the consideration of a stratum specific endpoint. In its simplest case, this means that the analysis of the effect of therapy in the overall cohort will be on a different endpoint than the analysis for the therapy effect in the subcohort. If the endpoint for the effect of therapy on the overall cohort has a greater incidence rate, the statistical power for the subgroup analysis will increase.

This new multiple endpoint strategy is one that can empower the subgroup analysis and the trial itself, but if a steady hand is not at the helm, the trial can be piloted into hazardous and dangerous waters. Clearly, the two different endpoints must be chosen with great care, with concentrated attention on the interpretation of these joint analyses. The publication of a design manuscript to educate the research community would be a very worthwhile activity in this case. Of course, the regulatory community, when appropriate, should be a full participant in the development of the analysis plan.

Some will cogently argue that it is difficult enough to interpret the effect of therapy within a traditional subgroup analysis without the introduction of the influence of a different endpoint. Equally clear is the observation that the wanton, undisciplined choice of an endpoint for the subgroup stratum analysis will completely undermine the confirmatory hypothesis test on which it is based. However, if the endpoint can be prospectively, carefully, and sensitively selected, the subcohort analysis will strengthen and not weaken the overall research endeavor, and the worthless arguments can be defeated.

11.5.1 Choosing the Subcohort Endpoints

The choice of the endpoint for the overall cohort and that of the subcohort analysis remains a delicate matter. Consider a clinical trial that is designed to have a confirmatory analysis for the effect of the randomly allocated intervention on each of the entire research cohort and a prospectively defined, proper subcohort. What we require are two endpoints that measure the same disease process. The endpoint to be evaluated within the subcohort should have a greater incidence rate, since this analysis will contain the fewest patients.

This is analogous to the situation in which we developed the underlying theory for the construction of a combined endpoint from several component endpoints.[2] Our examination of this issue then revealed that, in choosing endpoints that measured the same underlying pathophysiology, we were most concerned about two characteristics: (1) coincidence and (2) homogeneity of therapy effect. If the component endpoints commonly occurred in the same patients, and all available evidence suggested that the randomly allocated therapy would be effective for each of these endpoints, then the combined endpoint that is assembled from these component endpoints would be a useful reflection of the effect of therapy on the disease process of interest.

This line of reasoning suggests that we might use the theory from Chapters 7 and 8 to develop a combined endpoint from component endpoints, and then apply these endpoints to two prospectively developed analyses. The first of these analyses would be the effect of therapy in the entire cohort on one of the component endpoints; the second would be the effect of therapy in the smaller subcohort on the more frequently occurring combined endpoint. The notion of dependency and differential allocation of type I error would also be brought to bear in this circumstance to conserve the FWER.

11.5.2 Example

The following illustrates this principle: consider the design of a controlled clinical trial whose goal is to assess the effect of a randomly allocated medication on the occurrence of atherosclerotic cardiovascular disease in patients with isolated systolic hypertension (ISH) where ISH is defined as DBP < 90 mm Hg and SBP (SBP) greater than 140 mm Hg. Patients will be selected and then randomized to receive either control therapy or active medication to control their elevated SBP. The investigators are, of course, interested in demonstrating the effect of therapy in all randomized participants. The endpoint in which they have the greatest interest is the cumulative incidence rate of fatal/nonfatal stroke However, the investigators also have a particular interest in examining the effect of therapy in patients who have borderline ISH, which is defined in this clinical trials as patients whose SBP is be-

---

[2] These topics were discussed in Chapters seven and eight..

tween 140 mm Hg and 150 mm Hg. These investigators are interested in executing a confirmatory analysis in this subcohort.

However, upon first examination of this complex issue during the design phase of the trial, this goal appears unreachable. The investigators believe that resources will not be available to carry out their planned evaluation. Since the trial provides scarcely enough power (80%) for the analysis of the effect of therapy in the entire cohort, there will be inadequate power available to assess the effect of therapy within any of the subgroup strata for the occurrence of fatal/nonfatal stroke. The investigators, retaining their prospective wish to carry out a confirmatory subgroup analysis, therefore clearly state in the protocol during the design phase of the study that they are interested in examining the effect of the trial's intervention in this low ISH subgroup stratum. The first evaluation of sample size assumes that the analysis of the effect of therapy in the SBP subcohort will be the same as that of the entire cohort. The investigators determine that the minimum effectiveness of the intervention worth detecting is a 20% reduction in the incidence of the endpoint. For this first evaluation, no attempt is made to control the familywise error probability (Table 11.4).

Table 11.4. Sample size computation with one subgroup: Scenario 1.

Primary analyses	Cohort	Cumulative control group event rate	Efficacy	Alpha (two-tailed)	Power	Sample size
Fatal/nonfatal stroke	Total	0.070	0.20	0.050	0.90	12,649
Fatal/nonfatal stroke	SBP subcohort	0.050	0.20	0.050	0.90	18,053

This first examination provides an initial impression of the sample sizes required for each of the two analyses. It is somewhat surprising that the required number of patients is greater (rather than the same) for the analysis of therapy in the SBP subcohort when compared to the required number of participants for the overall cohort. However, an examination of the cumulative event rate of fatal/nonfatal stroke in the two analysis groups answers this question. Since the SBP subcohort is defined as 140 mm Hg < SBP ≤ 150 mm Hg, which is at the lower end of SBPs for patients recruited to this study, the event rate experienced by these patients is lower than for the overall cohort as a whole. Thus, not only is the number of patients to be included in the subcohort analysis smaller, we see that the control group event rate is lower as well. This is a combination of influences that only serves to lengthen the odds against the execution of a confirmatory analysis in the SBP subcohort.

In fact, it is precisely this issue of endpoint event rates that the investigators first tackle. During this phase in the design of the experiment, the investigators replace the primary endpoint of fatal/nonfatal stroke in the SBP cohort with the endpoint of fatal/nonfatal stroke + fatal/nonfatal MI. The choice of this composite endpoint is a reasonable one. The two component endpoints of this combined endpoint (fatal/nonfatal stroke and fatal/nonfatal MI) are both produced by the same underlying pathophysiologic mechanism and commonly occur in the same patients.

In addition, the effect of antihypertensive therapy is anticipated to produce an important clinical reduction in the cumulative incidence of each of these evaluations. Thus, the new endpoint satisfies the two requirements of an effective and useful combined endpoint. In addition, and most importantly in this scenario, the greater incidence rate of this combined endpoint produces a substantial reduction in sample size for the evaluation of therapy in the SBP subcohort (Table 11.5).

Table 11.5. Sample size computation with one subgroup: Scenario 2.

Primary analyses	Cohort	Cumulative control group event rate	Efficacy	Alpha (two-tailed)	Power	Sample size
Fatal/nonfatal stroke	Total	0.070	0.20	0.050	0.90	12,649
Combined endpoint*	SBP subcohort	0.135	0.20	0.050	0.90	6144

*Fatal/nonfatal stroke + fatal/nonfatal MI.

The investigators now set out to control the FWER, ξ. They begin with an asymmetrical allocation of the type I error rate for each of the two analyses, providing most of the type I error rate for the effect of therapy in the overall cohort, with only 0.015 allocated for the primary analysis in the SPB subcohort (Table 11.6).

Table 11.6. Sample size computation with one subgroup: Scenario 3.

Primary analyses	Cohort	Cumulative control group event rate	Efficacy	Alpha (two-tailed)	Power	Sample size
Fatal/nonfatal stroke	Total	0.070	0.20	0.035	0.90	13,833
Combined endpoint*	SBP subcohort	0.135	0.20	0.015	0.90	8065

*Fatal/nonfatal stroke + fatal/nonfatal myocardial infarction.

The reduction of the test-specific α level for each of the two primary analyses has predictably increased the required sample size of the clinical trial. However, this computation does not take dependence between the statistical hypothesis tests into account.

This issue of dependence between these two statistical hypothesis tests is a consideration that must be carefully deliberated because of the complexity of the circumstances. There are two separate factors that must be addressed in this situation. The first is the dependence between the two statistical hypothesis tests; a dependence that is based on the fact that the analyses of one contains a fraction of the patients in the other. The second issue is that the endpoints are related. Nevertheless, this consideration comes down to two factors, coincidence and homogeneity of therapy effect.

In Chapter 7, coincidence was measured as the degree to which the component endpoint appeared in the combined endpoint. In those situations, the same patients were evaluated for each of these endpoints, i.e., each analysis was carried out on the same cohort, but the endpoints that were evaluated were related but different. We expressed this concept in the dependency measure as

$$D_e = c_e \left[1 - (1 - c_e)(1 - h_e) \right].$$ (11.5)

However, the situation is somewhat different in the present circumstance because only a fraction of the patients are evaluated for the effect of therapy in the subcohort as will be analyzed in the initial cohort. We stated earlier in this chapter that when there are two statistical hypothesis tests in which the endpoints are the same, but the cohorts overlap, we can express the dependency parameter as

$$D_s = c_s^2 \left[2 - c_s \right].$$ (11.6)

In our current situation, we have two statistical hypothesis tests in which (1) the cohorts are not identical, but merely overlap, and (2) the endpoints are similar but not identical in the two analyses. The combination of these factors does not increase, but decreases the degree of dependence between the two statistical evaluations. We now express this concept as follows. In a clinical trial that is testing the effect of a randomly allocated intervention in which a primary analysis is to be carried out on a subcohort that uses a combined endpoint and a second primary analysis is to be carried out on the entire cohort using a component endpoint, then the dependency parameter between the two statistical hypotheses may be computed as

$$D = D_e D_s.$$ (11.7)

In the case of the SBP trial, assume the therapy effect is homogenous for the combined endpoint of fatal/nonfatal stroke + fatal/nonfatal MI and the component endpoint of fatal/nonfatal stroke. The investigators anticipate that 40% of patients who meet the criteria for a fatal/nonfatal stroke + fatal/nonfatal MI will have the fatal/nonfatal stroke. From $D_e = c_e \left[1 - (1 - c_e)(1 - h_e) \right]$ we can compute $D_e = 0.40$.

In addition, the investigators anticipate that 50% of all patients recruited into the study will meet the SBP criteria for the subcohort, or $D_s = 0.375$. Thus $D = (0.40)(0.375) = 0.15$. The result of this final computation is incorporated into the sample size computation[3] and can be incorporated into the sample size computation (Table 11.7).

---

[3] The details of this incorporation are described in chapter 5, section 5.9.

Table 11.7. Sample size computation with one subgroup: Scenario 4.

Primary analyses	Cohort	Cumulative control group event rate	Efficacy	Alpha (two-tailed)	Power	Sample size
Fatal/nonfatal stroke	Total	0.070	0.20	0.035	0.90	13,833
			$D = 0.15$			
Combined endpoint*	SBP subcohort	0.135	0.20	0.016	0.90	7974

*Fatal/nonfatal stroke + fatal/nonfatal MI.

In order to meet the investigators' concern that no more than 60% of the patients recruited will be in the SBP subgroup stratum of interest, the decrease the power of the combined endpoint evaluation in the SBP subcohort from 90% to 85% (Table 11.8). If the trial is designed using the computations and underlying thought process as contained in Table 11.8, the investigators will be able to carry out two confirmatory evaluations: (1)the effect of therapy in the entire cohort; and (2) the effect of therapy within the SBP subcohort.

Table 11.8. Sample size computation with one subgroup: Scenario 5.

Primary analyses	Cohort	Cumulative control group event rate	Efficacy	Alpha (two-tailed)	Power	Sample size
Fatal/Nonfatal stroke	Total	0.070	0.20	0.035	0.90	13,833
			$D = 0.15$			
Combined endpoint*	SBP subcohort	0.135	0.20	0.016	0.85	6950

*Fatal/nonfatal stroke + fatal/nonfatal MI.

The conclusion from this study should be straightforward, eased by the care taken in the choice of the combined and singleton endpoints for the two analyses. Since each of the two endpoints is a clinically accepted manifestation of atherosclerotic cardiovascular disease exacerbated by chronic hypertension, the conclusion of the effect of the therapy in either the overall cohort or the SBP subcohort will be unambiguous. Even if there was no evidence of an effect of therapy in the overall cohort, the identification of an effect of therapy in the reduction of atherosclerotic disease as measured by fatal/nonfatal stroke + fatal/nonfatal MI in the subcohort would represent a strong, confirmatory finding.

However, this second confirmatory evaluation does not come cheaply. The number of patients in the confirmatory subcohort is considerable. Also, there is the additional burden represented by the requirement of one more endpoint determination. In the initial trial design, when there was only one endpoint; every patient who was believed to have experienced a stroke during the course of the study had to be carefully evaluated in order to decide if that patient's event met the prospectively determined definition of a stroke for the trial. We now add to that considerable effort the additional task of assessing patients for the occurrence of a fatal or nonfatal

MI. Defined criteria for this new evaluation must be in place prospectively, and the logistics of the evaluation of these additional events must be embedded into the clinical trial's logistical mechanism.[4] This new workload can be a substantial drain on the trial's resources.

11.5.3 Dependency Parameter's Minimal Impact

In the previous example, there were a series of design decisions that led to the confirmatory subgroup evaluation. Of the various prospective adjustments made by the investigators to the sample size computations, including the implementation of a combined endpoint event rate in the subcohort, the differential allocation of the α error rate, the inclusion of the measure of dependence, and the adjustment of the statistical power, certainly the least influential procedure was the use of dependence. A comparison of α error rates in Tables 11.6 and 11.7 for the evaluation of the effect of therapy on the SBP subcohort reveals that the test-specific α error rate for the SBP cohort before dependence between the statistical hypotheses was invoked was 0.015; after dependence was invoked, it only increased to 0.016—certainly a minimal (if not negligible) impact. While this effect did not negate the impact of the choice of the combined endpoint for the SBP subcohort analysis, its role in promoting the confirmatory evaluation was minimal.

The reason for this minimal dependence effect is that the combined impact of using both (1) a different endpoint for each of the two hypothesis tests and (2) non-identical cohorts between the two confirmatory analyses produced a great reduction in the dependence parameter. In the next section we will discuss a procedure in which this dramatic discounting does not take place. However the point of the current exercise is that, with careful consideration, managing two separate endpoints (one for the overall cohort and a second for the subgroup stratum of interest) poses no conceptual, interpretative, or insurmountable logistical difficulty in a clinical trial.

11.6 Differential Event Rate

One of the difficulties in designing a clinical trial that will produce a confirmatory hypothesis test for the effect of therapy is the paucity of endpoint events. It is therefore useful to choose an endpoint whose incidence rate is so large that enough endpoint events are produced in an achievable sample size. In the previous section, we produced this rate by choosing a composite endpoint for the subcohort evaluation. However, this step may not be necessary in some settings. There are commonly occurring clinical trial situations in which the event rate for the subcohort of interest is greater than the event rate for the same endpoint in the overall research cohort.

In the previous section, we observed the reverse of this phenomenon. In the design of a clinical trial which examined the effect of a randomly allocated intervention on the occurrence of clinically significant atherosclerotic cardiovascular

---

[4] This additional burden may be lightened by the likelihood that measurement of the cumulative incidence rate of fatal/nonfatal MI was considered as a secondary endpoint.

disease, the SBP subcohort, in which the investigators had a prospectively stated interest was defined as patients whose SBP was between 140 mm Hg. and 150 mm Hg. Since this SBP level is in the lower range of SBPs for patients who had isolated systolic hypertension, the event rates for atherosclerotic disease were lower in the subcohort, making it even more difficult to execute a confirmatory evaluation of the effect of therapy in this group of patients. If the investigators had chosen a subcohort of patients with greater elevations in SBP, the event rate for fatal/nonfatal stroke would have been higher. Nevertheless, the investigators chose not to focus on this higher range of blood pressure because they had no special, prospective interest in it apart from their interest in the overall cohort.

However, there are other clinical trial circumstances in which there is prospective interest in a higher risk subcohort. Certainly the recent appearance of the concern of a different effect of therapy in African-American versus non-African-American patients is a setting in which the differential rate of events might be embedded into the experimental design. In fact there has been increasing regulatory pressure to evaluate the effect of therapy in ethnic and gender minority groups in general.

The first difficulty in carrying out accurate evaluations of the effect of a therapy within a randomized clinical trial in ethnic and gender minorities is the relative inability of these trials to successfully recruit patients from these populations. To help rectify this situation, the FDA has drafted regulations that provide guidance to the pharmaceutical industry concerning the appropriate representations of ethnic minorities and women in clinical trials. Specifically, Section 115(b) of the Food and Drug Modernization Act of 1997 (FDAMA) required the agency to "review and develop guidance, as appropriate, on the inclusion of women and minorities" [3]. According to its preamble, the Rule is intended to alert sponsors as early as possible to demographic deficiencies in enrollment that could lead to avoidable deficiencies that appear later in the subsequent New Drug Application (NDA) submission.

The FDA has taken additional steps to encourage ethnic minority recruitment in clinical trials. The Demographic Rule (February 11, 1998, Final Rule, investigational new drug (IND) applications and new drug applications (NDA)) requires private sponsors of clinical trials that are to be submitted to the FDA to, among other things, tabulate in their annual reports the numbers of subjects enrolled in clinical studies for drug and biological products according to age, group, gender, and race. This increased regulatory oversight of the inclusion of gender and ethnic minority in clinical trial reflects a sense of the poor recruitment of these underrepresented patient populations in research programs. This emphasis has led in part to increased recruitment of minority populations in both privately sponsored [17] and publicly sponsored [4] clinical trials. In fact, a trial involving solely African-American patients is currently under way [5], [6].

The second issue is of course the interpretative difficulties that are inherent in the traditional interpretation of subgroup analyses, for which we now develop an alternative. This development will follow that of Moyé and Powell [7].

11.6.1 Event Rate Differences

Subgroup cohorts of interest can have event rates that are anticipated to be different than the event rates in the overall cohort. These acknowledged differences can be embedded into a clinical trial design, producing a confirmatory subcohort evaluation.

One example of this different experience is in CHF in African-Americans. There is no question that atherosclerotic event rates are greater in African-Americans than others. [5] African-Americans are more likely to have such contributory risk factors as hypertension, diabetes and left ventricular hypertrophy than Caucasians. This amplifies the already increased prevalence of CHF among African-Americans. While 4.8 million Americans have CHF [8], CHF is more prevalent in African-Americans then in non-African-Americans. A recent examination of the age-adjusted prevalence of heart failure in patients who are twenty years of age or older revealed that CHF occurred more commonly in African-American patients, even after stratifying by gender. In addition, hospitalization for CHF is more common among African-Americans [9, 10, 11]. Finally CHF is believed to be more rapidly progressive in African-Americans then non-African-Americans, [12] with symptoms of CHF developing at an earlier age in African-American patients.

This has been observed in clinical trials as well. The Survival and Ventricular Enlargement Study [SAVE] [5] evaluated the effect of the ACE-i captopril in patients with left ventricular dysfunction but without symptoms of CHF. In an examination of the placebo group, 28.1% of non-Caucasian patients died during the course of the trial versus 24.3% of Caucasian patients. In that same trial, 48.3% of non-Caucasian patients died of a death that was believed to be of cardiovascular etiology, or had CHF that required either ACE-i therapy or hospitalization, or suffered a recurrent MI. Caucasian patients experienced this event 39.2% of the time.

If the investigator has a prospective interest in examining the effect of therapy in a subcohort whose endpoint event incidence rate is greater than that of the overall cohort, this difference in the event rate can be incorporated in the research design to help produce a confirmatory analysis in the evaluation of the effect of therapy in the subcohort. We will demonstrate the utility of this approach through an illustration of the design of a clinical trial. In this study, the investigators are interested in evaluating the effect of therapy to reduce morbidity and mortality in patients who have been diagnosed with CHF. The investigators will recruit patients with CHF, randomly allocating them to receive either the active intervention or the control group therapy. The trial's designers are interested in assessing the effect of the intervention on the cumulative total mortality rate; this will be one of the primary analyses of the study. However, in addition to this first evaluation, the investigators have a strong, prospectively declared interest in determining if there is an effect of the intervention in African-American patients with CHF. As a first evaluation of the requirements of the design of this complicated clinical trial, the trial designers examine the sample size requirement for this study (Table 11.9).

---

[5] This information on the ethnic prevalence of atherosclerotic disease was contributed by Dr. Anita Deswal.

Table 11.9. Sample size computation with one subgroup: Scenario 1.

Primary analyses	Cohort	Cumulative control group event rate	Efficacy	Alpha (two-tailed)	Power	Sample size
Total mortality	Total	0.150	0.20	0.050	0.90	5444
Total mortality	African-American	0.150	0.20	0.050	0.90	5444

The anticipated cumulative mortality rate for the placebo group in this clinical trail is 15%, and the investigators are interested in demonstrating that the intervention produces a 20% reduction in this event rate. The statistical hypothesis test is that under the null hypothesis, the cumulative mortality rates are equal, and under the alternative hypothesis, these rates are not equal. At this preliminary stage of the design of the clinical study, there is no attempt yet to control the FWER, and the statistical power is assumed to be 90%. With no difference in the design parameters of this study for the evaluation of the effect of therapy in either the total cohort or in the African-American subcohort, the required sample sizes are of course the same.

However, the investigators understand that the cumulative mortality rate for African-Americans will be substantially greater than the anticipated death rate in the overall cohort. A fair depiction of this circumstances for African-American patients with CHF requires that the trial designers use the best, most accurate estimate of the event rate in these patients, just as they will use the best estimate of the total mortality rate for the overall cohort. Thus the investigators assume that while the overall research cohort will experience a 15% cumulative mortality rate over the course of the trial, African-American patients will experience a 25% cumulative incidence rate of this endpoint. The incorporation of this assumption into the sample size calculation for the effect of the randomly allocated intervention produces a substantial reduction in the required sample size for the evaluation of the effect of therapy in this cohort (Table 11.10).

Table 11.10. Sample size computation with one subgroup: Scenario 2.

Primary analyses	Cohort	Cumulative Control Group Event Rate	Efficacy	Alpha (two-tailed)	Power	Sample size
Total mortality	Total	0.150	0.20	0.050	0.90	5444
Total mortality	African-American	0.250	0.20	0.050	0.90	2922

The next stage of the analysis development for this clinical trial is for the investigators to begin a prospective conservation of the type I error rate. The overall FWER of 0.05 is divided between the two primary analyses (Table 11.11). From a strict sample size consideration, the allocation of the FWER appears to be a step backward. For the overall cohort, controlling the familywise error level increases the sample size from 5444 to 6172, an increase of 13%. Decreasing the test-specific α error probability from 0.050 to 0.020 increases the sample size for the analysis of the effect of therapy in the African-American cohort by 24%, from 2922 to 3620. The larger sample sizes certainly increase the cost of the experiment; however, this is a necessary step if the investigators are to be empowered to execute confirmatory statistical hypothesis tests.

The impact of dependency between the two statistical hypothesis tests is now considered. The investigators anticipate that approximately one-half of the entire cohort will be African-American. This produces $c_s = 0.50$. As pointed out earlier, the selection of the measure of therapy homogeneity must be carried out carefully. If the investigators choose $h_s = 1$, then they are assuming that the effect of therapy will be the same in each of the African-American subcohort and the entire cohort.

Table 11.11. Sample size computation with one subgroup: Scenario 3.

Primary Analyses	Cohort	Cumulative control group event rate	Efficacy	Alpha (two-tailed)	Power	Sample size
Total mortality	Total	0.150	0.20	0.030	0.90	6172
Total mortality	African-American	0.250	0.20	0.020	0.90	3620

Since the purpose of the evaluation of the effect of therapy in the ethnic subcohort is to assess the heterogeneity of therapy, it would be misleading to assume the homogeneity of therapy was great merely to induce an artificially high dependence measure. However, to choose a value of $h_s = 0$ is equally inappropriate, since African-Americans make up both the subcohort of interest and approximately 50 % of the overall cohort. We will proceed with the simplifying assumption that $h_s = c_s$, permitting the following computation for the dependency parameter D_s:

$$
\begin{aligned}
D_s &= c_s^2 \left[2 - c_s \right] \\
&= 0.50^2 \left[2 - 0.50 \right] \\
&= 0.50^2 \left[2 - 0.50 \right] = 0.375.
\end{aligned}
\tag{11.8}
$$

The sample size for the effect of therapy in the African-American subcohort can now be computed incorporating the notion of statistical hypothesis test dependency (Table 11.12).

Table 11.12. Sample size computation with one subgroup: Scenario 4.

Primary analyses	Cohort	Cumulative control group event rate	Efficacy	Alpha (two-tailed)	Power	Sample size
Total mortality	Total	0.150	0.20	0.030	0.90	6172
			$D = 0.375$			
Total mortality	African-American	0.250	0.20	0.024	0.90	3482

A further reduction in the minimum required sample size for the African-American subcohort can be achieved by reducing the power for this analysis from 90% to 80% (Table 11.13).

Table 11.13. Sample size computation with one subgroup: Scenario 5.

Primary analyses	Cohort	Cumulative control group event rate	Efficacy	Alpha (two-tailed)	Power	Sample size
Total mortality	Total	0.150	0.20	0.030	0.90	6172
			$D = 0.375$			
Total mortality	African-American	0.250	0.20	0.024	0.80	2671

However, the sample sizes produced in Table 11.13 reveal that the ratio of African-American to the entire subcohort is not 50% but $2671/6172 = 43\%$. This is contrary to the assumption that the investigators made earlier in the sample size computation when they assumed $c_s = 0.50$. To correct this, D_s should be computed again with $c_s = 0.43$. This will produce from (8.11) $D_s = 0.29$ and the final sample sizes can be calculated (Table 11.14).

Table 11.14. Sample size computation with one subgroup : Scenario 5

Primary analyses	Cohort	Cumulative control group event rate	Efficacy	Alpha (two-tailed)	Power	Sample size
Total mortality	Total	0.150	0.20	0.030	0.90	6172
			$D = 0.29$			
Total mortality	African-American	0.250	0.20	0.023	0.80	2713

The concordant execution of the clinical trial with the design parameters as provided in Table 11.14 would lead to confirmatory analyses for the effect of the randomly allocated intervention on total mortality for each of the entire research cohort and the African-American subcohort.

11.7 Differential Efficacy

In the previous section, the investigators reduced the required minimum sample size of the analysis of the effect of therapy in the African-American subcohort by recognition of the observation that African-American patients with CHF experience a greater total mortality rate than others. It is important to note that the investigators did not "make up" this greater event rate—they merely recognized that a greater rate existed and made use of this fact. However, one design parameter that investigators do have complete control over is the efficacy of the study. The investigators choose this measure of effect size, being guided by the twin concerns of research community standard and resource constraints, for the execution of the clinical trial. In this section we will focus on efficacy selection.

11.7.1 The Relationship Between Efficacy and Sample Size

The effect size is the expected difference in the endpoint event rates between the control and active groups in the clinical trial. Clinical trial designers commonly confront the relationship between the effect size and sample size, on the one hand, and the relationship between effect size and community standard on the other. Each of these relationships must be understood if investigators are to wield this potent efficacy tool effectively without sacrificing the research design they seek to strengthen.

Efficacy is the measure of effect that is derived from the clinical trial. If the primary analysis in the clinical trial is the effect of therapy on a dichotomous endpoint, e.g., total mortality, then the efficacy of the therapy is commonly defined as the % reduction in the event rate produced by the therapy. For example, if the cumulative total mortality rate is 15% in the control group, and 12% in the active group of the clinical trial, then the efficacy is $(0.15 - 0.12)/0.15 = 0.20$ or 20%. If the sample was collected with strict adherence to the inclusion and exclusion criteria of the study, and the clinical trial was executed concordantly, then this 20% reduction seen in the primary analysis will be an accurate measure of what could be anticipated in the population.[6] The strength of the finding is further enhanced by the observation that the efficacy produced in the sample is very unlikely to be due to chance alone.

Thus, in order to make the most persuasive argument to the medical and regulatory communities, the effect size must be both clinically meaningful and statistically significant.[7] A clinically meaningful but statistically insignificant finding would be, for example, a 30% reduction in total mortality attributable to the therapy

---

[6] Different samples from the same population will produce different estimates of the effect size. While this random, sample-to-sample variability can be measured by the standard deviation of the effect size, it is more commonly reflected in the 95% confidence interval for the effect size.

[7] This assumes, as we will assume throughout the chapter, that the clinical trial was concordantly executed.

but producing a p-value of 0.35. Another example would be a large reduction in total mortality associated with a p-value of < 0.05 produced in an exploratory analysis. In neither case should the medical or regulatory community be persuaded that the effect size in the population of thousands (and sometimes, millions) of patients who were not included in the sample will be close to that seen in the sample. On the other hand, a statistically significant, but clinically insignificant effect size (e.g., the demonstration that an anti-lipid therapy reduces LDL cholesterol by 1 mg/dl in the average patient; $p = 0.03$) is a finding demonstrating that, while it is likely that the population will see this effect in the sample, the effect is negligible and not worth the cost of (or adverse event experience produced by) the medication[8]. In a well-designed study, the clinical significance and statistical significance of the primary analyses will match.

It is clear that the magnitude of the efficacy or effect size has an impact on the sample size required for the clinical trial. Consider a clinical trial that is being designed to assess the effect of a randomly allocated intervention on the total mortality incidence rate. The investigators are interested in detecting a reduction in the total mortality rate from the control group mortality rate of 15%. The α error probability for this study will be 0.05, and the power is 90%. Using the formula derived in Appendix D, and substituting the type I error rate, the type II error rate, and the control group event rate into this formulation[9], we find that the total number of patients required for the trial can be written as a function of the sample size, i.e.

$$N = \frac{1}{e}\left[\frac{238}{e} - 98\right] - 21 \tag{11.9}$$

and we can plot the required sample size as a function of the efficacy e (Figure 11.2).

Not only does the sample size decrease with increasing efficacy, but the decrease is dramatic.[10] This relationship has important consequences for sample size design and so must be considered carefully. As the sample size of the trial increases, so too does the clinical trial's ability to precisely detect smaller differences between the event rates of the treatment and control group. The only treatment effects that small clinical trials can identify (everything else being equal) are large effects; these experiments with smaller samples are in general unable to capture differences in the event rates between the two groups in clinical trials that exist in the population. We might think of the relationship between effect size and sample size as one of magnification. Just as the ability to distinguish between small features of objects increases with the magnifying ability of a microscope, so too does the ability to discern small differences between the control group and treatment group event experiences increase with the sample size of the trial. The resolving ability of the clinical trial increases for larger sample sizes.

---

[8] Or, as someone once said "a difference, to be a difference, must make a difference."

[9] This calculation is provided in detail at the end of this chapter.

[10] Technically, the sample size decreases not linearly, but quadratically. It decreases with the *square* of the efficacy.

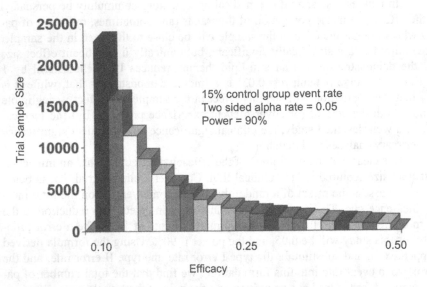

Figure 11.2. Reduction in the sample size as the efficacy of the Intervention increases.

Thus, just as it is best to first determine the correct level of magnification before one chooses the microscope lens to use, the investigator must first determine the size of the treatment effect in the population that they would like their sample to detect before they choose the sample size for the trial. They must choose the sample size carefully. Choosing a sample size that is too big is not only wasteful,[11] but it expends needless effort to identify insignificantly small clinical effects with great but ultimately unhelpful precision. Choosing a sample size for the clinical trial that is too small, on the other hand, denies the investigators the required precision to identify efficacy levels of clinical interest (Figure 11.3).

11.7.2 Choosing an Efficacy Level

This development is the rationale for the selection of efficacy determination. The investigations should first identify the efficacy level of clinical interest and then choose the sample size that allows this efficacy level to be identified with statistical significance, where the statistical error levels are chosen in accordance with acceptable a priori type I and type II error probabilities.

This approach of first determining the efficacy level that is of clinical interest begs the question of exactly how should this choice should be made. We should first begin with some notation. We will describe the efficacy level that is

---

[11] Wasteful not just in time and money, but in the inconvenience and inadvertent harm that is done to patients who volunteer their time to contribute to the scientific process.

chosen by the investigators for their clinical trial (i.e., the efficacy on which the trial's sample size is based) as the *design efficacy*. The typical advice that is given to investigators is that the design efficacy should be the minimum effect of the intervention that would justify its use in the population. This smallest efficacy of clinical significance we will define as the *minimum clinical efficacy*.

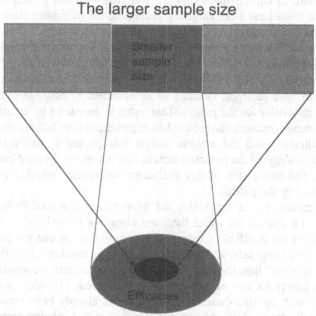

Figure 11.3. The larger sample has the resolving power to detect the smaller efficacy.

One of the rationales for this selection procedure is the concern that if an efficacy level that is larger than the minimum clinical efficacy is chosen, the sample size based on this larger efficacy level will be smaller. This smaller sample size will potentially fail to capture a smaller but clinically significant efficacy level that appears in the population (we will discuss this concept in some detail later in this chapter).

This observation has important implications for subgroup analyses. As we stated earlier in this chapter, the sample size constraints for the evaluation of the effect of therapy within a subgroup are profound. This observation, taken together with the discussion of the previous paragraph suggests that, everything else being equal, the effect of therapy within a subcohort that will be identifiable will not be a small effect but a large effect. To the degree that this large effect is greater than the minimum clinical efficacy, the evaluation of the effect of therapy within the subgroup cohort may be impaired. However, as we will soon see, the minimum clinical efficacy, much like the control group event rate, can vary from subgroup cohort to subgroup cohort.

In a profession whose professional creed is "First, do no harm," the clinical trial investigators are obligated to first assess the possible problems the therapy can cause in patients who choose to volunteer for their study. These problems include financial hardship as well as the occurrence of undesirable side-effects reasonably believed to be associated with new intervention. In addition, the current standard of care of the disease for which the medication may be indicated must also be considered. The minimum clinical efficacy is identified after a joint assessment of this standard of care, medication cost, and adverse event profile has been completed. Once these have been carefully evaluated, the minimum clinical efficacy is chosen as the efficacy level that balances these three factors.

It is no coincidence that this decision process mirrors the deliberation that the practicing physician undertakes with her patient as the two of them carefully consider the use of a new medication for the treatment of the patient's condition. Each of them have the right to make an independent assessment of the value that medication may offer for the patient. That value is measured by assessing the quality of the disease treatment the patient has experienced thus far, the financial burden of that medication and the adverse events that patient is likely to experience. Against this is weighed the potential benefit that the use of the medication offers for the patient. The conclusion of this evaluation determines whether the medication should be used by the patient.

Consider, for example, that the intervention is a medication that is proposed to treat a disease for which there are already a panoply of medications. The combination of the available therapies that are already in use are beneficial, well understood, relatively safe, and inexpensive. In this situation where the standard of care is "acceptable," then the new medication must demonstrate substantial efficacy in order to justify its use in this clinical environment in which practitioners are comfortable with the risk–benefit balance that has already been created by the established medications. If, in addition, the medication that is being proposed is costly and/or has a new and serious adverse event profile, the efficacy threshold for the medication must be even higher in order to preserve the risk–benefit balance .

On the other hand, consider a clinical trial that is evaluating a medication for the treatment of a condition that has a poorly tolerated standard of care (an example would be acquired immuno-deficiency syndrome). Assume that the new medication that the investigators wish to evaluate in a controlled clinical trial has a low frequency of adverse events, and that these adverse events are easily recognized and treated. Let us also assume that the financial cost of this medication is small. In this case, the demonstration of overwhelming efficacy by this medication would not be required by the medical community to justify the use of this compound in patients. A risk–benefit assessment would suggest that the demonstration of moderate efficacy by this therapy would be all that was required to offset the low risk and cost associated with its use. This does not imply that a larger effect size is undesirable; clearly the greater the effect size, the greater the attractiveness of the intervention. However, smaller effect sizes would lead to the use of this medication as well.

Thus, the minimum clinical efficacy is the resultant sense of the medical and regulatory communities about the effectiveness level of the medication that is required to offset both the adverse events and the cost of the medication while simultaneously considering the current standard of care for the disease. The more dangerous and more costly the medication, the greater the minimum clinical efficacy must be.[12]

11.7.3 Matching Clinical and Statistical Significance

Ideally, the clinical significance of the effect of a medication and the statistical significance of that medication should coincide in a clinical trial. Surprisingly, this is not often the case when the clinical trial is being designed.

It will be useful to examine the relationship between efficacy and the ability of the clinical trial to detect the effect of interest—we may most directly do this by examining how the p-value of the difference between the control and treatment groups is related to the efficacy of the study. Consider a clinical trial that is designed to execute one primary analysis; the effect of the randomly allocated intervention on the cumulative incidence of the total mortality rate. The total mortality rate in the placebo group is 20%. After considerable discussion, the investigators choose *a minimum* clinical efficacy of 15%. In this study, the investigators prospectively choose a two-sided type I error rate of 0.05 and a power of 90%. The required sample size of the trial based on these event rates is 7040. If the event rate in the placebo group is accurate, then it is actually possible for us to graph the p-value of the result versus the efficacy of the trial (Figure 11.4).

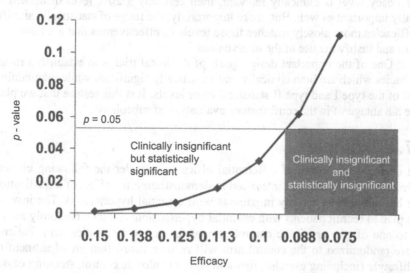

Figure 11.4 Shaded region reveals clinically insignificant efficacies with statistical significance.

---

[12] This assumes that the scientists have some reliable information about the safety profile of the intervention to be tested in the study.

Of course, the investigators expect that if they were to identify in their sample an efficacy of 15% (which is the efficacy that they expected), and if the trial was concordantly executed, then they would find a statistically significant difference between the total mortality rates of the treatment and control groups. However, Figure 8.4 reveals that in this clinical trial that was designed to discern an efficacy of 15% small efficacies become statistically significant as well. For example, an efficacy of 12.5% produced a p-value of 0.007, and an efficacy as small as 10% produces a p-value of 0.033. If the investigators had chosen the 15% efficacy level because if was the minimum efficacy level that would justify the use of the medication, then it appears that efficacies which do not justify the use of the medication would also be statistically significant in their clinical trial.

In a very real sense, this demonstration that statistical significance corresponds with clinical insignificance reveals an inefficiency in trial design. Some improvement might be offered by redesigning the study so that the region of clinical significance overlaps with the region for which statistical significance is identified. Consider an alternative approach to the plan of this study in which this clinical trial was prospectively designed to detect an efficacy of not 15% but 20%. One immediate consequence is that the size of the study has now decreased from 7040 to 3875. This change reduces the ability of the investigators to detect small levels of benefit that will be produced by the therapy. However, recall that the minimum clinical efficacy of the medication is 15%; the detection of efficacy levels smaller than this minimum are of no clinical importance and need not be identified with statistical significance. The efficacy levels that are statistically significant with this smaller sample size are levels of from 20% down to 15% (Figure 11.5). If a 15% efficacy level is clinically relevant, then certainly a 20% level of benefit is clinically important as well. But, more importantly, the range of statistically significant efficacies more closely matches those levels of effectiveness that are clinically relevant and justify the use of the intervention.

One of the important design goals of a clinical trial is to establish a range of efficacies which are both clinically and statistically significant while maintaining control of the type I and type II statistical error levels. It is this feature that we plan to take advantage of in the confirmatory evaluation of subcohorts.

11.7.4 Example

As an example of the use of differential efficacy, consider the following clinical trial design. Investigators are interested in demonstrating the effect of a medication which has antiplatelet activity in patients with essential hypertension. The investigators plan to recruit patients with essential hypertension, and then randomly assign them to one of two arms; the control arm or the active medication arm. Patients who are randomized to the control arm will receive instruction on adjustment of their lifestyle (including exercise, diet and sodium chloride control, smoking cessation, and stress management). They will then have their essential hypertension managed using a standard antihypertensive regimen e.g., [4]. These control group subjects will also receive a placebo pill that they must take each day.

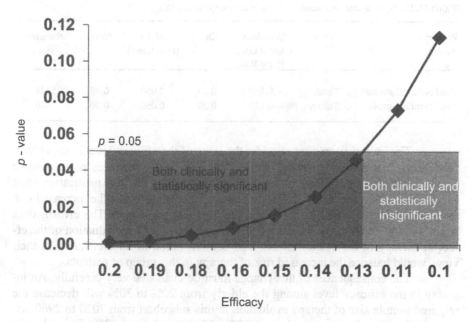

Figure 11.5. Statistically significant results are now matched with clinically significant effects.

Patients who are randomized to the active treatment arm receive control group therapy plus, instead of the placebo, the antiplatelet agent which they must take every day for the duration of the trial. The trial designers believe that they will be able to recruit up to 5000 patients for this trial.

The primary endpoint of this study will be the combined endpoint of fatal and nonfatal stroke. However, the antiplatelet agent is known to be associated with a different constellation of adverse events in elderly patients (including but not limited to, bleeding). The investigators have a prospective interest in demonstrating that the benefits of antiplatelet therapy justifies its use in this higher risk subcohort. Thus they prospectively design two primary analyses in this study: (1) the effect of the antiplatelet agent on the cumulative incidence rate of fatal/nonfatal stroke in the entire cohort, and (2) the effect of the antiplatelet agent on the fatal/nonfatal stroke rate in the elderly cohort.

The investigators have assumed a control group cumulative event rate of 15%. The cumulative incidence rate of fatal/nonfatal stroke is estimated to be 12%, somewhat lower in the elderly. This difference is a reflection of the fact that the distribution of the causes of death is different among the elderly than it is in the entire subcohort. An initial examination of the efficacy issue in the total cohort leads the investigators to the assessment that the minimum clinical efficacy is 20%. For their first evaluation, the trial designers assume that the minimum clinical efficacy is the same for the elderly subcohort. Thus, this initial examination produces a larger sample size for the subset of patients who are elderly (Table 11.15).

Table 11.15. Sample size computation with one subgroup: Scenario 1.

Primary Analyses	Cohort	Cumulative Control Group Event Rate	Efficacy	Alpha (two -tailed)	Power	Sample size
Fatal/Nonfatal stroke	Total	0.150	0.20	0.050	0.90	5444
Fatal/Nonfatal stroke	Elderly	0.120	0.20	0.050	0.90	7020

The investigators next consider the issue of the efficacy level in the elderly subcohort. In this vulnerable population, the medication produces more adverse events in older patients. Thus the level of benefit produced by this medication must be greater for this subcohort of elderly patients in order to offset the increased risk associated with the use of the medication in the older population. The investigators begin with the intention of increasing the efficacy level for the evaluation of the effect of therapy in the elderly cohort. The demonstration of 30% efficacy, in their view, would balance the increased risk of therapy in this group of patients.

The consequences of this change must be evaluated very carefully. An increase in the efficacy level among the elderly from 20% to 30% will decrease the required sample size of therapy evaluation in this subcohort from 7020 to 2960, assuming the type I error remains at 0.05 and the power is 90%. This change, however, does not imply that efficacy levels less than 30% will not be statistically significant. Continuing to focus our attention of the elderly subcohort, if the sample size of the subcohort analysis is 2960 patients (1480 patients randomized to each group), and the event rate in the control group is an accurate reflection of the population event rate, then statistical significance is retained for efficacy levels down to 20%. Thus, the investigator statement that they wish to identify an efficacy level of 30% is really a statement that they desire to demonstrate that the efficacy is greater than 20% with statistical significance. Therefore, designing the subcohort evaluation of the effect of therapy for a 30% efficacy level decreases the sample size for the elderly subcohort analysis while simultaneously aligning the range of statistically significant levels of effectiveness with the clinical significant range. This efficacy range of greater than 20% justifies the use of the anitplatelet agents in this subcohort that is known to be more vulnerable to side-effects of the medication (Table 11.16).

The investigators now turn to allocating the type I error rate between the two subcohorts in order to conserve the FWER at 0.05. They allocate the majority of the type I error probability to the analysis of the effect of the antiplatelet intervention on the cumulative incidence rate of fatal/nonfatal stroke. The balance of the α error rate is allocated to the analysis of the therapy's effect on the same endpoint in the smaller elderly subcohort (Table 11.17).

Table 11.16. Sample size computation with one subgroup: Scenario 2.

Primary Analyses	Cohort	Cumulative Control Group Event Rate	Efficacy	Alpha (two -tailed)	Power	Sample size
Fatal/Nonfatal stroke	Total	0.150	0.20	0.050	0.90	5444
Fatal/Nonfatal stroke	Elderly	0.120	0.30	0.050	0.90	2961

Table 11.17. Sample size computation with one subgroup: Scenario 3.

Primary Analyses	Cohort	Cumulative Control Group Event Rate	Efficacy	Alpha (two -tailed)	Power	Sample size
Fatal/Nonfatal stroke	Total	0.150	0.20	0.035	0.90	5954
Fatal/Nonfatal stroke	Elderly	0.120	0.30	0.015	0.90	3887

Consideration of hypothesis test dependency can now be embedded into this developing analysis structure. Recall that in subgroup analyses, we recommended that the homogeneity of the therapy measure and the coincidence measure should be identical and equal to the proportion of the total cohort that comprises the elderly subcohort. This is approximately 50%. Thus, the dependency parameter is $D_s = c_s^2 [2 - c_s] = 0.375$ which produces a small reduction in the sample size required for the analysis in the elderly subcohort (Table 11.18).

Table 11.18. Sample size computation with one subgroup: Scenario 4.

Primary Analyses	Cohort	Cumulative Control Group Event Rate	Efficacy	Alpha (two -tailed)	Power	Sample size
Fatal/Nonfatal stroke	Total	0.150	0.20	0.035	0.90	5954
				D= 0.375		
Fatal/Nonfatal stroke	Elderly	0.120	0.30	0.018	0.90	3744

Finally, the power is reduced to the minimum acceptable power for each of the analyses, producing a further sample size reduction (Table 11.19).

Table 11.19. Sample size computation with one subgroup: Scenario 5.

Primary Analyses	Cohort	Cumulative Control Group Event Rate	Efficacy	Alpha (two -tailed)	Power	Sample size
Fatal/Nonfatal stroke	Total	0.150	0.20	0.035	0.80	4509
				D= 0.375		
Fatal/Nonfatal stroke	Elderly	0.120	0.30	0.018	0.80	2895

11.8 The Differential Use of Event Precision

One final technique that will be developed in this chapter to embed a subcohort confirmatory analysis into a clinical trial is the use of a different standard of precision.

11.8.1 Sample Sizes for Continuous Endpoints

Thus far in this chapter we have focused on the evaluation of the effect of therapy on a dichotomous endpoint. However, it is certainly acceptable and permissible to have an endpoint that is not just measured in a 0–1 fashion but is instead measured over a continuous scale (e.g., LVEF). The evaluation of the effect of the randomly allocated intervention on the change in blood pressure, for example, or the change in urine output are common examples of the use of the continuous endpoint.

The sample size computation that is required to identify the effect of therapy to produce a change in a continuous endpoint is different (and actually simpler) than that for the dichotomous endpoint that was derived in Appendix E. Consider a clinical trial that has as its clinical hypothesis that the effect of the randomly allocated therapy will change the prospectively defined continuous outcome by d_t units, and that the expected change in the control group is d_c units, where $d_t \geq d_c$. In this case, the efficacy of the therapy may be written as $\Delta = d_t - d_c$. If the hypothesis test is to be carried out with a two-sided type I error rate of α and a power of $1-\beta$, then the required sample size (total number of subjects in the active group plus the total number of subjects in the placebo group is

$$N = \frac{4\sigma_D^2 \left[Z_{1-\alpha/2} - Z_\beta \right]^2}{\Delta^2},$$

(11.10)

where Z_c is the cth percentile value from the standard normal distribution. We will focus on the variability of the difference in the continuous measure from baseline to the end of the study, σ_D, commonly referred to as the standard deviation of the difference. Inspection of formula (11.10) reveals that the sample size increases as the standard deviation increases. This is intuitive since the larger the standard deviation, the greater the variability of the continuous measure that is due to sampling error. Since more observations are required for greater precision, more patients are required to offset the large sampling error.

11.8.2 Cohort-Dependent Precision

The tact that we will take in this section is to design the subcohort evaluation so that the standard deviation of the difference, σ_D is smaller in the subcohort than in the overall cohort. This might be most easily done by taking the measurement differently in the subcohort of interest, with an instrument that has more precision. Thus, two instruments would be used in this trial to measure the endpoint. The first instrument of acceptable but average precision would be used in subjects who are not part of the subcohort of interest. The second would be measured in subjects who are part of the cohort.[13] This design could be costly, since no doubt the more precise measurement would be more expensive.

As an example, consider a clinical trial that is designed to evaluate the effect of a new oral hypoglycemic agent on HbA1c levels in patients with type II diabetes mellitus. Patients for this study have been previously diagnosed with type II diabetes mellitus and have HbA1c levels between 9% and 12% at baseline. These patients are randomized to either the control group or the active therapy group. Patients who are randomized into the control group receive instructions on appropriate, sustainable measures of exercise and diet control. In addition to their current therapy for plasma glucose control, they receive a placebo pill. Patients in the active group receive the same therapy as the control group, but, the placebo pill is replaced with the new oral hypoglycemic therapy.

The endpoint for this study is the change in HbA1c level. It is anticipated that, although there will be a decrease in the HbA1c in the control group, the reduction in HbA1c that the active therapy group experiences should be greater. The investigators believe that they must demonstrate that there is at least a 1% greater decrease in the HbA1c in the active group when compared to the change in the control group. In addition, the investigators are particularly interested in the experiences of patients who are already on exogenous insulin to control their diabetes mellitus, and a major goal of this trial is the demonstration of the effect of the new oral hypoglycemic agents in these patients who require insulin therapy. Thus, there are two primary analyses for this trial. In order of importance, they are the effect of therapy on the change in HbA1c on insulin dependent type II diabetic patients and, secondly, the effect of therapy on HbA1c levels in patients with type II diabetes mellitus regardless of their background therapy. The initial evaluation of sample size is carried out with a two-sided α error rate of 0.05, power of 90% (Table 11.20).

---

[13] This design demonstrates the logistical necessity of prospective specification of the patients who are members of the subcohort. Without being able to identify the subgroup status of these patients at the time of randomization, it would be impossible to know to whom to give the more precise measurement.

Table 11.20 Diabetes study with a single subcohort: Scenario 1.

Primary Analyses	Cohort	Standard deviation of the difference	Delta	Alpha (two -tailed)	Power	Sample size
Change in HbA1c	Insulin Rx	1.70	1.00	0.050	0.90	121
Change in HbA1c	Total cohort	1.70	1.00	0.050	0.90	121

The standard deviation of the change in HbA1c for each group is estimated as 1.70, producing a sample size of 121 patients for each of the analyses. However the investigators recognize that most patients with type II diabetes mellitus do not require exogenous insulin therapy and these patients may be somewhat more difficult to find. They therefore invest in a new mechanism to measure HbA1c. This new device permits a more accurate determination of this level, decreasing σ_D from 1.70 to 1.25. This is a more expensive HbA1c evaluation, but it will reduce the required number of patients who need insulin for management of their diabetes mellitus for the trial (Table 11.21).

Table 11.21 Diabetes study with a single subcohort: Scenario 2.

Primary Analyses	Cohort	Standard deviation of the difference	Delta	Alpha (two -tailed)	Power	Sample size
Change in HbA1c	Insulin Rx	1.25	1.00	0.050	0.90	66
Change in HbA1c	Total cohort	1.70	1.00	0.050	0.90	121

The investigators now proceed to manage the FWER for the trial. They choose to allocate type I error rates such that the assessment of the effect of the therapy in the insulin-dependent patients retains the preponderance of the type I error rate. The α error rate for the subcohort evaluation is set at 0.04, with 0.01 remaining for assessment of the effect of therapy in the total cohort (Table 11.22).

Table 11.22 Diabetes study with a single subcohort: Scenario 3.

Primary Analyses	Cohort	Standard deviation of the difference	Delta	Alpha (two -tailed)	Power	Sample size
Change in HbA1c	Insulin Rx	1.25	1.00	0.040	0.90	70
Change in HbA1c	Total cohort	1.70	1.00	0.010	0.90	172

By dividing the type I error in this fashion, the investigators are able to keep the required number of patients requiring insulin therapy low. In essence they are willing to recruit more non-insulin requiring type II diabetic patients because these patients not requiring insulin are easier to recruit.

An adjustment for dependence produces $D = 0.375$ and a small decrease in the number of required patients for the study (Table 11.23).

Table 11.23 Diabetes study with a single subcohort: Scenario 4.

Primary Analyses	Cohort	Standard deviation of the difference	Delta	Alpha (two -tailed)	Power	Sample size
Change in HbA1c	Insulin Rx	1.25	1.00	0.040	0.90	70
				$D = 0.375$		
Change in HbA1c	Total cohort	1.70	1.00	0.012	0.90	166

Finally, the sample size for the study is reduced by decreasing the power for the evaluation of the effect of therapy in the overall cohort from 90% to 80% (Table 11.24),

Table 11.24 Diabetes study with a single subcohort: Scenario 5.

Primary Analyses	Cohort	Standard deviation of the difference	Delta	Alpha (two -tailed)	Power	Sample size
Change in HbA1c	Insulin Rx	1.25	1.00	0.040	0.90	70
				$D = 0.375$		
Change in HbA1c	Total cohort	1.70	1.00	0.012	0.80	130

Thus, the investigators have designed a study that keeps the required number of insulin-dependent type II diabetic patients small, but preserves the confirmatory analysis within this subcohort. This was accomplished by the investigators' choice to invest financial resources into an improved measure of the endpoint of the study, reducing the standard deviation of this endpoint, and reducing the required sample size for the subcohort of interest.

11.9 Conclusions

Subgroup analyses are most likely here to stay in the evaluation of clinical trials. As long as physicians focus on the treatment of individual patients with their unique and distinguishing characteristics, they will attempt to use those characteristics to aid them in the prediction of a therapy effect. This effort should not be belittled, for it is an honest attempt to reduce the number of unknowns in the prediction of an individual patient's response to treatment. This understandable need will continue to stoke the subgroup analysis fire.

It is also more likely than not that the majority of subgroup analyses will continue to be carried out as either secondary evaluations in clinical trials or exploratory evaluations. Thus the guidelines put forward by Yusuf will continue to be predominant for these evaluations—the best estimate of the effect of a therapy within a subgroup in such an analysis is the effect of the therapy that was seen in the overall cohort. These subgroup evaluations can suggest but not confirm the answers to questions about the risks and benefits of a randomly allocated therapy within a clinical trial.

This chapter has outlined tools and procedures by which subgroup evaluations may be confirmatory. The techniques that were advanced are consistent with our overall theme of the primacy of prospective design and the importance of controlling the FWER. Their product is the invigorated ability of a clinical trial to provide confirmatory analyses not just for the effect of therapy in the overall cohort of a clinical trial, but for the effect of therapy within the subgroup stratum of interest as well.

However, these procedures do not come for free, and this chapter has not provided an easy or casual solution to the subgroup analysis issue in clinical trials. The illustrations provided here do not impair the requirement for the disciplined nature of confirmatory subgroup analysis; instead, they amplify it. The planned subgroup evaluations must be considered very carefully. There must be a biologically plausible rationale that leads the investigators to focus on the response of the subgroup stratum to the clinical trial's intervention. The investigators must give careful consideration the initial type I error allocations, and they must think through the possible implications of the trial's findings.

As demonstrated in the examples of this chapter, the size of the subgroup is commonly on the order of 40% to 60% of the total cohort sample size for the confirmatory analyses to be executed successfully. In some cases, the size of the overall trial must be adjusted. These procedures certainly cannot be carried out for every subgroup of interest in the study. After careful study, one or perhaps two subgroups can have confirmatory analyses prospectively embedded in the trial. The remaining subgroup analyses can be traditionally executed and interpreted in an exploratory light. Also interpretation of trial results must jointly consider prospectively planning the manner of trial execution (concordant or discordant), effect size with its standard error, confidence intervals, and p-values. The focus of this manuscript is on the p-value component, but this focus does not detract from the primacy of the joint interpretation.

In addition, we must remember that many subgroups can be misinterpreted because subgroup membership may merely be a surrogate for another less obvious factor that determines efficacy. The investigator must consider this possible explanation for her subgroup specific effect in her interpretation of the analysis.

Finally, serious deliberation must be given to the importance of the subcohort evaluation. The choice of an endpoint that is different from that used to assess the effect of therapy in the overall cohort must be addressed. In addition, any distinction between the efficacy level required in the subgroup stratum of interest must be carefully justified to a sometimes skeptical medical and regulatory community. Finally, the increased cost of the trial in human, logistical, and financial resources are considerable. Confirmatory subgroup analyses, like well-designed clinical trials, should not be undertaken likely.

Problems

1. What are the requirements for a confirmatory subgroup analysis in a clinical trial?

2. How can the use of two separate endpoints in a clinical trial, one for the analysis of the effect of therapy in the overall cohort, and the second for the evaluation of the effect of therapy in the prospectively specified subgroup stratum of interest, be justified?

3. Why is the incorporation of dependency argument have less of an impact in assigning type I error levels a priori to subgroup analyses than in other circumstances (e.g., combined endpoints)?

4. Why is the overall measure of dependency between two hypothesis tests, one that uses a singleton endpoint of a combined endpoint for gauging the effect of therapy in the overall cohort and the second that evaluates the effect of therapy in the combined cohort, reduced and not increased by the use of the combined endpoint?

5. A clinical trial is being designed to test the effect of an intervention on the occurrence of a clinical event. Assume that the intervention will produce a 25% reduction in the occurrence of the primary endpoint. Also assume that the type I error for this evaluation is 0.05 (two sided) and the power is 80%. Let there be two candidate primary endpoints for the trial. The first candidate, C_1 has a cumulative endpoint event rate of 10%. The second candidate endpoint C_2 occurs with a 20% cumulative event rate. Show that there is a 45% reduction in the sample size for the entire two armed trial if the cumulative event of the primary endpoint is C_2 and not C_1. What are the implications for the construction of a confirmatory analysis for the subgroup analysis based on one as opposed to the other of these two primary endpoint candidates.

6. Why is the use of an efficacy level choice to reduce the sample size of a clinical trial been historically disparaged?

7. In the setting of a clinical trial, what is the difference between minimum clinical efficacy, and minimum statistical efficacy? What difficulties occur in clinical trial interpretation when the ranges of these two values do not substantially overlap?

8. What is cohort-dependent precision? What are the financial implications of a clinical trial that incorporates this procedure?

9. Why might it be important for the investigators in a clinical trial, who choose to carry out a confirmatory subgroup analysis, to first publish a preceding design manuscript in which they lay out the details of their research plans?

Note

The purpose here is to briefly demonstrate that the sample size formula can be written as a function of the control group event rate and the efficacy. Assume that a randomized, controlled clinical trial is being executed to test the effect of a medication to reduce the total mortality rate. Then recall from Appendix D that we saw

$$N = \frac{2\left[p_c\left(1-p_c\right)+p_t\left(1-p_t\right)\right]\left[Z_{1-\alpha/2}-Z_\beta\right]^2}{\left[p_c-p_t\right]^2} \tag{8.14}$$

where

N = number of placebo patients + number of active group patients
α = Type I error rate
β = Type II error rate
Z_c = the cth percentile from the standard normal probability distribution
P_c = cumulative primary endpoint event rate in the placebo group
P_t = cumulative primary endpoint event rate in the active group.

Our goal is to rewrite (8.14) in terms of the efficacy. Recall from section 8.7.6 that we wrote efficacy as

$$e = \frac{p_c - p_t}{p_c}. \tag{8.15}$$

Then $p_t = (1-e)p_c$, $p_c - p_t = p_c e$ and we can rewrite (8.14) as

$$N = \frac{2\left[p_c\left(1-p_c\right)+\left(1-e\right)p_c\left(1-\left(1-e\right)p_c\right)\right]\left[Z_{1-\alpha/2}-Z_\beta\right]^2}{\left[p_c e\right]^2} \tag{8.16}$$

and we only need to provide further simplification to a portion of the numerator of (8.16), namely $p_c\left(1-p_c\right)+\left(1-e\right)p_c\left(1-\left(1-e\right)p_c\right)$. This is

$$
\begin{aligned}
p_c\left(1-p_c\right) &+ \left(1-e\right)p_c\left(1-\left(1-e\right)p_c\right) \\
&= p_c\left[\left(1-p_c\right)+\left(1-e\right)\left(1-\left(1-e\right)p_c\right)\right] \\
&= p_c\left[1-p_c+\left(1-e\right)-\left(1-e\right)^2 p_c\right] \\
&= p_c\left[\left(2-e\right)-p_c\left(1+\left(1-e\right)^2\right)\right].
\end{aligned} \tag{8.17}
$$

Substituting the last line of expression (8.17) into the numerator of (8.16) reveals

$$N = \frac{2p_c\left[(2-e)-p_c\left(1+(1-e)^2\right)\right]\left[Z_{1-\alpha/2}-Z_\beta\right]^2}{\left[p_c e\right]^2}. \tag{8.18}$$

If we now assume that $\alpha = 0.05$ for a two-sided hypothesis test (i.e., $Z_{1-\alpha/2} = 1.96$), 90% power (i.e., $Z_\beta = -1.28$) and the control group event rate is 15% (i.e., $p_c = 0.15$) we may reexpress (8.18) as

$$N = \frac{3.15\left[(2-e)-0.15\left(1+(1-e)^2\right)\right]}{0.0225e^2}, \tag{8.19}$$

and further simplification reveals

$$N = \frac{1}{e}\left[\frac{238}{e}-98\right]-21. \tag{8.20}$$

References

1. Grundy, S.M. (1998). Statin trials and goals of cholesterol–lowering therapy. *Circulation* **97**:1446–1452.
2. Moyé, L.A., Deswal, A. (2001). Trials within trials; confirmatory subgroup analyses in controlled clinical experiments. *Control Clinical Trials.***22**:605–619.
3. Food and Drug Modernization Act of 1997. Public Law;105–115; 21 USC 355a; 111 Stat. 2295 (November 21, 1997).
4. Davis, B.R., Cutler, J.A., Gordon, D.J., Furberg, C.D., Wright, J.T., Cushman, W.C., Grimm, R.H., LaRosa, J., Whelton, P.K., Perry, H.M., Alderman, M.H., Ford, C.E., Oparil, S., Francis, C., Proschan, M., Pressel, S., Black, H.R., Hawkins, C.M. for the ALLHAT Research Group. Rationale and design for the antihyertensive and lipid lowering treatment to prevent heart attack trial (ALLHAT) (1996) *Hypertension Journal.***9**:342–360.
5. Franciosa, J.A., Taylor, A.L., Cohn, J.N., Yancy, C.W., Ziesche, S, Olukotun, A., Ofili, E., Ferdinand, K,, Loscalzo, Z.J., Worcel, W. for the A–Heft Investigators. (2002). African–American heart failure trial: rationale, design, and methodology. *Journal of Cardiac Failure* **8**:128–135.
6. Taylor, A.L., Cohn, J.N., Worcel, M., Franciosa, J.A. for the A-Heft Investigators (2002). The African–American Heart Failure Trial: Background, rationale, and significance. *Journal of the National Medical Association* **94**:762–769.

7. Moyé, L.A., Powell, J.H. (2001). Evaluation of Ethnic Minorities and Gender Effects in Clinical Trials:Opportunities Lost and Rediscovered. *Journal of the National Medical Association* **93***(suppl):* 1–6.

8. American Heart Association (2002) 2002 Heart and stroke statistical update, American Heart Association. Dallas, Tex. *American Heart Association*.

9. Alexander, M., Grumbach, K., Remy, L., Rowell, R., Massie, B.M. (1999). Congestive heart failure hospitalizations and survival in California: Patterns according to race/ethnicity. *American Heart Journal* **137**:919–927.

10. Bourassa, M.G., Gurne, O., Bangdiwala, S.I., Ghali, J.K., Young, J.B., Rousseau, M., Johnstone, D.E., Yusuf, S. (1993). Natural history and patterns of current practice in heart failure. The Studies of Left Ventricular Dysfunction (SOLVD) Investigators. *Journal of the American College of Cardiology.***22**(4 Suppl A):14A–19A.

11. Alexander, M., Grumbach, K., Selby, J., Brown, A.F., Washington, E. (1995) Hospitalization for congestive heart failure. Explaining racial differences. *Journal of the American Medical Association* **274**:1037–1042.

12. Yancy, C.W. (2000). Heart failure in African–Americans: a cardiovascular engima. *Journal of Cardiac Failure* **6**:183–186.

Chapter 12

Multiple Analyses and Multiple Treatment Arms

This chapter elaborates upon the ability of investigators to draw confirmatory conclusions from a clinical trial that consists of a control group and multiple treatment arms. After a review of the literature, a combination of the differntial apportionment of the type I error rates and the use of dependent hypothesis testing will be applied to the multiple testing issue that naturally arises from the mutliple treatment arm scenario. No new mathematical tools are developed, and several examples of clinical trials under design are provided to demonstrate the applicability of the procedures that we have developed in this book.

12.1 Introduction and Assumptions

Thus far in this text, we have focused on a clinical trial that has two arms; a control arm and a single treatment arm. The incorporation of additional treatment arms within clinical trials provides a new opportunity to the clinical trial designers. As reviewed in Chapter 3, both the clinical trial investigators and the trial's sponsor require efficient experimental design. In a clinical trial with a control group and a single treatment group, this drive for efficiency can produce multiple primary analyses with multiple, prospectively defined primary endpoints. In addition, as developed in Chapters 8 to 11, this efficiency can be improved by the execution of multiple confirmatory analyses from among various, prospectively defined subgroup cohorts.

The inclusion of a second treatment group can enhance the productivity of the clinical trial by providing supplemental information about a different characteristic of the active therapy. As an example, the second treatment arm might be a different dose of the therapy; this approach would shed light on the dose-response relationship between the randomly allocated intervention and the prospectively defined endpoint. Alternatively, the additional treatment arm could be the combination of the new therapy with another agent, illustrating the degree to which the two compounds interact.

However, with the inclusion of added treatment arms comes the responsibility for the effective evaluation of the resulting data. A central thesis of our discussions thus far has been that the investigators' intellectual discipline must increase with the number of possible analyses. This rigor serves these scientists well as they work to determine the small number of confirmatory analyses on which the conclusions of their trial will rest. In this chapter, we will use the tools developed thus far in this text to develop confirmatory analyses from clinical trials with multiple treatment arms.

In order to maintain our focus on the application of multiple testing to the unique characteristics of clinical trials with multiple treatment arms, we will continue with the same assumptions that have been the foundation of our discussions in the second half of this book, i.e., that the trial is well-designed in each of its other aspects and that it is concordantly executed. Under these circumstances, the effect size, effect size estimates, confidence intervals and p-values derived from the primary analyses are trustworthy and provide useful information that can be applied to the population from which the research sample was obtained.

12.2 Literature Review

There have been many discussions in the literature of the appropriate analysis of clinical trials that have multiple treatment arms. Before we begin our development, a brief survey of the available methods is in order.

One commonly occurring scenario in which multiple testing arises from clinical experiments that have several treatment arms is what statisticians refer to as the "analysis of variance." In this setting, there are K treatment groups to be evaluated; each of these groups represents a treatment group to which patients are randomly allocated. If the primary endpoint in this scenario is a continuous one (e.g., change in DBP from baseline to the end of the study), then a question that is commonly asked is, "Which of these treatment groups have effect sizes that are different from the control group?" The analysis of variance procedure addresses this question by first asking if there are any significantly different effects among any of these K results. This question is answered by a single statistical test. If that hypothesis test does not reject the null hypothesis, then work ceases. However, if the null hypothesis is rejected, then the question of which of the K treatments that were evaluated are statistically different from one another must next be addressed.

One useful testing procedure that may be implemented in this setting is the Student-Neuman-Keuls (SNK) test [1]. It is a very straightforward procedure to execute. If there are K treatment groups in a clinical trial, the worker must first rank the effect sizes from smallest to largest. After this has been accomplished, the investigator compares the largest mean to the smallest mean using a simple t test with a percentile value from a specially produced table[1]. If there is a significant difference between these two means, the investigator then compares the next largest mean with the next smallest. This process continues until there are no significant differences. Tukey has provided an adaptation of this procedure [2], which appears in standard textbooks [3]. His result is similar to that from the SNK test; the only difference is that the critical value to be used to judge significance between the means is different.

The presence of a control group, and the need to compare the results of each of the intervention groups to those of the control group, is one of the features that often distinguishes the analysis of a prospectively defined, continuous outcome variable in a clinical study from the analysis of variance. Dunnett's test [4], [5] can

---

[1] Such a table can be found in [1], pp. 587–590.

be very helpful in this setting. Dunnett's test is similar to the SNK test in that its basis is a t statistic. Simply, if there are K treatments and a single control group, and each treatment result is to be tested against the control group result, then there are K hypothesis tests to be carried out. Dunnett computed the appropriate percentile value of the t distribution to use in carrying out these hypothesis tests [6]. One major advantage of the Dunnett procedure is that it permits the investigator to determine which specific comparisons are to be made. Thus the investigator can choose the exact comparisons she wants to make, following the triage procedures that were outlined in Chapter 4. A fine example of the use of the Dunnett procedure in a clinical trial setting is the AntiHypertensive and Lipid Lowering Heart Attack Trial (ALLHAT) [7]. Cheung and Holland have extended the results of Dunnett to include an evaluation of all comparisons between the multiple treatment groups in the trial [8].

There has been additional work on the evaluation of the multiple testing problem in research efforts with more than one treatment group. Ping–Yu and Dahlberg [9] adapt the SNK approach to derive sample size estimates for clinical trials with multiple treatment arms in the setting in which the investigator wishes to identify the "best" treatment, i.e., the treatment which produces a result which is the furthest (among the K treatments studied) from the control group result. Alternative statistical testing procedures in the clinical trial setting in which there are multiple treatment arms have been explored, but the best results are often obtained by making assumptions that may not be defensible for a clinical trial[2]. The performance of these procedures is frequently inferior to the Bonferroni based test [10], but the evaluation can be complex [11], [12].

If the investigator is not interested in carrying out formal statistical inference, but is instead focused on the generation of confidence intervals for the results of each of the K treatment groups, then [13], [14] demonstrate the computations required to generate these multiple confidence intervals. Two stage procedures, in which the investigators carry out two sets of randomizations have been studied as well [15]. The orthogonal contrast test of Mukerjee et al. can be useful if one presumes no treatment arm is worse than the control group [16].

When the treatment involves different doses, one is commonly interested in identifying the lowest dose that produces an effect, and researchers have explored procedures to identity the optimal test [17], [18], [19]. In addition, interim monitoring approaches for clinical trials with multiple endpoints have been suggested as well [20].

12.3 Treatment Versus Treatment

One of the simplest and common motivations for investigators to prospectively include multiple treatment arms within their clinical trial is the situation in which the primary analyses of the study will: (1) compare the effect of therapy of each of the treatment arms to the effect seen in the placebo or control group arm; and (2) the effect of therapy in at least some of the treatment arms will be compared to each

---

[2] One such assumption is that the results of the multiple endpoints of a clinical trial follow a multivariate normal probability distribution.

other. The tools that we have developed thus far in this text will serve us well in the design of this study.

Consider the following illustration: a clinical trial is being designed to study the ability of several treatments to reduce the clinical consequences of chronic mild elevations in DBP. The purpose of this study is to evaluate the effect of two new pharmacologic therapies on the long-term treatment of this disorder. Each of these new therapies (therapy A and therapy B) has been convincingly demonstrated to reduce blood pressure effectively; however these blood pressure reduction studies were of short duration (approximately six months of follow-up time), that precluded the precise estimation of the effects of these therapies on atherosclerotic events. Therapy A has a moderate ability to reduce blood pressure, and its use is associated with a well-understood adverse event profile. The blood pressure lowering capability of therapy B is superior to that of therapy A; however, the use of therapy B has been associated with a rare, adverse event, anasarca.

The control group for this study will consist of patients who are randomized to diuretic therapy, a well-accepted standard for the control of blood pressure. The only primary endpoint of the study will be the cumulative incidence rate of cardiovascular disease, defined as the combined endpoint of fatal cardiovascular death, nonfatal MI, or nonfatal stroke[3]. All patients will be followed until the end of the study and the average follow-up time for the trial is anticipated to be 5 years.

Patients who have DBPs between 90 and 100 mm Hg will therefore be randomized to one of three groups; control group therapy, therapy A, or therapy B. Every recruited patient will begin an educational program to learn of the important role of each of a balanced diet, a regular exercise program, smoking cessation, and stress reduction in controlling essential hypertension. This message will be emphasized both during the follow-up period and during regularly scheduled counseling sessions. Each patient's randomized therapy will be titrated so that their DBP is maintained below 85 mm Hg. The investigators believe that this treatment goal will be easily accomplished for each of the medications, obviating the requirement for alternate therapy.

The investigators now focus on the statistical hypothesis tests that they wish to carry out. They decide that they must compare each of the two new therapies to the control group, and then compare the results of therapy A to those of therapy B. This involves three different hypothesis tests over which the FWER must be controlled.

The investigators also recognize that the three statistical hypothesis tests that they wish to carry out involve overlapping sets of patients (e.g., the control group is used in two of the evaluations) and the endpoint is the same for each of the evaluations. This suggests that embedding hypothesis test dependency into their clinical trial analysis plan may be a useful procedure. In addition, these scientists will keep in mind that there may be some justification for modifying the efficacy threshold for at least one of these hypothesis tests.

---

[3] Many secondary endpoint analyses will also be executed in accordance with our definition of these in Chapter 4 and in agreement with the principles of composite endpoint analysis that were described in Chapter 7.

To begin consideration of the analysis plan for this study, the investigators begin with a simple calculation of the sample size that would be required for each of the three analyses (Table 12.1).

Table 12.1. Alpha allocation example with composite endpoint: First design scenario.

Primary analyses	Cumulative comparitor group event rate	Efficacy	Alpha (two-tailed)	Power	Sample size
A versus control	0.080	0.20	0.05	0.95	13,553
B versus control	0.080	0.20	0.05	0.95	13,553
A versus B	0.064	0.20	0.05	0.95	17,208

Even though the clinical trial will have three groups, each sample size is based on a two-group analysis, since these two group analyses correspond to the prospectively asked scientific questions. The investigators believe that the cumulative event rate for the prospectively defined, combined, primary endpoint of this trial will be 0.080. The cumulative event rate used in the third primary analysis of therapy A versus B. is lower since the comparator group in this evaluation is not the control group, but is therapy A. Since the investigators believe that patients in therapy group A will experience 1 - 0.20 = 80% of the events as those patients recruited to the control group, the event rate for the comparator group in the therapy A versus therapy B evaluation is (0.80)(0.08) = 0.064.[4] This lower event rate is the reason for the increased sample size requirement for the therapy A versus therapy B comparison. No attempt has been made to control the FWER yet in this early phase of the analysis plan development.

In this first computation, the investigators have assumed that the efficacy of therapy is assumed to be 20% for each of these three primary analyses. However, this assumption requires close examination. Recall that the adverse event burden for therapy B, including the rare but serious event of anasarca, is greater than that of therapy A. Thus, patients who are to be exposed to the possibility of this serious side-effect for therapy B should be the beneficiaries of greater efficacy in order to balance the risk-benefit assessment for this therapy. Therefore, an argument that the efficacy threshold for the evaluation of the effect of therapy B versus the control group is greater than that for the evaluation of therapy A versus the control group is admissible. Similar consideration might be given to the therapy A versus therapy B comparison. However, this evaluation is already planned to demonstrate a 20% re-

---

[4] Of course if therapy A does not decrease the cumulative event rate, the patients randomized to therapy A will experience more events, and the resultant sample size for the therapy A versus therapy B evaluation will be lower, all other things being equal. However, it is perhaps safer to make the conservative assumption that the cumulative event rate in the therapy A group will be smaller than that of the control group sample size calculations.

duction in the cumulative risk of fatal and nonfatal cardiovascular disease below that produced by therapy A, an intervention that itself is believed to be effective. Thus, the comparison of the effect of therapy for treatment A and B already reflects the concept that a greater benefit must be produced by therapy B to offset the greater risk associated with its use (Table 12.2).

Table 12.2. Alpha allocation example with composite endpoint: Second design scenario.

Primary analyses	Cumulative comparitor group event rate	Efficacy	Alpha (two-tailed)	Power	Sample size
A versus control	0.080	0.20	0.05	0.95	13,553
B versus control	0.080	0.25	0.05	0.95	8447
A versus B	0.064	0.20	0.05	0.95	17,208

The investigators next allocate the type I error rate in such a way as to control the FWER (Table 12.3). These trial designers are less willing to run the risk of the occurrence of a misleading finding of superiority of therapy B to therapy A in the therapy A versus B comparison, a decision that reduces the maximum acceptable type I error in this evaluation.

Table 12.3. Alpha allocation example with composite endpoint: Third design scenario.

Primary analyses	Cumulative comparitor group event rate	Efficacy	Alpha (two-tailed)	Power	Sample size
A versus control	0.080	0.20	0.020	0.95	16,449
B versus control	0.080	0.25	0.020	0.95	10,251
A versus B	0.064	0.20	0.010	0.95	23,590

The investigators now grapple with the notion of dependent statistical hypothesis testing. Recall from Chapter 5 that we could compute the test-specific α level α_2 for a second statistical hypothesis test, given the familywise error ξ, the test-specific α error rate for the first hypothesis test α_1, and the dependency parameter D using

$$\alpha_2 = \min\left[\alpha_1, \frac{\xi - \alpha_1}{(1-\alpha_1)(1-D^2)}\right].\tag{12.1}$$

Analogously, from Chapter 6, we could compute α_3, the test-specific α error rate for a third statistical hypothesis test as

$$\alpha_3 = \min\left[\alpha_2, \frac{1 - \dfrac{1-\xi}{[1-\alpha_1]\left[1-\alpha_2\left(1-D_{3|1,2}^2\right)\right]}}{1-D_{3|1,2}^2}\right],\tag{12.2}$$

where $D_{2|1}$ is the dependency measure between the first and second hypothesis test, and $D_{3|1,2}$ is the measure of dependency for the third statistical hypothesis test, given the occurrence of the first two. Recall also that a useful formulation for the dependence parameter D was

$$D = c\left[1 - (1-c)(1-h)\right],\tag{12.3}$$

where c is the estimate of coincidence, and h is the estimate of therapy homogeneity.[5] Therapy homogeneity in this circumstance is a measure of the degree to which the effect of therapy is known to be the same for each of the three hypothesis tests. One could understandably argue that since the mechanism of action of the drugs (i.e., the reduction in blood pressure) is believed to reduce mortality and morbidity by the same mechanism, there is substantial homogeneity of therapy effect, suggesting a larger value of h. However since the control group itself represents an active modality for reducing blood pressure, any effect of therapy A or therapy B on the primary endpoint of the study above and beyond that produced by the control group would be mediated by either (1) the unique manner by which each of the agents reduces blood pressure or (2) by some other mechanism separate and apart from blood pressure reduction. Thus an assumption about therapy effect homogeneity is tightly linked to the clinical hypothesis to be tested. After pondering these considerations, the investigators, choose to take the most conservative tack of assuming no homogeneity of effect, or $h = 0$. Thus, (12.3) reduces to

$$D = c^2.\tag{12.4}$$

Proceeding, in order to compute $D_{2|1}$, the investigators must know the degree to which the cohorts involved in each of the two hypothesis tests: (1) control therapy

---

[5] This formulation is also discussed in Chapter 5.

versus therapy A; and (2) control therapy versus therapy B overlap. Let n_c be the number of control group patients, n_A be the number of patients randomized to treatment A and n_B be the number of patients randomized to treatment B. Then we will estimate $c_{2|1}$ as $c_{2|1} = \dfrac{n_C}{n_C + n_A}$. Analogously, we can compute $c_{3|1,2}$ the measure of coincidence that appears in the formulation for $D_{3|1,2}$ as

$$c_{3|1,2} = \frac{n_A + n_B}{n_A + n_B + n_C} \tag{12.5}$$

For the moment, we will assume that an equal number of patient have been randomized to the three groups. Thus $c_{2|1} = 0.50$ and we can compute $D_{2|1} = c_{2|1}^2 = 0.25$. Analogously, from (12.5), $c_{3|1,2} = 0.667$ and $D_{3|1,2} = c_{3|1,2}^2 = 0.44$. In a further effort to embed conservatism into this evaluation, the investigators let $D_{2|1} = D_{3|1,2} = D_m = \min(D_{2|1}, D_{3|1,2}) = 0.25$. Recall from Chapter 6 that in this case

$$\alpha_3 = \min\left[\alpha_2, \frac{[1-\alpha_1][1-\alpha_2(1-D_m^2)] - [1-\xi]}{[1-\alpha_1][1-\alpha_2(1-D_m^2)][1-D_m^2]}\right]. \tag{12.6}$$

The results of (12.1) and (12.6) are embedded in the next sample size estimate (Table 12.4).

Table 12.4. Alpha allocation example with composite endpoint: Fourth design scenario.

Primary analyses	Cumulative comparitor group event rate	Efficacy	Alpha (two-tailed)	Power	Sample size
A versus control	0.080	0.20	0.020	0.95	16,449
		$D_m = 0.25$			
B versus control	0.080	0.25	0.020	0.95	10,251
A versus B	0.064	0.20	0.012	0.95	22,860

Finally, the trial designers reduce the power to the minimum required for the therapy A versus therapy B comparison.

Table 12.5. Alpha allocation example with composite endpoint: Fifth design scenario.

Primary analyses	Cumulative comparitor group event rate	Efficacy	Alpha (two-tailed)	Power	Sample size
A versus control	0.080	0.20	0.020	0.95	16,449
		$D_m = 0.25$			
B versus control	0.080	0.25	0.020	0.95	10,251
A versus B	0.064	0.20	0.012	0.80	14,875

The recruitment of 24,000 subjects (approximately 8,000 into each of the control group, therapy A group, and therapy B group) is sufficient to meet the requirements of the investigators in the theapy A versus control and the therapy A versus therapy B comparisons. Fewer patients are required for the therapy B versus control statistical hypothesis test.

A less conservative approach that the investigators could take would be for them to assume a nonzero value for the homogeneity of therapy effect. If the investigators assumed that the homogeneity of therapy effect variable $h = 0.50$, then they would calculate that $D_{2|1} = 0.50 \ [1 - (1 - 0.50)(1 - 0.50)] = 0.375$. Analogously, they would compute $D_{3|1} = 0.67 \ [1 - (1 - 0.50)(1 - 0.50)] = 0.502$, and $D_m = 0.375$, the minimum of these two quantities. Table 12.5 could then be recomputed from this alternative set of assumptions (Table 12.6).

Table 12.6. Alpha allocation example with composite endpoint: Alternative design scenario

Primary analyses	Cumulative comparitor group event rate	Efficacy	Alpha (two-tailed)	Power	Sample size
A versus control	0.080	0.20	0.020	0.95	16,449
		$D_m = 0.38$			
B versus control	0.080	0.25	0.020	0.95	10,251
A versus B	0.064	0.20	0.014	0.80	14,496

The effect of the assumption of a homogeneity effect has been to increase the prospectively set α error level for the therapy A versus therapy B comparison from 0.012 to 0.014, decreasing the required number of patients for therapy A versus therapy B. evaluation from 14,875 to 14,496.

12.4 Dose–Response Effects

Another important research consideration that investigators face in the design and analysis of clinical trials is the desire to obtain information concerning the relationship between the intervention dose (or intervention duration) and the effect of the therapy on the prospectively stated primary endpoint. This information can be used to support the argument that the randomly allocated therapy is causally related to the disease endpoint.[6] If the clinical trial is being presented within the context of an application to the FDA for consideration of product approval, the FDA may require that this dose–response information be obtained within a pivotal clinical study. This request is likely to occur if these regulatory officials believe that sufficient biologic gradient data is not available in earlier phase II studies. An example of a pivotal study which focused on measuring the relationship between dose of therapy and the response to therapy is the NitroDur trial [21] discussed in Chapter 4.

While data concerning the dose-response relationship between the randomly allocated intervention and the prospectively delineated endpoint in a clinical trial can be critical, this need generates a new difficulty for the study designers. We will demonstrate this difficulty by example. Assume that investigators design a clinical trial that consists of a placebo group and three intervention group arms. This trial has a single prospectively designed clinical endpoint—total mortality. Each of the three treatment groups in this clinical trial expose the patient to a different, randomly allocated dose of the intervention.

In this trial, the effect of therapy can be evaluated by comparing the results of each of the three treatment group arms to that of the placebo group. Each of these evaluations would assess whether that dose of the intervention substantially and significantly reduces the cumulative incidence of the total mortality rate when compared to placebo therapy. Within the regulatory setting, it is quite possible that these assessments would serve as the basis for an indication for the use of the intervention at the effective doses. These three evaluations would be followed by a comparison of each of the three active therapy arms to each other in a pairwise fashion. This latter set of evaluations is the analysis that examines the degree to which increasing doses of the medication produces a greater therapy effect.

The difficulty with this approach is the requirement of as many as six different statistical tests. Unfortunately, the burden of controlling the familywise error for these six evaluations while maintaining reasonable test-specific type I error rates can be overwhelming.

One approach that can reduce some of the statistical testing required in this setting is to replace the last three pairwise active therapy dose comparisons with a single analysis that evaluates the dose-response relationship. There are well-established statistical procedures that permit this evaluation—one such commonly accepted procedure is regression analysis. Regression analysis is an analytical tool that can be easily incorporated into our evaluation plan for multiple comparisons. The use of regression analysis would reduce the number of required hypothesis tests from six to four.

---

[6] The usefulness of establishing the dose–response relationship is discussed in Appendix A.

Consider the situation of investigators who wish to design a clinical trial that will evaluate the effect of five different doses of a medication when compared to placebo therapy. The purpose of this investigation is to demonstrate that the therapy produces a reduction in C reactive protein (CRP) levels. After it has been established that each patient has met the clinical trial's inclusion and exclusion criteria, patients will be randomly allocated to placebo therapy or one of the five doses of the active therapy, and followed for 6 months.

We can identify the doses of active therapy as T_1, T_2, T_3, T_4, T_5 and associate the treatment group assigned to a given dose by the dose itself (i.e., group T_1 is the group that was randomly assigned to active therapy dose T_1). In addition, we will identify that group of patients randomly assigned to receive placebo therapy as group P. In this circumstance, there are 15 possible statistical pairwisehypothesis tests that the investigators could actually carry out in this research effort, a number that precludes any realistic attempt to control the familywise error level in the process of producing confirmatory hypothesis tests all of them. The investigators therefore proceed by prospectively identifying a small number of hypothesis tests in which they have the greatest interest.

Recalling that the purpose of this experiment is to identify specific, active therapy doses that are effective in reducing the CRP concentration, the scientists first focus on two pairwise comparisons. The first is T_1 versus C. This comparison establishes whether the lowest dose of the medication produces a CRP concentration that is substantially and significantly different from that of the placebo group. If therapy T_1 is not effective, then a useful lower bound on the dose-response curve has been located. On the other hand, if T_1 does reduce the CRP concentration, then perhaps a nonhomeopathic starting dose for the compound has been identified.

The second pairwise comparison of interest is a comparison of the change in CRP level observed in those patients taking the greatest dose of therapy to placebo; T_5 versus C. One might reasonably anticipate that there will be more adverse events associated with this highest therapy dose—clear evidence of efficacy should be demonstrated in order to establish a risk–benefit balance that would justify this degree of exposure. On the other hand, the identification of no therapy benefit would provide an important new perspective about the overall effectiveness of therapy[7].

However as useful as these two evaluations are, they do not directly address the biologic gradient (dose–response) issue. The investigators therefore prospectively decide to carry out regression analysis to quantify the relationship between the dose of the medication and the CRP concentration. The independent variable of interest in this regression model is the dose of therapy, of which there are six (including the control group). The dependent variable is the change in CRP concentration (follow-up CRP concentration – baseline concentration).

---

[7] A circumstance in which a low dose of an agent would produce a benefit that is not seen with a higher dose of an agent is the use of insulin therapy in a patient with newly diagnosed type I diabetes. Clearly, low to moderate levels of insulin would reduce the likelihood of death by preventing diabetic ketoacidosis or nonketotic hyperosmolar coma, but higher doses of insulin would produce profound hypoglycemia and resultant death.

The investigators are therefore poised to carry out three confirmatory statistical hypothesis tests. The first two of these tests identify the effect of therapy at each of its lowest and highest dosages when compared to the control group[8]. The final hypothesis test formally evaluates the dose-response relationship between therapy dose and CRP level.

The investigators are now poised to assess the test-specific type I error levels for each of these confirmatory tests. As an initial evaluation, these investigators choose to allocate type I error for each of the three confirmatory statistical hypothesis tests they envision that they will carry out (Table 12.7). In this assessment, the investigators choose to allocate the majority of the type I error rate to the comparison of the effect of the lowest dose of the randomly allocated therapy to the control group. The smallest type I error level is allocated to the evaluation of the presence of a linear trend. However, the investigators can modify these initial α allocation rates in the design phase of the trial by considering the issue of statistical hypothesis test dependency.

Recall from Chapters 5 and 6 that we can reduce the test-specific α error rates for different hypothesis tests by taking into account the degree to which the occurrence of a type I error in one hypothesis test provides information about

Table 12.7. Alpha allocation with dose response focus:
First design scenario.

Primary analyses	Alpha (two-tailed)
T_1 versus C	0.030
T_5 versus C	0.015
Linear trend	0.005

the occurrence of a type I error for an additional statistical hypothesis test. These computations were based on the dependency parameter D, which itself was formulated from a consideration of the degree to which (1) the subjects and endpoints were the same in each of the hypothesis tests and (2) therapy homogeneity or the evidence that the medication would produce the same effect in each of the different analyses. Thus far in this chapter, that relationship has focused on the degree to which the same subjects have been used in each hypothesis test. However, in the current situation in which we are evaluating different doses of the same medication, it is appropriate to consider the impact of the homogeneity of therapy factor in the computation of the measure of dependency. This is because the same therapy is being evaluated against the same endpoint.

---

[8] Since they do not directly gauge the degree to which one active dose's effect is greater than that of another active dose, the two comparisons T_1 versus C and T_5 versus C do not in and of themselves provide direct evidence of a dose-response relationship.

We will first consider the measure of dependence between the statistical hypothesis tests T_1 versus C and T_5 versus C. Again, we will use the formulation

$$D = c[1 - (1 - c)(1 - h)] \tag{12.7}$$

from Chapter 5. The parameter c measures the degree of coincidence between the two hypothesis tests. We can estimate this by the % of observations in the T_1 versus C comparison that are also used in the T_5 versus C evaluation. Let n_c be the number of observations in the control group, and let n_i be the number of subjects randomized to the ith treatment group, $i = 1$ to 5. Then we will define $c = \dfrac{n_c}{n_c + n_1}$. If we assume for the moment that equal numbers of patients are recruited to each of the six arms of this study, then $c = 0.50$. Assume also that $h = 0.50$. Then, using (12.7) we find that $D = 0.50\,[1 - (1 - 0.50)(1 - 0.50)] = 0.375$. Incorporating this into Table 12.7 provides a revised estimate of the test-specific α error rate for the T_5 versus C. comparison (Table 12.8). The use of (12.1) reveals that $\alpha_2 = 0.024$. Thus, if the investigators were planning to carry out only two hypothesis tests, setting $\alpha_1 = 0.030$ and $\alpha_2 = 0.024$ would completely exhaust the FWER of 0.05, leaving no type I error level for the evaluation of the effect of therapy for the linear trend.

Table 12.8. Alpha allocation with dose response focus: Second design scenario.

Primary analyses	Alpha (two-tailed)
T_1 versus C	0.030
$D_m = 0.375$	
T_5 versus C	0.024
Linear trend	?

Thus, the clinical trial designers must make one more conservatory adjustment; they can either reduce the type I error for the T_1 versus C comparison, or they can reduce the α error rate for the T_5 versus C comparison. Recall that in the computation of these FWERs, the first hypothesis test for which a test-specific α error is chosen is the statistical test that has the maximum α error rate assigned. (i.e., $\alpha_1 \leq \alpha_2 \leq \alpha_3$)[9]. The investigators choose to reduce the type I error rate for the

---

[9] This does not imply that the statistical tests must be evaluated in any specific order at the end of the trial. They may evaluated in any sequence the investigators choose as long as the type I error rates have been prospectively assigned.

evaluation of the effect of T_5 versus C on the CRP concentration, thereby freeing up some of the type I error rate for the linear trend analysis (Table 12.9).

Table 12.9. Alpha allocation with dose response focus:
Third design scenario.

Primary analyses	Alpha (two-tailed)
T_1 versus C	0.030
$D_{2|1} = 0.375$	
T_5 versus C	0.020
Linear Trend	0.004

It now remains to attempt to conserve additional type I error for the linear trend analysis. We begin with a computation of the dependency parameter in this circumstance. The measure of coincidence c may be written as

$$c = \frac{n_C + n_1 + n_5}{n_C + n_1 + n_2 + n_3 + n_4 + n_5} = 0.50 . \qquad (12.8)$$

We will use an estimate of therapy homogeneity of 0.75. Then we may compute D as $D = 0.50\,[1 - (1 - 0.50)(1 - 0.75)] = 0.438 = D_{3|1,2}$. Inserting this value of the dependency parameter into (12.2) allows the investigators generate a new type I error level for the linear effect statistical evaluation (Table 12.10).

Table 12.10. Alpha allocation with dose response focus:
Fourth design scenario.

Primary analyses	Alpha (two-tailed)
T_1 versus C	0.030
$D_{2|1} = 0.375$	
T_5 versus C	0.020
$D_{3|1,2} = 0.475$	
Linear trend	0.005

However, additional conservation of the type I error rate can be achieved by the unequal apportionment of sample size. Since an important component of the calculation of the test-specific type I error rate is the dependency parameter, and the dependency parameter is a function of the number of patients allotted to the different therapy groups in the clinical trial, the group sizes can have an important effect on the type I error allocations through the dependency parameter.

There is also an additional motivation for the use of unequal sample sizes. The investigators' interest in the examination of the possibility of a linear trend between CRP levels and therapy dose will require them to carry out straight line regression. In this regression, the dependent variable will be the CRP levels and the independent variable will be the therapy dose. In this regression analysis, each patient contributes their CRP level and the therapy dose to which they were randomly assigned. The focus of the investigators' attention in this regression analysis is on the estimate of the slope of this line, since the magnitude of the slope is a direct reflection of the strength of association between the randomly allocated therapy dose and the change in CRP concentration. Thus, the investigators will require the most precise estimate of this slope available. This desire translates into designing this clinical trial so that the variance of the slope estimate is as small as possible. A standard result from regression analysis is that the estimate of the slope may be written as

$$\frac{\sigma^2}{\sum_{i=1}^{n}\left(x_i - \bar{x}\right)^2},$$

(12.9)

where the expression $\sum_{i=1}^{n}\left(x_i - \bar{x}\right)^2$ is the measure of the variability of the randomly assigned therapy doses in the entire trial. The task commonly facing statisticians is to minimize this type of variability. However, in this circumstance, the goal is not to minimize $\sum_{i=1}^{n}\left(x_i - \bar{x}\right)^2$ but to minimize (12.9) a task that requires maximizing the expression $\sum_{i=1}^{n}\left(x_i - \bar{x}\right)^2$. This quantity is maximized by choosing the randomized doses in the trial so that they are as widely separated as possible. Mathematically, the minimum value of the variance of the slope estimate is achieved by randomly allocating the therapy in this trial such that half of the patients receive the minimum dose (i.e., the control therapy) and the other half receive the maximum therapy (T_5). The investigators cannot go to this extreme, but they do choose to do a partial optimization by placing more patients on doses T_1 and T_5. For example, let 90% of the subjects be randomly assigned to either the control group, active group therapy dose T_1, or active dose therapy T_5, with the remaining number of patients allocated to therapy doses T_2, T_3, and T_4. Then, if $c = 0.90$, then one can compute $D = 0.90\,[1 - (1 - 0.90)(1 - 0.75)] = 0.878 = D_{3|1,2}$ Table 12.11).

Table 12.11. Alpha allocation with dose response focus:
Fifth design scenario.

Primary analyses	Alpha (two-tailed)
T_1 versus C	0.030
$D_{2\mid1} = 0.375$	
T_5 versus C	0.020
$D_{3\mid1,2} = 0.878$	
Linear trend	0.015

An alternative scenario would be along the following lines, in which the type I error rate was reduced for the T_5 versus C statistical hypothesis test (Table 12.12).

Table 12.12. Alpha with dose response focus:
Sixth design scenario.

Primary analyses	Alpha (two–tailed)
T_1 versus C	0.035
$D_{2\mid1} = 0.375$	
T_5 versus C	0.015
$D_{3\mid1,2} = 0.878$	
Linear trend	0.012

12.5 Conclusions

While the prospective design of multiple treatment group clinical trials has broadened the utility and efficiency of clinical trials, this expansion has come with the additional need to tightly control the FWER. To some extent the burden these α error concerns place upon investigators has stunted the development of these multiple treatment arm trials. Developments in the literature reveal the importance of bringing modern α error conservation tools to bear in the clinical trial with multiple treatment arms. The developments offered in the second half of this chapter have been an attempt to add to these procedures.

However, the importance of any of these statistical tools pales in comparison to the need for investigator knowledge, initiative, and imagination. It is unfortunately all to easy for the weight of fiscal and administrative restrictions to rain down on the scientist, washing away any spark of clinical design initiative with a cold shower of regulatory and financial reality. It is useful to keep in mind that the notion of a clinical trial, with the random allocation of patients to different therapy groups was itself considered a flight of undisciplined fancy 60 years ago. The imaginative scientist, treasuring her own ability to think anew, with vigor and innovation, will be fully able to adapt the tools reviewed and developed in this book to carry out the successful execution of a multiple armed clinical trial. Knowledge, ethics-based innovation, and a tight tether to reality remain the only requisites.

References

1. Dowdy, S., Wearden, S. (1991). *Statistics for Research. 2nd Ed*. New York, John Wiley.
2. Tukey, J.W. (1953). The problem of multiple comparsions. Department of Mathematics, Princeton University (manuscript).
3. Woolson, R.F. (1987). *Statistical Methods for the Analysis of Biomedical Data*. New York. John Wiley.
4. Dunnett, C.W. (1955). A multiple comparison procedure for comparing several treatments with a control. *Journal of the American Statistical Association*. **50**:1096–1121.
5. Dunnett, C.W. (1964). New tables for multiple comparisons with a control. *Biometrics* **20**:482–491.
6. Winer, B.J. (1971). *Statistical Principles in Experimental Design*. New York.McGraw Hill. pp.201–204.
7. Davis, B.R. Cutler, J.A., Gordon, D.J., Furberg, C.D., Wright, J.T., Cushman, W.C., Grimm, R.H., LaRosa, J., Whelton, P.K., Perry, H.M., Alderman, M.H., Ford, C.E., Oparil, S. Francis, C., Proschan, M., Pressel, S., Black, H.R., and Hawkins, C.M. for the ALLHAT Research Group (1996), Rationale and Design for the Antihypertensive and Lipid Lowering Treatment to Prevent Heart Attack Trial (ALLHAT). *American Journal of Hypertension* **9**:342–360.
8. Cheung, S.H., Holland, B. (1991). Extension of Dunnett's multiple comparison procedure to the case of several groups. *Biometrics* **47**:21–32
9. Ping-Yu, Dahlberg, S. (1995). Design and analysis of multiarm clinical trials with survival endpoints. *Controlled Clinical Trials* **16**:119–130.
10. Laska, E.M., Tang, K.I., Meisner, M.J. (1992). Testing hypotheses about an identified treatment when there are multiple endpoints **87**:825–831.
11. Berger, V. (2000). Pros and cons of permutation tests. *Statistics in Medicine*. **19**:1319–1328.

12   Berger, V.W., Lunneborg, C., Ernst, M.D., Levine, J.G. (2002). Parametric analyses in randomized clinical trials. *Journal of Modern Applied Statistical Methods* **1**:74–82.

13. Fung, K.Y., Tam, H. (1988). Robust confidence intervals for comparing seveal treatment groups to a control group. *Statistician* **37**:378–399.

14. Cheung, S.H., Chan, W.S. (1996). Simultaneous confidence intervals for pairwise multiple comparisons in a two-way unbalanced design.*Biometrics* **52**:463–472.

15. Thall, P.F., Simon, R., Ellenberg, S.S. (1989). A two-stage design for choosing among several experimental treatments and a control in clinical trials. *Biometrics.***45**:537–547.

16. Mukerjee, H., Robertson, T., Wright, F.T. (1987). Comparison of several treatment with a control using multiple contrasts *Journal of the American Statistical Association* **82**:902–910.

17. Williams, D.A. (1971). A test for differences between treamtnet measns when several dose levels are compared with a zero dose level. *Biometrics.***27**:103–117.

18. Ruberg, S.J. (1989). Contrasts for identifying the minimum effective dose. *Journal of the American Statistical Assocation* **84**: 816–822.

19. Tamhane A.C., Hochberg Y., Dunnett, C.W. (1996). Multiple test procedures for dose finding. *Biometrics* **52**:21–37.

20. Follmann, D.A., Proschan, M.A., Geller, N.L. (1994). Monitoring pairwise comparisons in multi-armed clinical trials. *Biometrics* **50**:325–336.

21. Pratt, C.M., Mahmarian, J.J., Borales-Ballejo, H., Casareto, R., Moyé, L.A. for the Transdermal Nitrogen Investigators Group (1998). Design of a randomized, placebo-controlled multicenter trial on the long-term effects of intermittent transdermal nitroglycerin on left ventricular remodeling after acute myocardial infarction. *American Journal of Cardiology* **81**:719–724.

Chapter 13
Combining Multiple Analyses

In this penultimate chapter, the tools that we have utilized and developed thus far will be combined into constructive arrangements. Specifically, we will show how the use of (1) differential α allocation, (2) combined endpoints, (3) prospective requirements of different levels of efficacy, and (4) confirmatory subgroup analyses can be prospectively blended into effective combinations that may be brought to bear in some unique and challenging clinical trial situations.

13.1 Introduction

In the study of multiple analysis issues in clinical trials, we have developed several different tools to control the familywise error level, while simultaneously allowing the investigator to carry out all of the analyses they wish to execute in their experiment. These tools work best when they are set upon the foundation of a comprehensive knowledge of (1) the disease process being studied and (2) an understanding of the potential benefits and adverse events associated with the intervention. The development of this pretrial compendium culminates in the prospective construction of the questions which the clinical trial will address.

However, the development of each of the multiple analyses implements in this text has been carried out in relative isolation. In these illustrative, but artificial, environments we have had the opportunity to observe the isolated effect of a particular multiple analysis device (e.g., the use of combined endpoint analysis) on the FWER of a clinical trial's analysis plan. However, as pointed out in Chapter 4, real clinical trial questions are multifaceted, requiring not just one tool, but a combination of multiple analysis instruments that permit the prospectively asked questions to be addressed. Therefore, the most effective use of these procedures is when we can wield them in innovative combinations.

Therefore, having completed the isolated development of our panoply of multiple analysis tools, we now focus on the combination of the use of these implements in interesting and rather unique clinical trial environments. No new mathematics will be required for, or will be developed in, this penultimate chapter, and there will be no in-depth analysis of the statistical calculations. Our focus will be on (1) developing the vision to recognize when a clinical trial designer is in a multiple analysis environment, or when a multiple analysis environment can be usefully created and (2) the application of the tools that we have developed thus far in informative combinations.

13.2 Creating a Multiple Analysis Environment

How could clinical trial designers not see when they are actually working within a multiple analysis environment? While this circumstance may be difficult to initially envision, the situation is an all-to-common occurrence. Specifically, nonrecognition takes place when investigators struggle to choose between two or more analyses under the false belief that they must settle on one and only one. Selecting one of these two analyses may be the common choice, but it can be inferior to incorporating both analyses.

Consider the following scenario: clinical investigators have developed a device that they believe will reduce the morbidity of patients who are in chronic atrial fibrillation (CAF). This intervention consists of destroying (a procedure described as ablation) the electrical pathways in the heart that are causing the aberrant cardiac rhythm. The ablation procedure requires a brief hospital stay, after which the patient is discharged to resume their normal activities. Patients with CAF will be admitted to this study and randomly allocated to receive the ablation therapy or standard therapy. All of the randomized patients will be followed for 1 year.

Since the death rate of patients with AF in this study is anticipated to be low, the investigators do not expect that there will be many patient deaths in the study. Consequently, these scientists do not anticipate that they will be in a position to measure the effect of the ablation therapy on the death rate. Physicians recognize that the major source of morbidity for these patients is their frequent need for hospitalization to control their arrhythmia. The investigators therefore settle upon two endpoints to measure the effect of the ablation therapy: (1) time to first hospitalization and (2) proportion of patients with more than four hospitalizations, defined here as AF burden.

The design of this clinical trial would appear to require no particularly inventive analytic approach, and the investigators begin with a brief outline of an analysis plan (Table 13.1).

Table 13.1. Preliminary design for ablation study.

Primary analyses	Cumulative control group experience	Efficacy	Alpha (two–tailed)	Power	Sample size
Time to hospitalization					
			D		
AF burden					

Table 13.1 is the shell of a design plan with which we have become comfortable in this text. The investigators would need to decide on the cumulative control group experience, the anticipated efficacy of therapy, the dependency parameter, the test-specific type I error rate, and the power of the study.

The new difficulty this study represents is that the ablation therapy is anticipated to increase the hospitalization rate in the initial postrandomization phase of the study for patients who undergo this procedure. This is because the ablation itself causes some initial, minor injury to cardiac tissue that increases the frequency of aberrant rhythms. This increase in dysrhythmic frequency produces an initially greater rate of hospitalization, and an increase in AF burden. The clinical trial designers expect that as this acute injury resolves, the episodes of chronic AF will decrease causing an amelioration of the hospitalization rate and the AF burden. Thus, they expect that this initial worsening of the patient's condition produced by ablation therapy will lead to a long-term improvement.

This post randomization, intervention-induced, short-term deterioration of the patient's condition will have an important impact on the magnitude of the effect of the ablation therapy in this study. If the investigators could ignore the initial, harmful, short term effect of the therapy (anticipated to be limited to the first two weeks of the study) they believe the resulting analysis would demonstrate the advantage of the therapy.

Recognition of this two-phase effect of the randomly allocated intervention produces important discussion concerning the analysis plan. A post hoc analysis that ignores the first two weeks of follow-up in determining the effect of ablation therapy would be an inferior strategy since the non-prospective nature of this type of evaluation generates untrustworthy estimators of effect sizes, standard errors, confidence intervals and p-values[1]. An a priori evaluation of the experience of patients that sets aside the patients' first 2 week experiences, while producing trustworthy estimators, would be appropriately criticized for ignoring events that many would argue should be included if the medical community is to gain a full and complete appreciation of the risks and benefits produced by the ablation therapy.

Rather than choose one and only one confirmatory analysis from these two alternatives, the investigators choose both. They decide to evaluate the effect of therapy for each of (1) the recurrence of hospitalization and (2) AF burden, and then plan to carry out two analyses on each endpoint. The first evaluation (described as the full analysis) examines the effect of therapy using the complete follow-up period, including the first 2 weeks after randomization. The investigators then prospectively plan a censored analysis, censoring (or removing from consideration) any hospitalization event that occurs in the first two weeks of the post randomization period (Table 13.2).

The investigators have identified four confirmatory analyses that they will execute at the conclusion of the ablation trial. Two of them evaluate the effect of ablation therapy on the cumulative hospitalization rate; the remaining two statistical hypothesis tests examine the role of this therapy in reducing the AF burden.

---

[1] The concept of untrustworthy estimators is discussed in Chapter 2.

Table 13.2. Preliminary design for ablation study.

Primary analyses	Cumulative control group experience	Efficacy	Alpha (two–tailed)	Power	Sample size
Evaluation of cumulative hospitalization rate			*0.035*		
Cum hosp rate: Full	0.500	0.25	0.025	0.90	769
			$D = 0.50$		
Cum hosp rate: Censored	0.450	0.30	0.014	0.90	714
			$D = 0.70$		
Evaluation of AF burden			*0.030*		
AF burden: Full	0.150	0.50	0.020	0.80	703
			$D = 0.80$		
AF burden: Censored	0.100	0.60	0.020	0.80	716

The role of dependency suffuses these four confirmatory evaluations. Since the same patients are involved in each of these two sets of analyses, and the endpoints are so closely related (in general, the greater the cumulative hospitalization rate, the greater the AF burden), high levels of dependency between the statistical hypothesis tests are justified. There is dependence between the evaluations of the effect of therapy on the cumulative hospitalization rate and the AF burden. There is also dependency within the two evaluations of the effect of therapy on the cumulative hospitalization rate and the AF burden analyses.

Note that the event rates and efficacies used in these analyses are a function of the analysis procedure (full or censored). In general, the censored analyses in this example involve lower event rates (since two weeks of follow-up are excluded). However, these same evaluations involve higher efficacy levels since the investigators anticipate greater effectiveness of the therapy when the first two weeks are excluded from evaluation.

In this circumstance, the investigators will be able to assess the effect of their therapy in its optimum period of effectiveness, while simultaneously addressing concerns of the medical and regulatory community about the difficulties imposed in the interpretation of the censored analysis. This is achieved by transforming the analysis issue from accepting only one hypothesis test as confirmatory into executing multiple confirmatory analyses while maintaining familywise type I error rate control.

It is easily anticipated that a regulatory agency would balk at giving multiple indications for an intervention when the confirmatory analyses are so tightly intertwined. However, it is important to note that the investigators and the clinical trial's sponsor are not interested in gaining multiple indications from the regulatory community for use of the ablation tool. The proposed analysis as it appears in Table

13.2 provides a full, prospectively designed evaluation of the intervention's efficacy in two relevant scenarios. Those who evaluate the results of the trial will have the opportunity to examine the effectiveness of the intervention using a metric that is less favorable to the therapy but more generally accepted (full analysis), while still being able to assess the therapy's effect in a less used but more favorable setting (censored analysis).

An alternative analysis has been presented [1].

13.3 Composite Endpoints Within Subgroups

A common justification for a clinical trial is to provide useful treatment guidelines that physicians may follow. While the investigators may be interested in a global effect of the randomly allocated intervention on the entire research cohort, there is particular interest in the response to therapy for patients who are in a predefined special subcohort.

A fine example of the need for this type of analysis is the evaluation of the role of cholesterol therapy in reducing the occurrence of atherosclerotic cardiovascular disease. In the mid-1990s, several studies demonstrated the impact of the HMG-CoA reductase inhibitors (commonly and colloquially known as the "statins") on both serum low-density lipid (LDL) cholesterol level reduction and the reduction in the occurrence of atherosclerotic cardiovascular disease. These studies, carried out in Scotland [2], Scandinavia [3], the United States [4], and Australia [5] all demonstrated the effectiveness of this new class of agents in reducing the incidence of clinical atherosclerotic disease. An important question that none of these studies was designed to address, however, was whether there was an important reduction in the incidence of clinical atherosclerotic disease in the patients whose baseline level of LDL cholesterol was the lowest. The answer to this question could have a direct impact on treatment guidelines for patients who may falsely believe that, because their risk of atherosclerotic disease is lower than that of patients with higher levels of LDL cholesterol levels, their risk is too low to require therapy.

Investigators interested in pursuing this avenue of research for their particular LDL cholesterol reducing agent then have two questions that they need to address. The first question is the overall effect of therapy in the entire recruited cohort of patients (global analysis). The second investigation requires an evaluation of the effect of therapy within that subcohort of patients whose LDL cholesterol levels are the lowest. This subcohort, prospectively defined and identified based on an examination of baseline variables constitutes a proper subgroup.[2]

The investigators recognize the importance of familywise type I error control, and see the difficulty in carrying out a confirmatory subgroup analysis, because of the relatively smaller number of patients that are available for the subgroup analysis. They will therefore use two prospectively defined endpoints for these evaluations. The first endpoint, which will be the measurement used to assess the global effect of therapy is fatal CAD consisting primarily of patients who have a fatal MI.

---

[2] As defined by Salim Yusuf and discussed in Chapter 9 of this text.

The endpoint for the subgroup evaluations will be related to, but different from, the endpoint for the primary analysis. The effect of therapy in the low LDL subgroup will be measured against the combined endpoint of fatal/nonfatal MI and fatal/nonfatal stroke. The greater cumulative incidence rate will permit a confirmatory analysis in this small subgroup.

Before they begin with the sample size, the investigators also choose to increase the required efficacy level for the evaluation of the effect of therapy for the subgroup analysis. This is because these patients in the subcohort of lower LDL levels are at lower risk of having an atherosclerotic event *ceteris parabus*. Exposing them to a new therapy places these relatively low-risk patients at a new risk for adverse events. The investigators believe that this risk can only be justified if the patients derive a greater efficacy from the compound. They therefore increase the efficacy for the lower LDL subgroup from 15% to 20% and complete their computation (Table 13.3). The event rate for the composite endpoint used in the lower LDL subgroup analysis is the reason that the event rate is greater than the event rate for the component endpoint that will be utilized for the global analysis. The power for each of the these two evaluations, although different from each other, is adequate.

Table 13.3. Design for cholesterol reduction trial.
Scenario 1

Primary analyses	Cumulative control group experience	Efficacy	Alpha (two–tailed)	Power	Sample size
Global analysis	0.120	0.15	0.035	0.90	13,988
		$D = 0.15$			
Low LDL subgroup	0.250	0.20	0.016	0.80	2941

The lower level of statistical hypothesis testing dependence implemented here is consistent with the arguments made in Chapter 11. Recall that the level of dependency is tightly linked to the degree of "overlap" between the statistical hypothesis tests under consideration. This overlap is measured by the proportion of the same patients that are used in each of the hypothesis tests, and the degree to which the endpoints used in the analyses measure the same pathophysiology. For the hypothesis tests in the current illustration, the proportion of patients used in the subcohort is a minority of patients that are evaluated in the entire cohort. In addition, the endpoint analysis variable for the global analysis is only one of four components of the combined endpoint. These observations along with the omnipresent need for conservatism in these considerations suggest that the level of dependency between the two statistical hypothesis tests should be low.

However, another methodologically acceptable design provides a different organization. If the investigators are required to keep the sample size for the low

LDL subcohort to less than 2500 patients, then the analysis design as detailed in Table 13.3 would not be acceptable. Alternative decisions about the type I error allocation provides a different collection of sample size computations (Table 13.4).

Table 13.4. Design for cholesterol reduction trial.
Scenario 2

Primary analyses	Cumulative control group experience	Efficacy	Alpha (two–tailed)	Power	Sample size
Low LDL subgroup	0.250	0.20	0.040	0.80	2331
		$D = 0.15$			
Global analysis	0.120	0.15	0.011	0.80	14,033

In this scenario, the test-specific type I error for the lower LDL subgroup has increased from 0.016 in Table 13.3 to 0.040, decreasing the required sample size for this subgroup from 2941 to 2331. However, the FWER ξ remains well controlled. This control is produced by decreasing the type I error level that will be used in the global analysis and thereby increasing its sample size. If patients in the lower LDL subgroup are truly difficult to recruit, then the scenario presented in Table 13.4 requires the investigators to recruit fewer of these hard to find patients and, consequently, more of the patients with higher LDL cholesterol levels. These latter patients require less work to recruit.

The differential efficacy assumption is a lingering concern for some scientists as they review these two designs outlined in Tables 13.3 and 13.4 for this clinical trial that evaluates the effect of therapy in reducing the occurrence of atherosclerotic disease. Unfortunately, but realistically, the utilization of greater efficacy has been commonly seen as a maneuver that sacrifices clinical reality for an achievable sample size. Viewed as a "back door" approach to reducing the required sample size of the analysis, it is a procedure that is commonly and understandably disparaged.

However, in this case, the requirement for increased therapy efficacy in the lower LDL subgroup is defensible. Assume that 1165 patients who are members of the lower LDL subgroup are recruited to each of the active group and the control group. If the event rate estimates in this trial are correct, then the investigators would expect 25% or 291 patients to have experienced the analysis endpoint in the control group. If the LDL cholesterol-reducing therapy produces a 20% reduction in the prospectively defined analysis endpoint, then 233 patients in the active group would experience the endpoint. The criticism that requiring 20% efficacy prevents the investigators from identifying lower, clinically significant levels of efficacy as statistically significant reductions is blunted by the observation that, if as many as 251 patients die in the active group, reducing the efficacy to 14%, the p-value for this evaluation would be 0.050, a level at the prospectively declared maximum type I error level for this analysis. This level of efficacy is greater than the 15% efficacy that the investigators hope to identify in the evaluation of the entire cohort in the global analysis. Thus the careful choice of an efficacy level for the effect of therapy in the lower LDL subgroup retains sensitivity to clinical significant efficacy levels while simultaneously being responsive to the requirement that patients who are at lesser risk of cardiovascular morbidity due to their lower LDL levels receive a greater benefit from therapy to offset the anticipated occurrence of adverse events.

13.4 Majority Subgroups in Clinical Trials

The previous example focused on the use of a confirmatory subgroup analyses when the subgroup of interest comprised a minority of the entire randomized cohort. However, multiple analysis procedures can be of importance when the subgroup of interest is the majority of the patients.

Consider the following example. In the wake of the concern expressed by the FDA about the execution of international clinical trials that must also provide evidence of benefit in the subcohort of randomized United States patients[3], a group of clinical trialists are interested in identifying the effect of therapy for patients who have CHF. They plan to recruit patients with NYHA class II/III heart failure and assign them to either the control group therapy or active group therapy. These patients will be followed for 2 years. There will be two prospectively declared endpoints for this study: (1) the cumulative total mortality rate and (2) the combined endpoint of cumulative total mortality plus + cumulative hospitalization rate.[4] In addition, the investigators require a set of confirmatory analyses for the effect of therapy in the United States population. There will therefore be four confirmatory evaluations in this study:

(1) The effect of therapy on the cumulative total mortality rate in all recruited patients, regardless of country (global cohort)
(2) The effect of therapy on the cumulative combined endpoint of total hospitalizations/total mortality event rate in the global cohort.
(3) The effect of therapy on the cumulative total mortality rate in only those patients recruited from the United States (United States cohort).
(4) The effect of therapy on the cumulative combined endpoint of total hospitalizations/total mortality rate in the United States cohort.

The investigators anticipate that, since the predominant regulatory need for their clinical trial is to meet the requirement of the US FDA, the majority of patients recruited for their study will be US patients. The trial designers are interested in demonstrating that therapy is effective for the reduction in the cumulative incidence of both prospectively declared endpoints. While they desire the same

---

[3] Reviewed in Chapter 10.
[4] As discussed in Chapter 7, the composite endpoint measures the first occurrence of either hospitalization or death. Thus, a patient who is hospitalized and subsequently dies is not counted as an endpoint twice.

demonstration in the global endpoint evaluation, the investigators' primary focus remains on the identified effect in US patients.

The investigators anticipate that the cumulative total mortality rate in the placebo group will be 15% in all patients regardless of country of randomization. A 25% cumulative rate for the combined endpoint of total hospitalizations and mortality is anticipated in the United States while the same endpoint is expected to occur at a lower rate in non US countries; the combination of these two rates will produce a global rate of 20%.

The dependency parameter will play a pivotal role in this research design. There are three dependency parameters that are required for this clinical trial's analysis. The first parameter, D_s, measures the dependency between the analysis carried out in the United States versus that executed in the entire global cohort. The second measure of dependency is the level of dependency between the analysis for the effect of therapy on total mortality and the effect of therapy on the combined cumulative incidence of total hospitalizations and total mortality. Focusing on the D_s first, recall from chapter 11 that we can write this parameter in terms of the co-incidence level c_s and the therapy homogeneity parameter h_s as

$$D_s = c_s \left[1 - (1 - c_s)(1 - h_s) \right]. \tag{13.1}$$

In chapter 11, we stated that h_s, which measures the degree to which the therapy will have the same effect in each of the research cohorts, must be selected with great care. If we choose $h_s = 1$, then we assume that the therapy's effect is the same in the US cohort as it is in the global cohort. However since the purpose of the evaluation of the effect of therapy in the subcohort is to provide a separate estimate of the effect in the US cohort, it would be a mistake to embed a presumed answer to this question within the dependence parameter. However, to choose a value of $h_s = 0$ is equally inappropriate. A reasonable choice in this circumstance is simply to let $h_s = c_s$. Thus, the homogeneity of therapy effect is governed by the degree to which the subcohort and the entire cohort contain the same patients. In this circumstance we demonstrated, in Chapter 11 that a reasonable approach to the computation of D_s is

$$D_s = c_s^2 \left[2 - c_s \right], \tag{13.2}$$

where c_s is the fraction of the overall cohort that is included in the subgroup stratum of interest. Since 85% of the entire cohort will be US patients, (13.2) reveals that $D_s = 0.75$.

The remaining two dependency parameters measure the degree to which the statistical test of the effect of therapy on the cumulative incidence of total mortality is related to the effect of therapy on the combined endpoint of total hospitalization/total mortality within each of (1) the US cohort and (2) the global cohort. We will proceed in a straightforward manner, first estimating this dependency parameter in the US cohort and then use the same procedure to estimate the required dependency for the analysis in all randomized patients. We again use

(13.1), rewritten here to reflect the fact that the difference between the analyses is not a difference in the analysis cohort (as in the previous paragraph) but a difference in the endpoints. This parameter we will call D_e, and write

$$D_e = c_e \left[1 - (1 - c_e)(1 - h_e) \right]. \tag{13.3}$$

In this circumstance, c_e is a measure of the degree to which the component endpoint total mortality occurs in the same patient. The coincidence between the occurrence of a death and the occurrence of the composite endpoint is high; the investigators estimate $c_e = 0.65$. However, homogeneity of therapy effect is believed to be very high ($h_e = 0.90$). Thus, the investigators compute

$$\begin{aligned} D_e &= c_e \left[1 - (1 - c_e)(1 - h_e) \right] \\ D_e &= 0.65 \left[1 - (1 - 0.65)(1 - 0.90) \right] = 0.65[1 - (0.35)(0.10)] \\ &= (0.65)(0.965) = 0.63. \end{aligned} \tag{13.4}$$

This estimate of D_e is applied to the global cohort evaluation as well. The investigators are now ready to complete the statistical component of the analysis plan of their trial (Table 13.5).

Table 13.5. Preliminary design for the international study.

Primary analyses	Cumulative control group experience	Efficacy	Alpha (two–tailed)	Power	Sample size
U.S. population			*0.045*		
Total mortality	0.150	0.20	0.030	0.90	6171
		$D_e = 0.63$			
Combined endpoint	0.250	0.25	0.026	0.90	2148
		$D_s = 0.75$			
Global population			*0.012*		
Total mortality	0.150	0.20	0.010	0.90	7708
		$D_e = 0.63$			
Combined endpoint	0.200	0.25	0.003	0.90	4097

The investigators control the familywise error level at 0.05, and allocate 0.045 to the analysis within the US cohort and 0.012 to the global analysis. The intra-cohort dependency parameter estimates D_e permit additional type I error rate conservation within the two research cohorts.

An additional level of conservatism can be introduced by estimating the dependency parameter D_m as the minimum of D_s and D_e (Table 13.6).

Table 13.6. Preliminary design for international study.
Conservative Analysis

Primary analyses	Cumulative control group experience	Efficacy	Alpha (two–tailed)	Power	Sample size
U.S. population			*0.04*		
Total mortality	0.150	0.20	0.030	0.90	6171
		$D_m = 0.63$			
Combined endpoint	0.250	0.25	0.017	0.90	2339
		$D_m = 0.63$			
Global population			*0.017*		
Total mortality	0.150	0.20	0.010	0.90	7708
		$D_m = 0.63$			
Combined endpoint	0.200	0.25	0.010	0.90	3422

Finally, adjustments in power reduce the difference in sample sizes required for each of the within-cohort analyses (Table 13.7).

Table 13.7. Preliminary design for the international study.
Conservative Analysis

Primary analyses	Cumulative control group experience	Efficacy	Alpha (two–tailed)	Power	Sample size
U.S. population			*0.04*		
Total mortality	0.150	0.20	0.030	0.80	4698
		$D_m = 0.63$			
Combined endpoint	0.250	0.25	0.017	0.99	3862
		$D_m = 0.63$			
Global population			*0.017*		
Total mortality	0.150	0.20	0.010	0.80	6050
		$D_m = 0.63$			
Combined endpoint	0.200	0.25	0.010	0.99	5527

13.5 Atherosclerotic Disease Trial Designs

In Chapter 3, we saw that efficiency was a prime motivator for the scientist to in-corporate multiple analyses within her clinical trial. The near prohibitive cost of clinical trials requires that as much information as possible be obtained from them to justify the trial's expense. Unfortunately, this drive for efficiency can lead to confusion concerning which of the many trial results are confirmatory and which are exploratory. Use of the procedures that we have described in this text can in-crease the confirmatory information that can be gained from a single trial without violating the tenets of good experimental methodology.

As an illustration, consider the following design of a cardiology clinical trial. The investigators are interested in assessing the effectiveness of a new class of anti-inflammatory agents in reducing the risk of atherosclerotic disease. The inves-tigators would like to learn if the use of this oral agent reduces the risk of atherosclerotic disease in the entire randomized cohort. However the investigators would like to delve deeper into the issue of risk modification. These clinical trial designers are interested in determining if the randomly allocated intervention will provide a benefit in patients who have different risks of developing atherosclerotic disease. They are not interested in whether the risk of disease modifies the effect of therapy;[5] instead. they simply want to know if the randomly allocated therapy effec-tively reduces atherosclerotic disease in low risk patients. Analogously, they seek the answer to the same question in patients who are at high risk of atherosclerotic disease. Finally, the trial designers are interested in evaluating the dose–response relationship that this randomly allocated therapy produces. The investigators envi-sion that there will be three treatment arms in this clinical trial: control group therapy, dose T_1 of the active intervention and dose T_2 of the active intervention where dose 1 < dose 2.

Thus, the investigators are interested in addressing three issues: (1) the overall effect of therapy in reducing future atherosclerotic disease, (2) the effect of therapy in each of a low risk and a high risk subcohort and (3) an assessment of the dose–response relationship of the effect of therapy and its impact on atherosclerotic disease. The investigators plan to recruit patients who are at risk of clinical morbid-ity and mortality from atherosclerotic disease, and randomly allocate them to one of three treatment arms: (1) placebo, (2) active intervention dose $T1$, or (3) active in-tervention dose T_2.

In order to carry out the analysis of the effect of the active intervention in patients who have different risks of future atherosclerosis, patients must undergo an assessment of this risk at baseline. Thus, while being screened for this study but be-fore they are recruited and assigned a randomly allocated therapy, each patient will have his or her risk of atherosclerotic disease assessed. Age, history of a prior MI or stroke in either the subject or the subject's parents will be obtained. The patient will be evaluated for the presence of hypertension, the presence of diabetes mellitus, and the presence of dyslipidemias. An assessment of the patient's lifestyle, specifically, their body weight, alcohol consumption, exercise pattern, and history of cigarette

---

[5] The evaluation of whether the patient's risk of a disease modifies the effect of therapy would be an interaction analysis. This approach is discussed in Chapter 11.

smoking will be obtained. The measurement of all of these factors will be used to gauge the patient's risk of future atherosclerotic disease, and patients will be categorized into one of three categories; low risk, moderate risk, and high risk. Only patients at low risk or patients at high risk of developing atherosclerotic disease will be recruited and randomized. The random allocation of therapy will be balanced within each of the low risk and high risk subcohorts. This last procedure will ensure that one-third of the patients get placebo therapy, one-third will receive dose 1, and one-third are randomized to dose 2 in each of the low-risk and high-risk subcohorts.

As the investigators work to incorporate these several analyses within a single clinical trial, they ponder whether they should use more than one endpoint in this analysis plan. The criteria that they must use for the choice of these endpoints begin with the requirement that the endpoints must be prospectively selected and they must each be an irrefutable measure of clinical atherosclerotic cardiovascular disease. Although many different analyses will be conducted as the experiment's conclusion, the confirmatory analyses that will specifically address the prospectively asked questions will concentrate on the findings on these prospectively identified endpoints. The investigators decide that the effect of therapy in the entire cohort will be based on the cumulative incidence of CAD death (primarily, fatal MI). The investigators anticipate that this endpoint will occur with a cumulative incidence rate of 12% in the placebo group over the course of the clinical trial.

The relatively low incidence rate of this endpoint makes it unsuitable for its use in the analysis of the effect of therapy in patients who are at either low risk or high risk of atherosclerotic disease. Although those at high risk of atherosclerotic disease would naturally be expected to have a greater rate of atherosclerotic morbidity and mortality (an observation of which these investigators will take full advantage as they design this clinical experiment), the relatively fewer number of patients available in this subcohort will vitiate any advantage the greater event rate will provide. Of course the circumstance is more extreme for patients who are in the low-risk subcohort. The combination of a relatively small number of patients and low event rates would make a confirmatory analysis with adequate statistical power even more difficult to execute in this low-risk subcohort.

Therefore, as a response to these subcohort analysis difficulties, the investigators prospectively declare the composite endpoint of fatal CAD death and nonfatal MI as the endpoint for which the effect of therapy in each of the low risk and high risk subcohorts will be assessed. Since the nonfatal MI component of this composite endpoint is itself a clear expression of atherosclerotic disease progression, the component endpoints of this combined endpoint are coherent, making the final composite endpoint interpretable.[6] Finally, the prospective declaration of this endpoint produces trustworthy estimators of effect size, their standard errors, confidence intervals, and p-values.

By choosing this combined endpoint, the investigators have substantially increased the logistical burden of the trial. The evaluation of the CAD endpoint required that the investigators review each death that occurred during the course of the trial and determine whether the death was a CAD death. For the evaluation of

---

[6] The principles that underlie the construction of a combined endpoint are discussed in Chapter 7.

the new nonfatal MI component, the scientists must (1) agree upon a definition of an MI and (2) examine the hospital records of all patients, in order to learn if an MI occurred. Since some MIs occur in the absence of symptoms, the investigators may decide to obtain annual electrocardiograms on all randomized patients. In this situation, the investigators would use electrocardiographic findings to supplement their clinical definition of an MI. The administrative, financial, and logistical difficulties imposed by the addition of the nonfatal MI component to the endpoint analysis represents one of the prices the investigators must pay to gain a confirmatory analysis within the two prospectively declared subcohorts of interest.

The evaluation, of the dose–response relationship requires what the investigators believe is a fairly subtle gradation of therapy effect magnitude. Not only will the subcohorts be relatively small, but the efficacy levels will also be low, a combination that increases the difficulty of executing an adequately powered confirmatory analysis. Therefore, these planned evaluations require an endpoint whose incidence rate is even greater than that of the composite endpoint of fatal CAD death + nonfatal MI. The investigators therefore prospectively create a second combined endpoint of fatal CAD death + nonfatal MI + fatal/nonfatal stroke. The fatal/nonfatal stroke component adds a new component of atherosclerotic disease to the endpoint, a component that will demand additional work to collect during the course of the trial. With full recognition of this complexity, the investigators then proceed with the analysis plan for the study (Table 13.8).

In this clinical trial which examines the effect of therapy on the occurrence of atherosclerotic cardiovascular disease, there are five statistical hypothesis tests. These five confirmatory hypothesis tests are divided into three classes that match the prospectively asked questions of the investigators: (1) the evaluation of the effect of therapy in the overall cohort, (2) the effect of therapy in each of the low risk and high risk subcohorts, and (3) the assessment of the dose–response relationship of the randomly allocated intervention. Type I error rates have been prospectively set for each of these classes of statistical hypothesis tests. For the effect of therapy in the overall cohort. the type I error rate is 0.025. The allocated type I error rate for the collection of hypothesis tests examining the effect of therapy for the low- and high-risk subcohorts is 0.020, the type I error rate for the dose–response evaluation is 0.008.

Table 13.8. Design for Cholesterol reduction trial: scenario 1.

Primary Analyses	Cumulative control group experience	Efficacy	Alpha (two–tailed)	Power	Sample size
Class 1					
Total cohort (CHD death)	0.120	0.15	0.025	0.90	17,398
		$D_1 = 0.25$			
Class 2					
subgroups		Available alpha	0.025		
Combined endpoint 1*		Allocated alpha	0.020		
Low risk	0.200	0.20	0.012	0.95	7362
		$D_s = 0.50$			
High risk	0.300	0.15	0.011	0.95	7948
		$D_2 = 0.30$			
Class 3					
Dose response		Available alpha	0.008		
Combined endpoint 2**		Allocated alpha	0.008		
Dose 2 versus dose 1	0.350	0.12	0.005	0.90	8351
		$D_{dr} = 0.50$			
Dose 1 versus placebo	0.350	0.12	0.004	0.90	8768

*CHD Death + nonfatal MI
**CHD death + nonfatal MI + nonfatal stroke.

The determination of the effect of therapy in the total cohort is straightforward. The endpoint for this analysis is CAD death, which is expected to occur with a cumulative mortality rate of 0.120. The investigators believe that they must demonstrate a 15% reduction in the incidence of this event in order to persuade the medical and regulatory community of the therapy's importance, and the power of this evaluation is to be 90%. The required sample size for this evaluation is 17,398 patients. The investigators anticipate that there will be some dependence between the effect of therapy in the overall cohort and the evaluation of the effect of therapy in the low risk and high risk subcohorts. However, this degree of dependency (signified by D_1 in Table 13.8) is very low for two reasons. First, the evaluation of the effect of therapy in the low- and high-risk subcohorts does not include all of the same patients as are included in the total cohort analysis. The second reason for the low level of dependency between the two statistical hypothesis tests is that the evaluation of the effect of therapy in the low-risk and high-risk subgroups uses a different endpoint (CAD death + nonfatal MI) than the CAD mortality endpoint used in the total cohort evaluation. As we saw in Chapter 11, the combination of these two influences serve as arguments to keep the level of dependency between the two classes of statistical hypothesis tests low.

The risk substrata assessments (Class 2 in Table 13.8) evaluate the effect of therapy in patients who are (1) at low risk and (2) at high risk of developing atherosclerotic disease. Specifically, the cumulative event rate of combined end-point 1 for low-risk patients on active therapy is compared to that endpoint's event rate for low-risk patients assigned to placebo therapy. The analogous comparison is made for patients who are classified as being at high-risk. There are two points that we need to make about the utilization of the CAD death + nonfatal MI combined endpoint to be used in risk substrata analyses. The first is that the event rate in each of the low-risk and high-risk subcohort evaluations is greater than the event rate used in the analysis of the effect of therapy in the total cohort evaluation. This is anticipated since the event rate of the composite endpoint is greater than that of the component endpoint used in the class I analysis. The second point is that, within the subgroup analyses, the anticipated endpoint incidence rate of high-risk patients as-signed to placebo therapy is greater than that of the low-risk, placebo-assigned patients. This is a natural consequence of the accurate assessment of the risk factors measured on each patient at baseline.

However, we must also note that the efficacy required of the low-risk pa-tients is greater than that designed into the evaluation of the effect of therapy in the high-risk patients. The occurrence of therapy-induced adverse events urged the in-vestigators to require greater efficacy from the randomly allocated therapy. This decision is an affirmative attempt by the investigators to confirm that they will not focus on the measurement of an efficacy level that is too low and therefore does not provide an adequate counterbalance to the occurrence of adverse events in these patients.

A higher level of dependency (D_s) is incorporated to reflect the depend-ency between the effect of therapy in the low-risk patients and the effect of therapy in the high-risk patients, primarily because the endpoint is the same between the two groups. Of the two evaluations, the evaluation of the effect of therapy for the low-risk group is assigned greater type I error than the effect of therapy within the high-risk substratum. Finally, power is high for each of the evaluations, increasing the likelihood that a finding of no therapy efficacy in either of the two evaluations in this concordantly executed trial accurately reflects the absence of efficacy in the population.

The difference between the endpoints that are used for (1) the evaluation of the effect of therapy in the subgroup evaluations and (2) the dose response as-sessments (which constitute the third class of confirmatory analyses in this clinical trial) require us to keep the measure of dependency $(D_2 = 0.30)$ low. Within class 3, there are two confirmatory statistical hypotheses that the investigators will carry out. The first is an evaluation of the ability of dose 2 to reduce the rate of athero-sclerotic morbidity and mortality above and beyond the effect of the lower dose 1. The second hypothesis test compares the effect of dose 1 to placebo. The antici-pated efficacies produced from these two hypothesis tests is realistically low; 12% for each test. As pointed out earlier, the investigators prospectively chose the com-bined endpoint of CAD death + nonfatal MI + nonfatal stroke for the dose-response determinations since they require an endpoint whose relatively frequent occurrence offsets the combination of lower levels of efficacy and type I error rates.

In this illustration, the combination of multiple analysis procedures per-mits five confirmatory analyses for the effect of randomly allocated intervention in this trial. If this trial is executed concordantly, then a finding that the study is positive for any of these five analyses permits the investigators to claim that the study is positive. Adequate statistical power is preserved for each of these analysis procedures, permitting the investigators to affirm that hypothesis tests that do not lead to null hypothesis rejection represent strong evidence for the absence of efficacy (as opposed to the finding that the result is merely uninformative, a conclusion that would be forced upon the investigators if the analyses were underpowered.) The low-efficacy levels and type I error rates that are required for the evaluations of the dose–response relationships in this study are offset by the greater frequency of the event rate of the composite endpoint for that analysis, resulting in sample sizes that are achievable.

However, the penetrating ability of this clinical trial design to simultaneously provide confirmatory answers (as opposed to speculative hypothesis generation) to multiple prospectively identified questions comes at a cost. The investigators are required to identify not just all patients who report a CAD death, but those patients that have had an MI or a stroke. The burden of accurately classifying all patients with regard to these morbidity measures certainly and, perhaps profoundly, increases the cost and difficulty of executing this study. At the conclusion of the study's design, when the benefits and costs of carrying out the trial are weighed, the investigators will have to determine for themselves whether enough scientific fruit will be produced from the research tree that requires so much attention and care.

13.6 Multiple Treatment Groups Revisited

In Chapter 11, we focused on the use of multiple analysis procedures in the circumstance of multiple treatment group clinical trials. The following is one final example of the use of these procedures in an innovative and unusual setting.

Recent work has focused on the ability to improve upon the current state of the art for the management of CHF. This has involved the evaluation of the use of angiotensin receptor blockers (ARB) in addition and in replacement of ACE-i therapy. Clinical investigators are interested in the evaluation of the benefits of the combined use of an ARB and an ACE-i in reducing mortality from CHF. They are also interested in identifying any additional advantage that an ARB offers above and beyond that of ACE-i therapy. The prospectively declared primary endpoint for this study is the cumulative total mortality rate. There are to be three treatment groups in this clinical trial; (1) established therapy + ACE-I (ACE-i only), (2) established therapy plus an ARB (ARB only) (3) established therapy + ACE-I + ARB (ACE-i/ARB).

The investigators recognize that the use of ACE-i is the established therapy for heart failure. One way this may be improved is to add ARB therapy to ACE-i therapy. An alternative would be to replace the ACE-i therapy with an ARB. However, since ARB therapy is already approved therapy for CHF, it is possible that the addition of ACE-i therapy may lead to an additional improvement in these patients' survival. These three questions may be stated as follows:

Question 1: Does the reduction in the total mortality rate observed in the ACE-
            i/ARB treatment group exceed that produced by either ACE-i alone or
            ARB alone?
Question 2: Does the use of an ARB in any form (i.e., as a replacement for, or
            combined with captopril) confer a survival advantage over that af-
            forded by captopril?)
Question 3: Does the mortality effect of the ARB exceed that of the ACE-i?

An example of such an analysis plan would require that the type I error rate be
prospectively allocated for each of the three analyses, and that each of these
analyses should be adequately powered. The evaluation of Question 1 requires a
comparison of the joint ACE-i/ARB group to the mortality effect that is observed in
the ACE-i alone and ARB alone group when these latter two groups are combined.
The answer to Question 2 requires a comparison of the combined effect of ACE-
i/ARB and the ARB alone group to the mortality experience of the ACE-i therapy
group. Finally, the investigators wish to compare the mortality experience of the
ARB group alone to the ACE-i group. Of course many other evaluations will be
executed using a variety of combinations of treatment group comparisons and
secondary endpoints. However the focus of the clinical trial is to identify
confirmatory conclusions to Questions 1 through 3 (Table 13.9).

Table 13.9. Design for angiotensin receptor blocker trial.

Primary analyses	Cumulative control group experience	Efficacy	Alpha (two–tailed)	Power	Sample size
		Familywise error rate = 0.05			
Analysis 1		Available alpha	0.300		
Q1: Combined vs. individual use	0.210	0.15	0.030	0.95	10,526
Total cohort					
		$D_1 = 0.44$			
Analysis 2		Available alpha	*0.026*		
Q2: Any use of ARB versus ACE-i		Allocated alpha	0.025		
Total cohort	0.210	0.15	0.020	0.95	11,406
		$D_1 = 0.44$			
Analysis 3		Available alpha	*0.006*		
Q3: Ind ARB vs. ind ACE-i		Allocated alpha	0.006		
ARB group and ACE-i group	0.210	0.15	0.006	0.95	12,155

    Patients will be followed for 3 years in this study. The investigators antici-
pate that the 3-year total mortality rate for patients in this trial will be 21%. The
investigators choose an efficacy level of 15%. However, a different efficacy level
selection will be made for Question 3. In this case, the investigators desire to demonstrate that the effect of the ARB will be essentially equivalent to that of the ACE-

i therapy. They therefore need to design this analysis so that the non-rejection of the null hypothesis is tantamount to equivalence of the two groups.

Table 13.9 provides the plan for the execution of three confirmatory analyses. The total sample size for this trial would be approximately 18,000, since Analysis 3 requires 12,155 patients, 6078 in each of the ARB-alone and ACE-i (alone) groups, and an additional 6078 patients would be recruited to the treatment group that is jointly exposed to the ARB and ACE-i. Analysis 1 will compare the total mortality rate for the joint therapy to the combined effect seen in the group exposed to ARB alone, and the group exposed to the ACE-i alone. A type I error of 0.03 is allocated for this evaluation. The dependency measure, D_1, reflects the observation, that since the sample patients are used in analysis 2 as were used in analysis 1, there is some overlap in the type I error between the two tests. Using the dependence argument that we developed in Chapters 5 and 6, the available type I error level is 0.026 for the remaining two analysis Of this 0.026 type I error level selected, 0.025 is chosen as the type I error rate for the second evaluation. However, the continued dependence between the third analysis and the first two analysis produces additional type I error conservation, leaving 0.006 type I error available for the third analysis. Note that these are not hierarchal analyses. They do not have to be carried out in any specific order. Also, because the type I error was allocated prospectively and the familywise type I error rate was controlled, these are each confirmatory analyses. Thus, the study is positive if any of the three analyses are positive.

An alternative analysis plan permits an expanded evaluation in Analysis I (Table 13.10).

Table 13.10. Design for angiotensin receptor blocker trial.

Primary analyses	Cumulative control group experience	Efficacy	Alpha (two–tailed)	Power	Sample size
Analysis 1		Familywise error rate = 0.05			
Q1: Combined vs. individual use		Allocated alpha	0.030		
Analysis 1A: Combined versus ARB	0.210	0.15	0.017	0.95	11,756
		$D_1 = 0.44$			
Analysis 1B: Combined versus ACE-i	0.210	0.15	0.016	0.95	11,833
		$D_1 = 0.44$			
Analysis 2		Available alpha	0.030		
Q2: Any use of ARB versus ACE-i		Allocated alpha	0.025		
Total cohort	0.210	0.15	0.020	0.95	11,406
		$D_1 = 0.44$			
Analysis 3		Available alpha	0.006		
Q3: Ind ARB versus. Ind ACE-i		Allocated alpha	0.006		
ARB group and ACE-i group	0.210	0.15	0.006	0.95	12,155

In this setting, the evaluations of Analysis 1, which had comprised a single evaluation, now require two evaluations. This leads to four confirmatory statistical hypothesis tests. These tests will each have maximum type I error rates of 0.017, 0.016, 0.020, and 0.006 respectively. Even though the sum of these error rates is greater than 0.05 (the sum is equal to 0.059), the FWER is conserved at 0.05 because of the overlap in the type I error events between these dependent statistical hypotheses. The sample size of the study has increased slightly to between 5500 and 6000 subjects for each of the three treatment groups.

References

1. Berger, V.W. (2002). Improving the information content of categorical clinical trial endpoints. *Controlled Clinical Trials* **23**:402–514.
2. Shepherd, J., Cobbe, S.M., Ford, I., et. al (1995). Prevention of CAD with pravastatin in men with hypercholesterolemia. *New England Journal of Medicine* **333**:1301–1307.
3. Scandinavian Simvastatin Survival Study Group (1994). Randomized trial of cholesterol lowering in 4444 patients with CAD: the Scandinavian Simvastatin Survival Study (4S) *Lancet* **344**:1383–9.
4. Sacks, F.M., Pfeffer, M.A., Moyé, L.A., Rouleau. J.L., Rutherford, J.D., Cole, T.G., Brown, L., Warnica, J.W., Arnold, J.M.O., Wun, C.C., Davis, B.R., Braunwald. E. (1996). The effect of pravastatin on coronary events after myocardial infarction in patients with average cholesterol levels *New England Journal of Medicine* **335**:1001–1009.
5. Long–Term Intervention with Pravastatin in Ischaemic Disease (LIPID) Study Group (1998). Prevention of cardiovascular events and death with pravastatin in patients with CAD and a broad range of initial cholesterol levels *New England Journal of Medicine* **339**:1349–1357.

Chapter 14
Conclusions: The Two-Front War

By describing useful research strategies in a fairly nonmathematical environment, it has been our goal to deepen the discernment and comprehension of physicians who are involved in clinical trials. We are cautiously optimistic that you as a clinical trialist now understand the nature of the multiple analysis issue and are empowered to successfully create the research design and analysis environment necessary to address the complicated problem of multiple analyses. Just as knowledge produces self-control and perseverance, it is our hope that superior understanding will rejuvenate intellectual discipline and consequently produce enhanced study designs.

When designing a clinical trial, we as investigators commonly feel that we are fighting (or are caught in the middle of) a two-front war. On the one side is the requirement that the research effort should be productive, bearing a rich bounty of valuable results. In order to comply with the expectation that the investigator's clinical trial should produce a satisfactory "return on investment," the investigator genuinely desires to collect all of the information that is available and that can be collected on every patient in their research cohort. The natural tendency to use the clinical trial's dataset to the fullest spawns many statistical hypothesis tests.

We have also seen that epidemiologic timber can be added to fuel the fire that is driving the multiple testing engine. There are fundamentally sound motivations for the inclusion of dose–response analyses, the assessment of the effect of therapy on different but related endpoints, and the evaluations of possible therapy action mechanisms. Investigators who, after all, are in the business of research because of their natural, intensely felt desire to learn, want to supply good answers to these good questions.

14.1 Compromise and Sampling Error

However, this drive to carry out expansive, inquisitive analyses is blocked by statistical concerns that make up the second front in the battle for the heart and mind of the investigator. The statistical concerns arise because we as investigators make a definite, though not formally recognized, compromise when we carry out research. We desire to study an entire population of patients in complete detail. For example, in a clinical trial studying a new heart failure therapy, we may wish to recruit all heart failure patients. However, logistical, financial, and ethical concerns preclude this effort. We therefore choose not to study the entire population of patients, but instead take a small sample from the large population. The process of drawing a sample helps on the one hand, but hurts on the other. The sample's availability offers the ability to carry out an executable research program on a relatively small number of subjects; however, the same process hurts by stealing from us the notion that we as investigators can identify population effects with certainty. The same population can produce different samples, and since these samples contain different patients with different experiences, each sample's results are different. Which sample is right? Sometimes the population produces, through the play of chance and the random aggregation of events, a sample that does not accurately reflect the therapy–outcome relationship of the population, even though the sample was selected randomly.

We do not directly identify or measure this sampling error when we are examining a randomized participant, or entering that patient's laboratoty results into a database, or computing a sample relative risk; we observe only the data. However, sampling error, like gravity, goes unseen but has powerful effects. The central contribution of statistics to health research in general, and to controlled clinical trials in particular, is its guidance on research result interpretation in the presence of sampling error. The successful application of statistics within clinical trials does not remove sampling error; sampling error is instead appropriately channeled into estimates of effect size, standard errors, confidence intervals, p-values, and power. However, this sampling error segregation is only successful when the underlying assumptions on which these estimators are built have been satisfied [1].

One of these critical assumptions is that the experiment must be executed concordantly (i.e., in accordance with its prospectively written protocol). The estimators are reliable only if they are produced within a research environment in which the only source of variability is the sample-to-sample variability of the endpoint data. This assumption is violated when the clinical trial's data choose the analysis plan, e.g., when there are mid-trial endpoint changes in response to a surprise finding in the growing dataset, or in the case of data dredging. In these cases, the sample doesn't just provide data for the endpoint, but exceeds this contribution by actually selecting the endpoint (e.g., choosing the only endpoint with a small p-value). In this circumstance, our commonly used estimators are no longer valid; they have become newly distorted by this additional source of endpoint selection variability. If we give too much credence to what these disoriented estimators tell us, then we as investigators will lose our way [2].

The issue raised by multiple testing is one of propagation of type I error. Since there is a chance that a false answer is provided by the sample to the question the investigator has asked, the likelihood that at least one false answer is produced by our sample increases with the number of questions we ask, just as the probability of obtaining at least one head in a sequence of tosses of a coin grows as we continue to flip the coin. This error is critical in assessing the impact of an intervention that we study in a clinical trial on the population from which the clinical trial's patients were obtained. Since the intervention will produce adverse events and most likely will have a financial cost associated with it, there must be some benefit that the intervention offers that will offset these disadvantages. The FWER, ξ is the likelihood of making at least one type I error among all of the hypothesis tests that the investigators carry out. ξ conveys to the investigators the likelihood that the therapy will not be effective in the population, i.e., that treated patients in that population will experience the adverse events of the medication, and pay the financial cost of the therapy, but not retain its benefits. The FWER must be accurately measured and tightly controlled to ensure that its level is kept to a minimum.

Thus, investigators may seem to be in an intolerable position. As they design their clinical trial, these scientists are quite naturally motivated to answer all of the relevant issues that their dataset can address. However, they are simultaneously tightly bound by the compelling statistical arguments to abstain from this desire. Thirsting for answers to their scientific question, they may feel like the parched man who, when at last he comes upon the fresh mountain river, responds with amazement when he is given only a tiny cup to collect the water that he requires. What water is caught in the small statistical thimble, while refreshing, does not completely satisfy, and he watches in amazement and disappointment as the rest of the (data) stream flows by unused.

14.2 The Handcuffs

Investigators often feel as though the statistical concerns that are contained in the careful design of their clinical trial "puts the handcuffs" on them. My goal has been to demonstrate the wealth of design tools that are available to the trialists, providing some of the keys to release (or at least loosen) their shackles. A first principle in this process is that no team of investigators should be denied or discouraged from analyzing any component of the dataset that they desire. The unique combination of inquisitiveness, insight, and intuition that investigators possess should be encouraged, not repressed. However, it is best if these analysis plans are triaged so that the interpretation of the results are clear. There are two levels of triage: (1) planning, and (2) error control.

Is the analysis to be prospectively planned or data driven? The major advantages of prospectively planned analyses are that the estimates of effect size, confidence intervals, standard errors are trustworthy. Data-driven analyses are commonly carried out and are frequently useful, and these exploratory analyses are commonly our first data based view of future research paths. However, because the promulgated analyses are essentially chosen by the data (i.e., the investigator was not obligated to report the result of the analysis, but chose to report it because of the magnitude and direction of the finding) that is itself contaminated with sampling error, the results of such analyses can be misleading. Nonprospectively planned, exploratory results should be carried out and reported, but they must be clearly labeled as exploratory. They require confirmation before they can be integrated into the fund of knowledge of the medical community.

The second level of triage during the design phase of the clinical trial is carried out among the prospectively planned analyses, dividing them into primary analyses or secondary analyses. Primary analyses are those analyses on which the conclusions of the trial rest. Each of the primary analyses will have a prospectively set type I error level attached to it in such a way that the familywise error does not exceed the community accepted level (traditionally 0.05). The trial will be seen as positive, null (no finding of benefit or harm), and negative (harmful result) based on the results of the primary analyses. It is critical to note that a clinical trial can have more than one primary endpoint. If appropriately designed, the study can be judged as positive, if any of those primary endpoints produces a p-value less than the test-specific α level for that hypothesis test.

Secondary endpoints do not control the familywise error, and each secondary analysis is typically interpreted at nominal 0.05 levels. Secondary analyses, being prospectively designed, produce trustworthy estimates of effect sizes and p-values. However, because secondary analyses do not control the familywise error, the risk to the population is too great for confirmatory conclusions to be based upon them. The role of secondary endpoints is to provide support for the primary endpoint findings, and not to serve as independent, confirmatory analyses. In the typical clinical trial, there are more exploratory analyses than there are prospectively declared endpoints, and more secondary endpoints than there are primary endpoints (Figure (14.1) This is consistent with the statement that a small number of key questions should be addressed, accompanied by careful deliberation on the necessity and extent of adjustment for multiple comparisons [3].

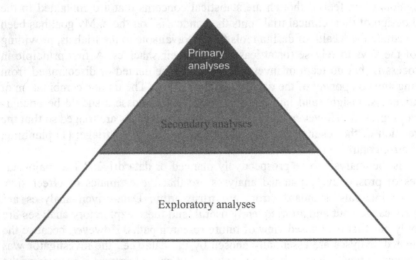

Figure 14.1. The role and relative number of analyses in a clinical trial.

Some would have us believe that innovative designs should permit analysis tools, such as data mining or exploratory findings to be accepted as confirmatory. The foundation on which this book rests is that innovative designs are readily available when we stay tightly tethered to the principles of experimental design that have been in place for over two hundred years. The purpose of this text has not been to show investigators how to do statistical analyses—you as an investigator will in all likelihood not be doing your own analyses. The purpose has been to demonstrate how confirmatory analyses that address the question at hand may be obtained. The first and most fundamental component for this is clinical knowledge and research discipline. Statistical methodology cannot make up for critical shortages in these two areas.

Several tools are available to the investigator as they allocate type I error rates among the primary analyses of their clinical trial. Among the first is the unequal allocation of type I error levels. The Bonferroni procedure provides equal allocation of the α error among the several primary analyses. This typically produces type I error levels that are too small for some of the analyses, in turn generating a sample size that is beyond the attainable. Investigators can allocate type I error selectively among the different primary analyses. The only rules that they are obligated to follow are that the allocation be made prospectively and that the type I error levels be made to conserve the familywise error level ξ.

We have also explored the notion of hypothesis test dependency for the conservation of the type I error between the different primary analyses. The review of available procedures and the development of a new procedure in this text gives the investigator the opportunity to more efficiently allocate type I error levels among the K primary analyses which may be related to each other. Whichever tool the investigator uses, it must be prospectively designed and conservatively implemented.

A formal examination of the use of combined endpoints reveals that these complicated implements are most effective when they (1) are clinically relevant, (2) are prospectively deployed, (3) are cohesive (i.e., the combined endpoint components measure related but distinct aspects of the same disease process, (4) are each ascertained precisely and with superior quality, and (5) are each reported. The notion of dependence between statistical hypothesis tests was especially useful here.

The application of these tools in turn demonstrated the utility of an alternative use of subgroup analyses. With the recognition that there are circumstances in which subgroup evaluations in controlled clinical trials need not be the evaluation of interactive effects, we found that the implements of (1) differential α allocation, and (2) the utility of combined endpoints were especially useful for the determination of whether a significant effect of therapy resided within a particular subcohort of interest. In this development, we engaged in a detailed evaluation of the role of efficacy of therapy in a clinical trial. The differential determination of efficacy is yet one more tool that the investigator can wield as she forges the design of her study.

It would be particularly useful to the disciplined investigator if the medical and regulatory community would revisit the notion of keeping the upper bound of the familywise error level at 0.05. All of the examples that we have explored in this book have been designed on the bedrock of the 0.05 boundary. However, as we saw in the Prologue, this "bedrock" is merely the loose stones of tradition. The 0.05 familywise error level is inadequate to the task of producing a realistic cap on the error of making at least one mistake due to sampling error. If investigators are willing to (1) triage their endpoints prospectively and (2) prospectively assign type I error to the primary analyses such that each test-specific α error is no greater than 0.05, then a prospectively computed familywise error level greater than 0.05 (e.g., 0.075 or 0.10) should be permissible. I have argued for this in the peer-reviewed literature [4], but have yet to discern any community movement to this idea.

Finally, we must remember that clinical trial standards are not static but instead represent a fluid evolution of research principles and execution. An examination of the clinical literature reveals that 200 years ago healthcare research was primarily, if not exclusively, case reports. This progressed to the appearance of the results of case series. The idea of a clinical trial with the use of randomization and a contemporaneous control group is relatively new, appearing only sixty years ago. During this process, mistakes have been made. A fair criticism of clinical trial methodology has been an over reliance on *p*-values. Unfortunately, confusion between confirmatory and exploratory analyses still reigns. Pocock [5] has correctly pointed out that concerns for multiplicity of type I error should be balanced. While we have not reached out destination, the development and maintenance of research discipline helps to ensure that we stay on the right path.

References

1. Moyé, L.A. (2000) *Statistical Reasoning in Medicine: The Intuitive P-value Primer*. Spinger– Verlag..
2. Moyé, L.A. (2001) Random Research. *Circulation*.**103**:3150–3.
3. Proschan, M.A, Waclawiw, M.A. (2000). Practical guidelines for multiplicity adjustment in clinical trials. *Controlled Clinical Trials*.**21**:527–539.
4. Moyé, L.A. (2000). A Calculus in Clinical Trials:Considerations and Commentary for the New Millenium. *Statististics in Medicine*.**19**:767–779.
5 . Pocock, S.J.. (1997). Clinical Trials with multiple outcomes: a statistical perspective on their design, analysis, and interpretation. *Controlled Clinical Trials* **18**;530–545.

Appendix A
Case Reports and Causality

A case report is simply a summary of the findings of an exposure–disease combination in a single patient and the communication of those findings to the medical community. Many times that communication contains insufficient information. In other circumstances, the data from this report can be voluminous and complex. This material can consist of a complete medical history comprising all symptoms and signs the patient had experienced, in addition to information both about the patient's treatment and their ultimate disposition. A case series is a collection of case reports, linked together by a common thread (e.g., all of the patients were seen by the same doctor, or all patients were exposed to the same agent e.g., diet drugs).

Case reports are somewhat paradoxical at the current stage of medical research and practice. Although the findings from case reports are commonly criticized by researchers, who utilize sophisticated mathematics and design methodology to examine exposure–disease relationships, carefully compiled case reports provide necessary observations from which clinicians and public health workers learn. Case reports remain the first data-based view of either a new disease or a potential cure for an established disease. Despite substantial criticism, it is undeniable that case reports and case series are among the most time-tested, and useful tools epidemiologists have at their disposal to alert clinicians and the public to a possible health problem.

For over 2000 years, the growth of medical knowledge has been fueled by the use and dissemination of case reports. Like fire, when used constructively, case reports are the fuel which has historically propelled medical progress. It is a device used first not by epidemiologists but by clinicians. This is not difficult to understand. Medical practice at its heart has been a single concerned individual struggling to decide what was best for his patient. This was an immensely solitary, burdensome experience, requiring wrenching decisions about an individual's care from an individual with incomplete knowledge. Often, regardless of the action the physician took their patient died. The one natural tool physicians had to distribute and thereby reduce the weight of the decision process was to share their experiences with one another. This shared experience is at the heart of the case report. A physician read (or listened to) the description of a patient with a particular combination of symptoms and signs from another physician, and learned that physician's interpretation of these findings and treatment of this patient. The physician then integrated this new external experience into his own fund of knowledge.

A good case report is based on careful observation. From the earliest of times, the evolution of clinical medicine and epidemiology was based on careful observation. The heart of this approach is best captured by Celsus (circa A.D. 25) who stated that "Careful men noted what generally answered the better, and then began the same for their patients" [1].

From that time on, and for the next 1800 years, through the Middle Ages, the Renaissance, the Industrial Revolution, and the Age of Discovery and Enlightenment, advances in clinical medicine occurred through the careful principle of observation and recording embodied in the case reporting systems. The discovery that gunshot wounds could be healed without the application of burning hot oil [2] demonstrated that case reports can uncover new information and overturn prior erroneous principles in medicine.

It wasn't until the nineteenth and twentieth centuries, after 1800 years of the evolution of case reports, that modern statistical and epidemiological tools evolved to the point of providing a new, more useful perspective to healthcare research. However, even after the advent of these case control studies, new diseases, appearing in unusual settings, were successfully identified and their cause established using the method of case reporting. Examples of the more spectacular uses of case report methods to establish the cause of disease would be:

(1)   An outbreak of a very rare form of bone cancer in young women watch-dial painters in the Chicago area in the 1930s. It was established that radium used to paint the watch dial was the cause [3].

(2)   From the 1930s to the 1960s, a chemical company dumped tons of mercury into Mina Mata Bay in Japan. Thousands of people living around the bay developed methyl mercury poisoning through the consumption of contaminated fish. The victims suffered from severe neurological damage, that later became known as Mina Mata Disease. Symptoms of this disorder include tingling sensations, muscle weakness, unsteady gait, tunnel vision, slurred speech, hearing loss, and abnormal behavior such as sudden fits of laughter. The establishment that toxic fish ingestion was the cause of mercury poisoning in the Japanese fishing village of Mina Mata in the 1950s was established through the scientific examination of case reports [4].

(3)   The use of case reports in establishing the cause of a disease was the findings of Lenz [5] that thalidomide ingestion by pregnant women causes the birth defects phecomelia and achondroplasia.

(4)   The demonstration that the acute, debilitating pneumonia inflicting a collection of veterans attending an American Legion convention in Philadelphia, Pennsylvania in 1976 was due to a heretofore unknown bacterium, *Legionella pneumophila*. Although clinical trial methodology was well accepted as a research tool at this time, case report methodology accomplished the identification of the cause and cure of this disease.

(5)   The identification of the relationship between tick bites and Lyme disease. There are over 16,000 cases per year of Lyme disease, but its cause went unrecognized until the 1990s.

Case reports in combination with careful observation and deductive reasoning to this day continue to provide important insight into the cause of disease. A major reason they continue to be essential in the presence of more sophisticated research techniques is because at their root, well-documented case reports use the best skills of epidemiology and clinical medicine—skilled observation and careful deductive reasoning. In each of these circumstances, the use of case reports successively and accurately warned the medical community of an exposure that caused a debilitating disease or a birth defect. Even though modern epidemiological models were available, these advanced tools were unnecessary for a clear view of the exposure–disease relationships in the aforementioned circumstances. The argument that sophisticated epidemiological studies are always required to build a causal argument for disease is defeated by these forceful examples from history.

The utility of case reports and case series has taken on a new sense of urgency in the healthcare issues of today. Case reports are critical in quickly identifying the causes of disease. Today, citizens of New York City and the surrounding environs are not asked to await the results of a large scale controlled clinical trial to provide conclusive evidence that the constellation of symptoms known as West Nile fever is caused by the West Nile virus, itself spread by a mosquito. The utilization of modern molecular techniques in concert with case reporting systems identified the link between the mosquito and the outbreak of disease in the northeastern United States. In Texas, the scientific community has not been required to wait for an epidemiological study to determine if the annual appearance of fever, malaise, convulsions, and coma are due to St. Louis encephalitis virus, spread by the mosquito. Careful, patient work by epidemiologists has correctly obviated a requirement for large epidemiological trials in these critical public health areas.

A.1 Causality Tenets

The fact that case reports are so useful in demonstrating the cause of a disease begs the question, What issues must be addressed in establishing that an exposure causes a disease? Essentially, efforts to understand and articulate the arguments necessary to construct a causality thesis have been long discussed and debated. In 1965, Hill [6] described the nine criteria for causality arguments in health care. These nine rules or tenets are remarkably and refreshingly devoid of complex mathematical arguments, relying instead on natural, honest intuition and common sense for the inquiry into the true nature of a risk factor–disease relationship. The questions Dr. Hill suggested should be asked make good sense. Are there many disease cases when the risk factor is present, and fewer disease cases when the risk factor is absent? Does a greater exposure to the risk factor produce a greater extent of disease? Other questions asked by Hill explore the "believability" of the relationship. Some of these are: Is there a discernible mechanism by which the risk factor produces the disease? Have other researchers also shown this relationship? Are there other such relationships whose demonstration helps us to understand the current risk factor–disease relationship? The nine precise Bradford Hill criteria are: (1) strength of association, (2) consistency, (3) specificity, (4) temporality, (5) biologic gradient, (6) biologic plausibility, (7) biologic coherence, (8) experimental evidence, (9) analogy.

1. Strength of association

This tenet requires that a greater percentage of patients who have been exposed to the risk factor develop the disease than patients unexposed to the risk factor. Although this is commonly addressed by epidemiological studies that produce relative risks or odds ratios, we will see later that, in very clear circumstances, with definable, predictable conditions, this can be satisfied with a case series.

2. Consistency with other knowledge

Consistency requires that the findings of one study be replicated in other studies. The persuasive argument for causality is much more clearly built on a collection of studies involving different patients and different protocols, each of which identify the same relationship between exposure to the risk factor and its consequent effect. There are numerous examples of collections of studies with different designs and patient populations, but that nevertheless successfully identify the same hazardous relationship between an exposure and disease. Identification of case series involving different series of patients in different countries and different cultures—yet each series producing the disease after the exposure would satisfy this criteria. Since research findings become more convincing when they are replicated in different populations, different studies that examine the same exposure–disease relationship and find similar results add to the weight of causal inference.

3. Specificity

The specificity of a disease is directly related to the number of known causes of the disease. The greater the number of causes of a disease, the more nonspecific the disease is, and the more difficult it is to demonstrate a new causal agent is involved in the production of the disease. The presence of specificity is considered supportive but not necessary, and epidemiologists no longer require that the effect of exposure to an agent such as a drug be specific for a single disease. However, the more specific the disease, the more useful the appearance of a case series. We will explore this issue later in this appendix.

4. Temporal relationship

Exposure must occur before the disease develops for it to cause that disease. A temporal relationship must exist in order to convincingly demonstrate causation. Protopathic bias (drawing a conclusion about causation when the disease process precedes the risk factor in occurrence) can result without appropriate attention to the condition. This criterion can be clearly satisfied by a case report that accurately documents that the exposure occurred before the disease.

5. Biologic gradient (dose response)

This assumes that the more intense the exposure, the greater the risk of disease. However, a dose–response relationship is not necessary to infer causation.

6. Biologic plausibility

There should be some basis in the scientific theory that supports the relationship between the supposed "cause" and the effect. However, observations have been made in epidemiological studies that were not considered biologically plausible at the time but subsequently were shown to be correct.

7. Biologic coherence

This implies that a cause–and–effect interpretation for an association does not conflict with what is known of the natural history and biology of the disease.

8. Experimental evidence

This would include in vitro studies, laboratory experiments on animals as well as human experiments. Experimental evidence also includes the results of the removal of a harmful exposure. These are termed challenge–dechallenge–rechallenge experiments

9. Analogy

This would include a similarity to some other known cause–effect association.

It is important to note in the application of these tenets that satisfaction of all nine is not required to establish to the satisfaction of the medical community that a causative relationship exists between the exposure and the disease. Hill himself stated:

> None of my nine viewpoints can bring indisputable evidence for or against the cause–and–effect hypothesis, and none can be required as a *sine qua non*.

The second, and somewhat surprising observation is that not a single one of these tenets requires that an epidemiological study (e.g., a case-control study) be executed to satisfy these tenets. It is even possible for a strength of association tenet to be satisfied by a well-chosen case series.[1] Some of the tenets were designed with a case report in mind. For example, the tenet of experimentation was developed to be satisfied by a challenge–dechallenge–rechallenge experiment.

There is no question that case reports can and indeed have been subject to criticism. In general, there are three main categories of criticisms of case reports. The first is that case reports and case series do not provide quantitative measures of the relationship between an exposure and a disease. While this is in general true, the historical examples of thalidmide exposure and birth defects, or toxic fish exposure and mercury poisoning demonstrate that, in selected instances, complicated mathematics are not necessary to provide clear evidence of a relationship between exposure and disease.

A second criticism of case reports is that they do not rule out other, competing causes of disease. The implication of this criticism is that case reports,

---

[1] If all of the disease occurs among the exposed, and the disease is simply not seen in the unexposed, a de facto infinite odds ratio is produced from the case series.

because they reflect a finding in one individual, cannot possibly be known to have its implications extended to a larger population. One cannot deny that the best minds in cardiology, epidemiology, and biostatistics believe that large, expensive clinical trials, despite the burden they place on healthcare resources, are required to evaluate the relationship between elevated cholesterol levels and MI's. Why aren't case reports sufficient for a causality argument in this setting?

This is a very useful criticism and requires further evaluation. In fact, case reports lose their utility when the disease has many causes. We call a disease cause-specific if it has one cause, and cause-nonspecific (or just nonspecific) if it has multiple causes. Examples of cause-specific diseases are (1) the occurrence of fetal phecomelia with maternal thalidomide ingestion, (2) malignant pleural mesothelioma and aspestos exposure and, (3) cinchonism that is unique to quinine exposure. In these circumstances, the identification of a disease that occurs only with the exposure defines the optimum utility of case reports. On the other hand, diseases such as atherosclerotic cardiovascular diseases have multiple contributing factors (genetics, obesity, cigarette smoking, diabetes, elevated lipid levels, and hypertension) requiring different data than that supplied in case reports to identify a new causative agent.

However, although it is clear that when a disease has many causes it can be difficult if not impossible to identify which cause was precisely the cause that excited the production of a disease in a given patient, one can often exclude other causes if there are only a few of them. Consider acute liver failure in the presence of diabetes. Acute liver failure does not occur as a well-known consequence of diabetes. If the common causes of acute liver failure can be removed as possibilities, the way is then open for establishing a new cause for the malady.

A.2 Do Case Reports Prove Causality?

A third and final criticism of case reports is the implication that by their very nature, case reports are unscientific. Consider the following quote from the Texas Supreme Court in the Havner decision:

> The FDA has promulgated regulations that detail the requirements for clinical investigations of the safety and effectiveness of drugs. 21 C.F.R. §314.126 (1996). These regulations state that "isolated case reports, random experience, and reports lacking the details which permit scientific evaluation will not be considered." Id. §314.126(e). Courts should likewise reject such evidence because it is not scientifically reliable.

This has led to the unfortunate interpretation that all case reports are not scientifically reliable. In fact, when case reports are isolated, random, and lacking in scientific detail, they make no useful contribution to our fund of knowledge about the risk-factor disease relationship. However, case reports can be clustered, specific, and provide great attention to detail, thereby imparting useful information about the relationship between a risk factor and a disease. A fine example of such a case report is that of Monahan [7], who provided a clear measurement of the effect of the two drugs, Seldane and Ketoconazole, and the occurrence of dangerous heart rhythms. This case report was obtained in scientifically controlled conditions, clarifying the mechanism by which the Seldane–Ketoconazole relationship could cause sudden death. Yet another example of the value of a case series was the identification of 24 patients in the upper Midwest United States by Heidi Connolly who had both exposure to the diet drug fenfluramine (fenphen) and heart value damage [8]. These case reports were not isolated but clustered[2]. Important detail was provided concerning the patients' medical history and exposure to the drugs. The patients underwent special studies of their hearts (echocardiography). In five cases, the heart valves themselves were recovered after the patients had undergone surgery and these heart valves were examined in a methodological, objective fashion. There was nothing unscientific about the evaluation of the patients in the Connolly case series. Although this study was followed by epidemiological studies, the findings of Connolly et al. and their implication that heart valve damage is caused by the fenfluramines have not been debunked.

Yet another example of the contribution of a scientific case control study was that of Douglas et al. [9], who demonstrated, again, under controlled, scientific settings, that the diet drug fenfluramine would consistently increase blood pressure in the pulmonary circulation of patients. This suggested that fenfluramine could be the cause of primary pulmonary hypertension. This study was followed by the case series of Brenot [10]. Although some have argued that this was not sufficient evidence for causality, the large epidemiological study that followed [11] validated the associations identified by the case report of Douglas or the case series of Brenot.

It is important to note that case reports have added value when they appear in the peer-reviewed literature. This is a sign that the study's methodology is consistent with the standard research procedures accepted by the scientific community. These articles must be given a greater priority than publications in non-peer-reviewed journals. Peer-reviewed journals also are superior to abstracts, that are themselves only brief, preliminary reports of non-peer-reviewed work.

The clear message from advances in scientific methodology is that good practice can produce useful results regardless of the methodology employed. While it is true that case reports, when shoddily documented or slovenly interpreted, will produce little of value, the criticisms are not specifically crafted for case reports but applicable as well to large epidemiological studies and placebo-controlled randomized clinical trials. Each of these scientific tools of investigation must be wielded carefully to be effective.

---

[2] Examples of important information provided by clustered case reports are those of Lyme disease and of the illness caused by the Hanta virus.

References

1. Bull, J.P. Historical development of clinical therapeutic trials. *Journal of Chronic Disease.*:218–248.
2. Malgaigne, LF. (1947). Weuvres Completes d'Ambrosise Paré, vol. 2. Paris, p. 127. Reported in Mettler, p 845.
3. Clark C. (1997). Radium Girls: Women and Industrial Health Reform, 1910–1935 Chapel Hill, University of North Carolina Press,.
4. Pepall, J. (1997). Methyl mercury poisoning: the Minamata Bay disaster. Copyright © International Development Research Centre, Ottawa, Canada .
5. Lenz, W. (1962). Thalidomide and congenital abnormalities. *Lancet* **1**:45.
6. Hill, B. (1953) Observation and Experiment. *New England Journal of Medicine* **248**:995–1001.
7. Monahan, B.P., Ferguson, C.L., Killeavy, E.S., Lloyd, B.K., Troy, J, Cantilena L.R. Jr. (1990). Torsades de pointes occurring in association with terfenadine use. *Journal of the American Medical Association* **264**:2788–90.
8. Connolly, H.M., Crary, J.L., McGoon, M.D., et al. (1997). Valvular heart disease associated with fenfluramine–phentermine [see comments] [published erratum appears in *New England Journal of Medicine* **337**:1783.
9. Douglas, J.G., et al., (1981). Pulmonary hypertension and fenfluramine. *British Medical Journal* **283**:881–3.
10. Brenot, F, et al (1993). Primary pulmonary hypertension and fenfluramine use [see comments]. *British Heart Journal* **70**:537–41
11. Abenhaim, L., et al.(1996). Appetite–suppressant drugs and the risk of primary pulmonary hypertension. International Primary Pulmonary Hypertension Study Group [see comments]. *New England Journal of Medicine* **335**:609–16.

Appendix B
Estimation in Random Research

B.1 Introduction

The purpose of this appendix is to document the assertion made in Chapter 2 that the random research paradigm perturbs our commonly used estimators in clinical trials. In Chapter 2, the motivation for the prospective identification of a research plan was developed from its foundations. In that chapter, we saw that the principle reason for the prospective choice of the analysis plan of a clinical trial was to keep that plan from being shifted, twisted, or otherwise altered by post-randomization events. Fixing the analysis plan during the design phase of the trial anchors it, keeping the plan unperturbed by the suggestions of trends presented by the incoming data stream. Central to this thesis is the acknowledgment that the urge to respond to incoming data can be irresistible: it is difficult for an inquisitive investigator to be unresponsive to the trends suggested by the incoming data.[1]

Without the existence of a firm tether on the analysis plan, this plan will be caught up in the trends produced by sampling error in the incoming data. Since the trends produced by sampling error are indistinguishable from the systematic trends in the sample that reflect population findings, the investigator will be uncertain as to what she is responding—a true effect or a spurious one. Like a feather caught up in the current of a stream, the analysis plan will be pushed, pulled, and twisted chaotically by random sampling error, in the end producing an unrecognizable and ungeneralizable result. Therefore, in a clinical trial that contains multiple analyses, the procedure that governs their interpretation must be specified a priori and must be rigorously designed if its results are to add to our corpus of knowledge about the disease under investigation.

As pointed out in Chapter 2, the estimators commonly used in statistics and epidemiology do not serve well when the analysis plan is chosen by the data. These estimators fail because they are constructed to function when the only variability is sampling variability—not analysis plan variability. The purpose of this appendix is to demonstrate the effect of one aspect of analysis plan variability—endpoint selection variability—on the estimator of an endpoint. In this demonstration, we will first identify the endpoint event rate in the circumstance of a fixed research paradigm (i.e., the endpoint was chosen prospectively and remained

---

[1] The proper place for summarization of these exploratory analyses is in the exploratory portion of the results section of the manuscript or presentation as discussed in Chapter 4.

unchanged), and then examine the event rate estimator in the random research paradigm. This demonstration will reveal that the estimator to be used in the random research paradigm is different than that derived for the fixed research setting. Since the best estimator for a situation is the estimator derived for that situation, fixed estimators should be avoided in the random research setting. Therefore, if only fixed estimators are available, the random research environment should be avoided.

B.2 Dichotomous Clinical Events

Assume a clinical trial is carried out to measure the effect of an intervention on a clinical event of interest (e.g., mortality). The trial has two arms, a placebo arm and an active arm. In order to examine the effect of therapy in this study, the cumulative event rate has to be computed in each of the control arm and the active arm and then compared across the two arms. This demonstration will derive the cumulative event rate in the placebo group in the fixed research paradigm, and then derive it for each of two random research paradigms, pointing out where sampling error exerts its influence.

B.2.1 Event Rate for the Fixed Research Paradigm

In the fixed paradigm, the endpoint is chosen prospectively, and the choice is not influenced by the data. Assume that the prospective choice for the endpoint in this study was total mortality. In the placebo group assume that there are n_c patients. Each of these patients n_c patients can either survive the trial or die during the trial. Let $i = 1, 2, \ldots, n_c$ index the n_c patients. Then describe the survival experience of each patient by x_i through the use of the following definition

$$x_i = 0 \text{ if the } i^{th} \text{ patient survives the trial,}$$
$$x_i = 1 \text{ if the } i^{th} \text{ patient dies during the trial.}$$
(B.1)

This is a useful device. For example, the number of patients who have died in the placebo group is simply $\sum_{i=1}^{n_c} x_i$. What we desire is an estimate of p_c, the cumulative proportion of patients who died in the control group.

In order to proceed, we invoke one of the simplest probability distributions to use, the Bernoulli distribution. The probability that $x_i = 1$, written as $P[x_i = 1] = p_c$. This can be written as

$$P[x_i] = p_c^{x_i} \left(1 - p_c\right)^{1 - x_i}$$
(B.2)

From expression (B.2) we see that $P[x_i = 0] = 1 - p_c$, and the $P[x_i = 1] = p_c$. This is where sampling error enters our consideration. By the beginning of the trial, we have chosen the endpoint of total mortality. However, we do not know which patients in the research sample will die. In our sample, patients x_1, x_{20}, and x_{103} could die. In another sample, x_1, x_{20}, and x_{103} could have survived, but x_{11}, x_{35}, x_{56}, and x_{190} will have died. This is the sample-to-sample variability: we do not know, and it is impossible to predict, which patients will die in each sample. However, once we have chosen the endpoint, the probability distribution governing the occurrence of that clinical endpoint is the same from sample to sample: $P[x_i] = p_c$.

This easy to use probability distribution nicely handles the straightforward value of x_i for each individual. However in this trial, we must focus on not just a single one of the x_i's but all of them jointly. This is because it makes sense to use the maximum information available, or all n_c patients in the control group, to estimate p_c. We do this by invoking the property of independence, i.e., knowledge of the death of one individual tells us nothing about whether another specific individual will survive the trial or not. For this we turn to the likelihood function $L\left(x_1, x_2, x_3, ..., x_n\right)$ which can be written as

$$L\left(x_1, x_2, x_3, ..., x_n\right) = \prod_{i=1}^{n_c} P[x_i]$$

$$= \prod_{i=1}^{n_c} p_c^{x_i} \left(1 - p_c\right)^{1-x_i} = p_c^{\sum_{i=1}^{n_c} x_i} \left(1 - p_c\right)^{n_c - \sum_{i=1}^{n_c} x_i},$$

(B.3)

and we write

$$L\left(x_1, x_2, x_3, ..., x_n\right) = p_c^{\sum_{i=1}^{n_c} x_i} \left(1 - p_c\right)^{n_c - \sum_{i=1}^{n_c} x_i},$$

(B.4)

Our job is to estimate p_c using our collection of placebo data $\left(x_1, x_2, x_3, ..., x_n\right)$. To accomplish this, we will maximize the likelihood function (B.4). The work proceeds smoothly if we first take the log of each side of (B.4)

$$\ln\left[L\left(x_1, x_2, x_3, ..., x_n\right)\right] = \ln\left[p_c^{\sum_{i=1}^{n_c} x_i} \left(1 - p_c\right)^{n_c - \sum_{i=1}^{n_c} x_i}\right]$$

$$= \sum_{i=1}^{n_c} x_i \ln[p_c] + \left(n_c - \sum_{i=1}^{n_c} x_i\right) \ln[1 - p_c].$$

(B.5)

We now take a derivative of each side of (B.5) with respect to p_c.

$$\frac{d\ln\left[L\left(x_1, x_2, x_3, \ldots, x_n\right)\right]}{dp_c} = \frac{d\left[\sum_{i=1}^{n_c} x_i \ln[p_c] + \left(n_c - \sum_{i=1}^{n_c} x_i\right)\ln[1-p_c]\right]}{dp_c}$$

(B.6)

$$= \frac{\sum_{i=1}^{n_c} x_i}{p_c} - \frac{\left(n_c - \sum_{i=1}^{n_c} x_i\right)}{1-p_c}.$$

We find the maximum by solving

$$\frac{\sum_{i=1}^{n_c} x_i}{p_c} - \frac{\left(n_c - \sum_{i=1}^{n_c} x_i\right)}{1-p_c} = 0$$

(B.7)

for p_c. Add the term

$$\frac{\left(n_c - \sum_{i=1}^{n_c} x_i\right)}{1-p_c},$$

to each side of (B.7), and cross multiply to find

$$(1-p_c)\sum_{i=1}^{n_c} x_i = p_c\left(n_c - \sum_{i=1}^{n_c} x_i\right),$$

$$\sum_{i=1}^{n_c} x_i - p_c\sum_{i=1}^{n_c} x_i = p_c n_c - p_c\sum_{i=1}^{n_c} x_i,$$

(B.8)

$$\sum_{i=1}^{n_c} x_i = p_c n_c,$$

$$p_c = \frac{\sum_{i=1}^{n_c} x_i}{n_c},$$

and we find that the best estimator p_c^* of the probability of death p_c based on our sample of data is

$$p_c^*(f) = \frac{\sum_{i=1}^{n_c} x_i}{n_c}$$

where $p_c^*(f)$ represents the estimator[2] for p_c under the fixed research paradigm.

B.2.2 Event Rates in Random Research

How does the derivation presented above change in the random research paradigm? We will modify the derivation provided in the previous section, but this time, the primary endpoint will not be chosen prospectively. Therefore, our goal will be to find $p_c^*(r)$, an estimator of the primary endpoint event rate under the random paradigm. We will change the experiment in the previous section in the following manner. Rather than there being one primary endpoint that was prospectively determined, let there be two endpoints (total mortality and stroke) competing to be the single primary endpoint. The investigator will choose one of these two endpoints as the primary endpoint based on the results of the study and compare the cumulative incidence rate of that endpoint across the two treatment groups. We will estimate the cumulative event rate in the placebo group under this random paradigm.

Beginning this development, we seen at once that we have an immediate departure from the derivation in the previous setting. In the fixed paradigm, we could define x_i as denoting whether the ith patient died or not. However, in this study, we are not sure which endpoint we will use as the primary endpoint, death or stroke. This uncertainty represents a new source of variability not present in the fixed research paradigm. One clear way to handle this is do define a new quantity, reflecting this additional source of endpoint variability. Define θ as the endpoint selection variable that we will allow to take only two values, one or zero. If total mortality is to be the selected endpoint, then $\theta = 1$. If stroke is to be the endpoint, then $\theta = 0$.

Once we know the value of θ we can proceed with the estimator. If, for example, we know that $\theta = 1$, then the primary endpoint is total mortality and we can define our estimator as

$$p_c^* = \frac{\sum_{i=1}^{n_c} x_i}{n_c}.$$

However, if $\theta = 0$, then the primary endpoint of the study will be the occurrence of a stroke, and we will find

$$p_c^* = \frac{\sum_{i=1}^{n_c} y_i}{n_c}$$

where y_i is defined as $y_i = 1$ if the ith patient had a stroke and $y_i = 0$ if the ith patient had no stroke during the course of the trial.

---

[2] This is called the *maximum likelihood estimator*, since it is the estimator that maximizes the likelihood of the observed data set. It turns out that this estimator is also unbiased and has the lowest variance of any other unbiased estimator.

The difficulty here is that, just as we do not know at the beginning of the clinical trial whether any particular patient will have an event during the course of the trial, we likewise do not know whether the total mortality endpoint or the stroke endpoint will be chosen as the primary endpoint of the study. In the fixed research paradigm, the number of primary endpoints was a function of sampling error. In this random paradigm the choice of the endpoint and the number of endpoints are both left to sampling error. One way for us to proceed is to admit that we don't know whether θ will take the value zero (stroke will be the primary endpoint) or the value one (total mortality endpoint will be the primary endpoint), and use probability to reflect this uncertainly. Thus we can define $P[\theta = 1] + P[\theta = 0] = 1$. In addition, we know that when $\theta = 1$, a good estimator for p_c is $p_c^* = \sum_{i=1}^{n_c} x_i \Big/ n_c$, and when $\theta = 0$, a good estimator for p_c is $p_c^* = \sum_{i=1}^{n_c} y_i \Big/ n_c$. Thus we can write $p_c^*(r)$ as $\sum_{i=1}^{n_c} x_i \Big/ n_c$ when $\theta = 1$ and $\sum_{i=1}^{n_c} y_i \Big/ n_c$ when $\theta = 0$. Thus

$$p_c^*(r) = \left[p_c^* \mid \theta = 0 \right] P[\theta = 0] + \left[p_c^* \mid \theta = 1 \right] P[\theta = 1]. \qquad (B.9)$$

But we know $\left[p_c^* \mid \theta = 0 \right]$: it is just the estimator of p_c when the primary endpoint of the study is stroke. Similarly, $p_c^* \mid \theta = 1$ is $\sum_{i=1}^{n_c} x_i \Big/ n_c$, the estimator of p_c when the primary endpoint of the study is total mortality. Substituting these quantities into (B.9) reveals

$$p_c^*(r) = \frac{\sum_{i=1}^{n_c} y_i}{n_c} P[\theta = 0] + \frac{\sum_{i=1}^{n_c} x_i}{n_c} P[\theta = 1] \qquad (B.10)$$

This can be written as

$$p_c^*(r) = \frac{\sum_{i=1}^{n_c} y_i}{n_c}\left[1 - P[\theta = 1]\right] + \frac{\sum_{i=1}^{n_c} x_i}{n_c} P[\theta = 1]$$

$$= \frac{\sum_{i=1}^{n_c} y_i}{n_c} + \left[\frac{\sum_{i=1}^{n_c} x_i}{n_c} - \frac{\sum_{i=1}^{n_c} y_i}{n_c}\right] P[\theta = 1] \qquad (B.11)$$

$$= \frac{\sum_{i=1}^{n_c} y_i + \left[\sum_{i=1}^{n_c} x_i - \sum_{i=1}^{n_c} y_i\right] P[\theta = 1]}{n_c}.$$

Examine the difference between the two estimators $p_c^*(f)$ and $p_c^*(r)$. For the fixed paradigm when total mortality was prospective selected, the estimator for the primary endpoint $p_c^*(f)$ in the placebo group was simply the proportion of patients in the placebo group who died. In this random paradigm, this more complicated estimator is the number of strokes plus a function of the difference between the number of deaths and the number of strokes divided by the total number of patients in that treatment group. We also must acknowledge at this point that we have no way to estimate P $[\theta = 1]$, a necessary quantity for the computation of $p_c^*(r)$. If we assume that we are just as likely at the end of the trial to choose total mortality as the primary endpoint as we would choose stroke as the primary endpoint,[3] then P$[\theta = 1] =$ 0.5 and the estimator under the random paradigm becomes

$$p_c^*(r) = \frac{\sum_{i=1}^{n_c} y_i + \frac{\left[\sum_{i=1}^{n_c} x_i - \sum_{i=1}^{n_c} y_i\right]}{2}}{n_c}. \qquad (B.12)$$

We must keep in mind that as peculiar as (B.12) appears, it is the appropriate estimator to use in the random research setting of this section. Thus, if at the end of this hypothetical clinical trial, there are 2200 patients randomized to the placebo group of the study, and 200 patients randomized to placebo therapy die, and 75 placebo patients have strokes, then $p_c^*(f) = \frac{200}{2200} = 0.091$, while

---

[3] This may be a completely unreasonable assumption. It is difficult to foresee what the likelihood is that, at the end of the trial, an analysis will demonstrate a mortality effect when the effect of therapy on the stroke endpoint is null. One of the difficulties of this paradigm is choosing and justifying the value of $P[\theta = 1]$.

$$p_c^*(r) = \frac{\displaystyle\sum_{i=1}^{n_c} y_i + \frac{\left[\displaystyle\sum_{i=1}^{n_c} x_i - \displaystyle\sum_{i=1}^{n_c} y_i\right]}{2}}{n_c} \tag{B.13}$$

$$= \frac{75 + \frac{(200 - 75)}{2}}{2200} = \frac{75 + 62.5}{2200} = 0.063.$$

In this setting, $p_c^*(r)$ is the preferred estimator, although its interpretation is extremely problematic. The random research estimator is a function of the difference between the number of patients who died in the study and the number of patients who suffered strokes. The clinical interpretation of this endpoint is very difficult, especially in light of the fact that a patient may have suffered a stroke and died. Note that $p_c^*(r)$ is only as accurate as our estimate of $P[\theta = 1]$ and that, unless we know that $P[\theta = 1] = 1$, $p_c^*(r) < p_c^*(f) = 0.091$. Obviously, test stastistics and p-values are also influenced by these considerations also.

Table B.1. Random research estimator of cumulative incidence. the primary endpoint.

$P[\theta = 1]$	Random estimator of the primary endpoint
0.00	0.034
0.10	0.040
0.20	0.045
0.30	0.051
0.40	0.057
0.50	0.063
0.60	0.068
0.70	0.074
0.80	0.080
0.90	0.085
1.00	0.091

The estimator increases as the probability that the mortality endpoint is chosen as the primary endpoint increases.

B.3 Hypothesis Testing

When we move from estimation to hypothesis testing, the implications of fixed and random paradigms continue to diverge. In the fixed research paradigm, we obtain an estimate of the cumulative mortality rate in the treatment group p_t^* for the n_t patients randomized to active therapy and construct the following test statistic to evaluate whether the population from which the sample was drawn contains differences in the mortality rates between those treated with control therapy and those treated with active group therapy.

$$\frac{p_c^* - p_t^*}{\sqrt{\frac{p_c^*\left(1-p_c^*\right)}{n_c} + \frac{p_t^*\left(1-p_t^*\right)}{n_t}}} \tag{B.14}$$

The test statistic in (B.14) is covered in standard introductory statistical textbooks and is easy to compute and understand. Part of the reason for its ease of use is that it is easy to find the variance of p_c^*, $Var\left(p_c^*\right) = {p_c^*\left(1-p_c^*\right)}\Big/{n_c}$. However, the variance computation is problematic for

$$p_c^*(r) = \frac{\sum\limits_{i=1}^{n_c} y_i \;+\; \left[\sum\limits_{i=1}^{n_c} x_i - \sum\limits_{i=1}^{n_c} y_i\right] P[\theta = 1]}{n_c},$$

which is the estimator derived under the random research paradigm. One reason for the difficulty is that deaths and strokes may not be independent of each other. The occurrence of a stroke may increase the likelihood of subsequent death, and of course, death precludes a following stroke. These relationships between the two endpoint complicates the interpretation of this endpoint. The test statistic for this random paradigm will be very difficult to construct, and more complex than that of the fixed research paradigm. Also, we continue to be bedeviled by the assessment of the $P[\theta=1]$, a quantity that must be estimated in order to calculate $p_c^*(r)$. In all likelihood, this quantity may have a variance attached to it as well, further deepening the enigma of random analysis.[4]

In this development, clearly the fixed paradigm with prospectively stated endpoints and analysis plan is preferred. Its estimators are easily constructed, intuitive, and lead to uncomplicated comparisons between the control and treatment groups in the clinical trial. However, if the random paradigm is to be employed estimators of event rates are complicated and difficult to interpret, and hypothesis

---

[4] Those who work in the Bayesian field recognize this problem, and often respond by placing a probability distribution on the value of $P[\theta = 1]$, e.g., a beta distribution. However, this maneuver is little help to us here, since this probability distribution will have parameters that would themselves require estimation and justification. Unfortunately, a deeper level of parameterization does not solve our problems, but instead pushes it further away.

testing can be burdensome. To best way to avoid these difficulties is to avoid the random paradigm.

Appendix C
Relevant Code of Federal Regulations

The following are excerpts from the *Code of Federal Regulations*, providing the language from which guidelines are generated for private industry as they develop therapeutic agents and devices. Two provisions are provided:

(1) Indications Section of the Label for Prescription Drugs, and
(2) Adequate and Well-Controlled Trials.

C.1 Indications for Prescritpion Drugs

Subpart B–Labeling Requirements for Prescription Drugs and/or Insulin
Sec. 201.57 Specific requirements on content and format of labeling for human prescription drugs.

(c) Indications and Usage.

(1) Under this section heading, the labeling shall state that:

(i)   The drug is indicated in the treatment, prevention, or diagnosis of a recognized disease or condition, e.g.,, penicillin is indicated for the treatment of pneumonia due to susceptible pneumococci; and/or

(ii)   The drug is indicated for the treatment, prevention, or diagnosis of an important manifestation of a disease or condition, e.g.,, chlorothiazide is indicated for the treatment of edema in patients with CHF; and/or

(iii)   The drug is indicated for the relief of symptoms associated with a disease or syndrome, e.g.,, chlorpheniramine is indicated for the symptomatic relief of nasal congestion in patients with vasomotor rhinitis; and/or

(iv)   The drug, if used for a particular indication only in conjuction with a primary mode of therapy, e.g.,, diet, surgery, or some other drug, is an adjunct to the mode of therapy.

(2) All indications shall be supported by substantial evidence of effectiveness based on adequate and well-controlled studies as defined in Sec. 314.126(b) of this chapter unless the requirement is waived under Sec. 201.58 or Sec. 314.126(b) of this chapter.

(3) This section of the labeling shall also contain the following additional information:

(i)   If evidence is available to support the safety and effectiveness of the drug
        only in selected subgroups of the larger population with a disease, syn-
        drome, or symptom under consideration, e.g.,, patients with mild disease
        or patients in a special age group, the labeling shall describe the available
        evidence and state the limitations of usefulness of the drug. The labeling
        shall also identify specific tests needed for selection or monitoring of the
        patients who need the drug, e.g.,, microbe susceptibility tests. Information
        on the approximate kind, degree, and duration of improvement to be an-
        ticipated shall be stated if available and shall be based on substantial
        evidence derived from adequate and well-controlled studies as defined in
        Sec. 314.126(b) of this chapter unless the requirement is waived under
        Sec. 201.58 or Sec. 314.126(b) of this chapter. If the information is rele-
        vant to the recommended intervals between doses, the usual duration of
        treatment, or any modification of dosage, it shall be stated in the ``Dosage
        and Administration'' section of the labeling and referenced in this section.

(ii)   If safety considerations are such that the drug should be reserved for cer-
        tain situations, e.g.,, cases refractory to other drugs, this information shall
        be stated in this section.

(iii)   If there are specific conditions that should be met before the drug is used
        on a long-term basis, e.g.,, demonstration of responsiveness to the drug in
        a short-term trial, the labeling shall identify the conditions; or, if the indi-
        cations for long-term use are different from those for short-term use, the
        labeling shall identify the specific indications for each use.

(iv)   If there is a common belief that the drug may be effective for a certain use
        or if there is a common use of the drug for a condition, but the preponder-
        ance of evidence related to the use or condition shows that the drug is
        ineffective, the Food and Drug Administration may require that the label-
        ing state that there is a lack of evidence that the drug is effective for that
        use or condition.

(v)   Any statements comparing the safety or effectiveness, either greater or
        less, of the drug with other agents for the same indication shall be sup-
        ported by adequate and well-controlled studies as defined in Sec.
        314.126(b) of this chapter unless this requirement is waived under Sec.
        201.58 or Sec. 314.126(b) of this chapter.

C.2 Adequate and Well-Controlled Trials

TITLE 21--Food and Drugs
Department of Health and Human Services

Part 314--Applications for FDA Approval to Market of a New Drug

Subpart D—FDA Action on Applications and Abbreviated Applications
Sec. 314.126 Adequate and well-controlled studies.

(a)   The purpose of conducting clinical investigations of a drug is to distin-
        guish the effect of a drug from other influences, such as spontaneous

change in the course of the disease, placebo effect, or biased observation. The characteristics described in paragraph (b) of this section have been developed over a period of years and are recognized by the scientific community as the essentials of an adequate and well-controlled clinical investigation. The Food and Drug Administration considers these characteristics in determining whether an investigation is adequate and well-controlled for purposes of Sction 505 of the act. Reports of adequate and well-controlled investigations provide the primary basis for determining whether there is "ubstantial evidence" to support the claims of effectiveness for new drugs. Therefore, the study report should provide sufficient details of study design, conduct, and analysis to allow critical evaluation and a determination of whether the characteristics of an adequate and well-controlled study are present.

(b) An adequate and well-controlled study has the following characteristics:

(1) There is a clear statement of the objectives of the investigation and a summary of the proposed or actual methods of analysis in the protocol for the study and in the report of its results. In addition, the protocol should contain a description of the proposed methods of analysis, and the study report should contain a description of the methods of analysis ultimately used. If the protocol does not contain a description of the proposed methods of analysis, the study report should describe how the methods used were selected.

(2) The study uses a design that permits a valid comparison with a control to provide a quantitative assessment of drug effect. The protocol for the study and report of results should describe the study design precisely; for example, duration of treatment periods, whether treatments are parallel, sequential, or crossover, and whether the sample size is predetermined or based upon some interim analysis.

Generally, the following types of control are recognized:

(i)　Placebo concurrent control. The test drug is compared with an inactive preparation designed to resemble the test drug as far as possible. A placebo-controlled study may include additional treatment groups, such as an active treatment control or a dose-comparison control, and usually includes randomization and blinding of patients or investigators, or both.

(ii)　Dose-comparison concurrent control. At least two doses of the drug are compared. A dose-comparison study may include additional treatment groups, such as placebo control or active control. Dose-comparison trials usually include randomization and blinding of patients or investigators, or both.

(iii)　No treatment concurrent control. Where objective measurements of effectiveness are available and placebo effect is negligible, the test drug is compared with no treatment. No treatment concurrent control trials usually include randomization.

(iv)   Active treatment concurrent control. The test drug is compared with
         known effective therapy; for example, where the condition treated is such
         that administration of placebo or no treatment would be contrary to the in-
         terest of the patient. An active treatment study may include additional
         treatment groups, however, such as a placebo control or a dose-
         comparison control. Active treatment trials usually include randomization
         and blinding of patients or investigators, or both. If the intent of the trial is
         to show similarity of the test and control drugs,the report of the study
         should assess the ability of the study to have detected a difference between
         treatments. Similarity of test drug and active control can mean either that
         both drugs were effective or that neither was effective. The analysis of the
         study should explain why the drugs should be considered effective in the
         study, for example, by reference to results in previous placebo-controlled
         studies of the active control drug.

(v)   Historical control. The results of treatment with the test drug are compared
         with experience historically derived from the adequately documented natu-
         ral history of the disease or condition, or from the results of active
         treatment, in comparable patients or populations. Because historical con-
         trol populations usually cannot be as well assessed with respect to
         pertinent variables as can concurrent control populations, historical control
         designs are usually reserved for special circumstances. Examples include
         studies of diseases with high and predictable mortality (certain malignan-
         cies) and studies in which the effect of the drug is self-evident (general
         anesthetics, drug metabolism).

(3) The method of selection of subjects provides adequate assurance that
they have the disease or condition being studied, or evidence of susceptibility and
exposure to the condition against which prophylaxis is directed.

(4) The method of assigning patients to treatment and control groups minimizes bias and is intended to assure comparability of the groups with respect to
pertinent variables such as age, sex, severity of disease, duration of disease, and use
of drugs or therapy other than the test drug. The protocol for the study and the report of its results should describe how subjects were assigned to groups. Ordinarily,
in a concurrently controlled study, assignment is by randomization, with or without
stratification.

(5) Adequate measures are taken to minimize bias on the part of the
subjects, observers, and analysts of the data. The protocol and report of the study
should describe the procedures used to accomplish this, such as blinding.

(6) The methods of assessment of subjects' response are well-defined and
reliable. The protocol for the study and the report of results should explain the variables measured, the methods of observation, and criteria used to assess response.

(7) There is an analysis of the results of the study adequate to assess the effects of the drug. The report of the study should describe the results and the analytic methods used to evaluate them, including any appropriate statistical methods. The analysis should assess, among other things, the comparability of test and control groups with respect to pertinent variables, and the effects of any interim data analyses performed.

(c) The Director of the Center for Drug Evaluation and Research may, on the Director's own initiative or on the petition of an interested person, waive in whole or in part any of the criteria in paragraph (b) of this section with respect to a specific clinical investigation, either prior to the investigation or in the evaluation of a completed study. A petition for a waiver is required to set forth clearly and concisely the specific criteria from which waiver is sought, why the criteria are not reasonably applicable to the particular clinical investigation, what alternative procedures, if any, are to be, or have been employed, and what results have been obtained. The petition is also required to state why the clinical investigations so conducted will yield, or have yielded, substantial evidence of effectiveness, notwithstanding nonconformance with the criteria for which waiver is requested.

(d) For an investigation to be considered adequate for approval of a new drug, it is required that the test drug be standardized as to identity, strength, quality, purity, and dosage form to give significance to the results of the investigation.

(e) Uncontrolled studies or partially controlled studies are not acceptable as the sole basis for the approval of claims of effectiveness. Such studies carefully conducted and documented, may provide corroborative support of well-controlled studies regarding efficacy and may yield valuable data regarding safety of the test drug. Such studies will be considered on their merits in the light of the principles listed here, with the exception of the requirement for the comparison of the treated subjects with controls. Isolated case reports, random experience, and reports lacking the details which permit scientific evaluation will not be considered.

(Collection of information requirements approved by the Office of Management and Budget under control number 0910-0001)

[50 FR 7493, Feb. 22, 1985, as amended at 50 FR 21238, May 23, 1985; 55 FR 11580, Mar. 29, 1990; 64 FR 402, Jan. 5, 1999]

Effective Date Note: At 64 FR 402, Jan. 5, 1999, Sec. 314.126 was amended in paragraph (a) by removing the word *sections* and adding in its place the word *section'* and removing the words *and 507* from the third sentence and by removing the words *and antibiotics* from the fourth sentence, effective May 20, 1999.

Appendix D

Sample Size Primer

The purpose of this appendix is to provide a brief discussion of the underlying principles in sample size computations for a clinical trial. In the process, one of the simplest and most useful formulas for the sample size formulations will be reproduced. These basic formulas are the source of the calculations in Chapters 4–9. First we will provide the solution, and proceed to a discussion which both motivates and derives the sample size and power formulas.

D.1 General Discussion of Sample Size

Assume that a clinical trial has been designed to measure the effect of a randomly allocated intervention on a prospectively defined primary endpoint. Let θ_c be the cumulative incidence rate of the primary endpoint in the control group and let θ_t be the cumulative incidence rate of the primary endpoint in the treatment group. Then the statistical hypothesis for the primary endpoint in this clinical trial is

$$H_0 : \theta_c = \theta_t \quad vs. \quad H_a : \theta_c \neq \theta_t. \tag{D.1}$$

Let Z_a be the ath percentile from the standard normal distribution. The investigators have chosen an a priori test-specific type I error level α, and the power of the statistical hypothesis test is $1 - \beta$. The hypothesis test will be two-sided. Let p_c be the cumulative incidence rate of the primary endpoint in the control group of the research sample, and let p_t be the cumulative incidence rate of the active group in the research sample. Then the trial size, or the sample size of the clinical trial,[1] N may be written as

$$N = \frac{2 \left[p_c (1 - p_c) + p_t (1 - p_t) \right] \left[Z_{1-\alpha/2} - Z_\beta \right]^2}{(p_c - p_t)^2}. \tag{D.2}$$

Analogously, the power of the study may be calculated as a function of N.

---

[1] This is the total number of patients in the study (number of patients in the placebo group plus the number of patients in the control group).

$$1-\beta = P\left[\,N(0,1) > Z_{1-\alpha/2} \;-\; \frac{p_c - p_t}{\sqrt{\dfrac{p_c\left(1-p_c\right)}{N/2} + \dfrac{p_t\left(1-p_t\right)}{N/2}}}\,\right]. \qquad (D.3)$$

There are many different treatises on sample size calculations in clinical trials. A representative group is [1], [2], [3], [4], [5]. Several of these sources discuss important and useful nuances of the sample size computation which are useful in complex clinical trial design. The focus of the discussion here, however, will be on the most basic sample size computation, since that formula demonstrates most clearly the influence of the design parameters of the study (cumulative primary endpoint event rate in the control group, the anticipated effect of the intervention, the magnitude of the statistical errors, and test sidedness) on the resulting sample size.

For these discussions, assume that patients are randomized to receive either a new intervention or to receive control group therapy. In this example, there is one primary endpoint that occurs with a cumulative event rate θ_c. In the intervention group the cumulative event rate for the primary endpoint is θ_t. The investigator does not know the value of θ_c since he does not study every patient in the population. He therefore selects a sample from the population and uses that sample to compute p_c, which will serve as his estimate of θ_c. If the clinical trial has been executed concordantly, then p_c is a good estimator of θ_c; this means that the investigator can expect that p_c will be close to the value of θ_c. Analogously p_t is the estimate from the investigator's sample of the cumulative incidence of the endpoint in the population θ_t. Thus, if the trial was executed according to its protocol (and not subject to the destabilizing influences of random research), then $p_c - p_t$ can be expected to be an accurate estimate of $\theta_c - \theta_t$. If the null hypothesis is true then $\theta_c - \theta_t$ will be zero and we would expect $p_c - p_t$ to be small. If the alternative hypothesis is correct, and the investigator's intuition that the therapy being tested in the clinical trial will reduce the cumulative event rate of the primary endpoint is right, then θ_c is much greater than θ_t, and $p_c - p_t$, the best estimate of $\theta_c - \theta_t$ will be large as well.

A key point in understanding the sample size formulation is the critical role played by the number of endpoint events produced by the sample. The research sample produces primary endpoints—the rate at which these endpoints are accumulated is directly linked to the cumulative event rate in the control group. This cumulative event rate therefore plays a central role in the sample size calculations. If the primary endpoint of a clinical trial is total mortality, then recruiting 1000 patients into the study provides no useful information for the evaluation of the effect of therapy on total mortality if at the end of the study none of the 1000 recruited patients die. The more primary endpoint events which occur during the course of the trial, the greater the volume of germane data available to answer the scientific question of whether the occurrence of those endpoint events are influenced by the intervention being studied. Therefore, the larger the cumulative control group event rate is, the greater the number of primary endpoint event rates that will be generated. The greater the rate at which primary endpoints are produced, the smaller the required sample size for the clinical trial will be, assuming that everything else (effect of therapy, test sidedness, magnitude of the statistical errors) is equal.[2]

A second measure which is critical in sample size considerations is the effectiveness of the therapy. This is often measured by the difference between the cumulative incidence rate of the primary endpoint in the population θ_c and the cumulative incidence of the primary event rate in the population if everyone in the population were to receive the treatment being studied in the clinical trial, θ_t. This difference is commonly referred to as "delta" or $\Delta = \theta_c - \theta_t$.[3] The greater the difference between θ_c and θ_t, then the fewer the number of patients required to obtain a reliable estimate of that difference.

To understand this principle, it may be helpful to think of the two primary sources of variability involved in the estimation of the treatment effect in a clinical trial. The test statistic used to test the statistical hypothesis that $\theta_c = \theta_t$ versus the alternative hypothesis that these events are not equal is

$$\frac{p_c - p_t}{\sqrt{Var[p_c - p_t]}}. \tag{D.4}$$

The first source of this variability is systematic; it is induced by the intervention being studied by the clinical trial and is an estimate of Δ. This variability is estimated by $p_c - p_t$ and resides in the numerator of (D.4). This is the "signal". The denominator of (D.4) is the second source of variability or the "noise"; it is an expression of the fact that, since the research is sample-based, estimates of $p_c - p_t$ will vary from sample to sample. Since this sampling variability "noise" should not be confused with the systematic, intervention-induced "signal" measured by $p_c - p_t$, this noise must be removed from the estimate of the therapy's effect. Therefore using these characterizations, the greater the signal to noise ratio, the larger the expression in (D.4) will be.

The greater the signal–to–noise ratio as represented by (D.4), the easier it is to detect a genuine population effect of the intervention. If the magnitude of $\theta_c - \theta_t$ is small in the population, then $p_c - p_t$ is also likely to be small. In this circumstance where the magnitude of the signal is small, the noise must be coincidently reduced to detect the weak signal with precision. One useful tool the investigator has to reduce the background noise is to increase N, the sample size of the clinical trial. Part of the genius of choosing the reliable estimate $p_c - p_t$ of $\theta_c - \theta_t$ is that this estimate's sampling variability decreases as the sample size increases.[4]

---

[2] Also known as the ceteris parabus assumption.
[3] Some times it is useful to refer to the percent reduction in events attributable to the therapy, otherwise known as the therapy's efficacy.
[4] This indispensable property of the estimates of effect size can be lost if the experiment is not executed concordantly (see Chapter 2).

D.2 Derivation of Sample Size

To compute the sample size for the clinical trial as outlined in this appendix, note that the test statistic

$$\frac{p_c - p_t - (\theta_c - \theta_t)}{\sqrt{Var[p_c - p_t]}} \tag{D.5}$$

follows a normal distribution. Under the null hypothesis that $\theta_c - \theta_t = 0$ reduces to

$$\frac{p_c - p_t}{\sqrt{Var[p_c - p_t]}}. \tag{D.6}$$

One useful way to think of this test statistic

$$(p_c - p_t) \Big/ \sqrt{Var[p_c - p_t]}$$

is as a normed effect size. Under the null hypothesis, we expect this normed effect size to have a mean of zero and a variance of one. It will follow the normal or bell shaped distribution. Then, the null hypothesis will be rejected when[5]

$$\frac{p_c - p_t}{\sqrt{Var[p_c - p_t]}} > Z_{1-\alpha/2} \tag{D.7}$$

or,

$$p_c - p_t > Z_{1-\alpha/2}\sqrt{Var[p_c - p_t]}. \tag{D.8}$$

We now consider what should have if the alternative hypothesis was true. In this case, we start with the definition of statistical power.

Power = Probability [the null hypothesis is rejected | the alternative hypothesis is true]

---

[5] This is not the only circumstance under which the null hypothesis will be rejected. It will also be rejected when harm is caused by the intervention or when $p_t - p_c$ is very much less than zero. However, in the sample size computation, attention is focused on the tail of the distribution in which the investigators are most interested.

The null hypothesis is rejected when the test statistic falls in the critical region or when $p_c - p_t > Z_{1-\alpha/2}\sqrt{Var[p_c - p_t]}$. The alternative hypothesis is true if $\theta_c - \theta_t = \Delta \geq 0$. This allows us to write

$$Power = 1-\beta = P\left[p_c - p_t > Z_{1-\alpha/2}\sqrt{Var[p_c - p_t]} \mid \theta_c - \theta_t = \Delta\right]. \qquad (D.9)$$

We now standardize the argument in the probability statement of (D.9) so that the quantity on the left follows a standard normal distribution. This requires subtracting the population mean effect under the alternative hypothesis (i.e., Δ) and dividing by the square root of the variance of $p_c - p_t$. These operations must be carried out on both sides of the inequality in the probability expression in (D.9) as follows.

$$1-\beta = P\left[\frac{p_c - p_t - \Delta}{\sqrt{Var[p_c - p_t]}} > \frac{Z_{1-\alpha/2}\sqrt{Var[p_c - p_t]} - \Delta}{\sqrt{Var[p_c - p_t]}}\right]$$

$$= P\left[\frac{p_c - p_t - \Delta}{\sqrt{Var[p_c - p_t]}} > Z_{1-\alpha/2} - \frac{\Delta}{\sqrt{Var[p_c - p_t]}}\right] \qquad (D.10)$$

$$= P\left[N(0,1) > Z_{1-\alpha/2} - \frac{\Delta}{\sqrt{Var[p_c - p_t]}}\right].$$

By the definition of a percentile value from a probability distribution, we can now write

$$Z_\beta = Z_{1-\alpha/2} - \frac{\Delta}{\sqrt{Var[p_c - p_t]}}. \qquad (D.11)$$

We are now ready to conclude this computation, by solving for N, the size of the trial. The sample size is embedded in the variance term in the denominator of expression (D.11).

$$Var[p_c - p_t] = \frac{p_c(1-p_c)}{n_c} + \frac{p_t(1-p_t)}{n_t}. \qquad (D.12)$$

where n_c is the number of patients to be recruited to the control group in the clinical trial and n_t is the number of patients to be recruited to the active group. The sample size or trial size is the total number of patients required for the experiment $= N = n_c + n_t$. If we assume that the number of patients in the control group will equal the number of patients in the treatment group, then $n_c = n_t = n$ and $N = 2n$. Then (D.11) can be rewritten as

$$Z_\beta = Z_{1-\alpha/2} - \frac{\Delta}{\sqrt{\dfrac{p_c(1-p_c)}{n} + \dfrac{p_t(1-p_t)}{n}}}. \qquad (D.13)$$

We only need solve this equation for n:

$$n = \frac{\left[p_c(1-p_c) + p_t(1-p_t)\right]\left[Z_{1-\alpha/2} - Z_\beta\right]^2}{\Delta^2}. \qquad (D.14)$$

The trial size $N = 2n$ may be written as

$$N = \frac{2\left[p_c(1-p_c) + p_t(1-p_t)\right]\left[Z_{1-\alpha/2} - Z_\beta\right]^2}{\Delta^2}. \qquad (D.15)$$

To compute the power we only need to adapt the following equation from (D.10),

$$1-\beta = P\left[N(0,1) > Z_{1-\alpha/2} - \frac{\Delta}{\sqrt{Var[p_c - p_t]}}\right] \qquad (D.16)$$

and rewrite the Var [p_c - p_t] to find

$$1-\beta = P\left[N(0,1) > Z_{1-\alpha/2} - \frac{\Delta}{\sqrt{\dfrac{p_c(1-p_c)}{N/2} + \dfrac{p_t(1-p_t)}{N/2}}}\right]. \qquad (D.17)$$

D.3 Example

If the experiment is designed for a two sided α of 0.05, 90 % power ($\beta = 0.10$), $p_c = 0.20$, and $\Delta = 0.03$, then $p_t = 0.17$. The trial size can be computed from

$$N = \frac{2\left[p_c(1-p_c) + p_t(1-p_t)\right]\left[Z_{1-\alpha/2} - Z_\beta\right]^2}{\left[p_c - p_t\right]^2}. \qquad (D.18)$$

Inserting the data from this example reveals

$$N = \frac{2\left[(0.20)(0.80)+(0.17)(0.83)\right]\left[1.96-(-1.28)\right]^2}{\left[0.20-0.17\right]^2} = 7024 \quad \text{(D.19)}$$

or 3512 subjects per group. If only 2000 subjects per group can be identified, the power can be formulated from

$$Power = P\left[N(0,1) > Z_{1-\alpha/2} - \frac{\Delta}{\sqrt{\dfrac{p_c\left(1-p_c\right)}{N/2}+\dfrac{p_t\left(1-p_t\right)}{N/2}}}\right] \quad \text{(D.20)}$$

and including the data from this example

$$Power = P\left[N(0,1) > 1.96 - \frac{0.03}{\sqrt{\dfrac{(0.20)(0.80)}{2000}+\dfrac{(0.17)(0.83)}{2000}}}\right] = 0.69. \quad \text{(D.21)}$$

References

1. Lachim, J.M. (1981). Introduction to sample size determinations and power analyses for clinical trials. *Controlled Clinical Trial* **2**:93–114.
2. Sahai, H., Khurshid, A. (1996). Formulae and tables for determination of sample size and power in clinical trials for testing differences in proportions for the two sample design. *Statistics in Medicine* **15**:1–21.
3. Davy, S.J., Graham, O.T.(1991). Sample size estimation for comparing two or more treatment groups in clinical trials. *Statistics in Medicine* **10**:3–43.
4. Donner, A. (1984). Approach to sample size estimation in the design of clinical trials – a review.*Statistics in Medicine* **3**:199–214.
5. George, S.L., Desue M.M. (1974). Planning the size and duration of a clinical trial studying the time to some critical event. *Journal of Chronic Disease* **27**:15–24.

References

Appendix E

Additional Dependent Hypothesis Testing Results

In Chapter 5, we developed the idea of dependency between statistical analyses in clinical trials. The evaluation of the level of dependency was determined prospectively by the investigators, and each of the statistical analyses would have a type I error allocated to them. Section 5.4 developed the principle of dependent hypothesis testing, and Sections 5.6 through 5.9 derived a measure of dependence between two statistical hypothesis tests in a clinical trial. Section 6.1 developed an analogous measure between three prospectively defined primary hypothesis tests. In section 6.2 we provided some formulations that apply to more than three dependent statistical primary analyses. This appendix provides the derivations of the results described in Section 6.2 and 6.3.

E.1 Derivation of Dependence for $K = 4$

The evaluation when there are four dependent hypothesis tests is a direct generalization of the consideration for $K = 2$ and $K = 3$. Continuing with the notation that we used in Chapter 5, we will assume here that there are four prospectively defined statistical hypothesis tests, H_1, H_2, H_3 and H_4. We define the variables T_1, T_2, T_3, and T_4 ,each of which will take on the value of one when a type I error has occurred, and, alternatively will become zero when no type I error has occurred. Then, as before, we have $P[T_1 = 1] = \alpha_1$, $P[T_2 = 1] = \alpha_2$, $P[T_3 = 1] = \alpha_3$, and $P[T_4 = 1] = \alpha_4$. We will also assume that $\alpha_1 \geq \alpha_2 \geq \alpha_3 \geq \alpha_4$ without any loss of generality. We may write the experiment wide type I error as

$$\xi = 1 - P[T_1 = 0 \cap T_2 = 0 \cap T_3 = 0 \cap T_4 = 0] \qquad (E.1)$$

This derivation proceeds analogously for the case of $K = 3$ presented in chapter five, and we will begin here as we began there with the identification of the relevant, joint probability. In this circumstance, that probability involves the four variables T_1, T_2, T_3, and T_4 and is writen as $P[T_1=0 \cap T_2=0 \cap T_3=0 \cap T_4=0]$. Start with the definition of conditional probability

$$P[T_4 = 0 \mid T_1 = 0 \cap T_2 = 0 \cap T_3 = 0] = \frac{P[T_1 = 0 \cap T_2 = 0 \cap T_3 = 0 \cap T_4 = 0]}{P[T_1 = 0 \cap T_2 = 0 \cap T_3 = 0]} \qquad (E.2)$$

This conditional probability is the probability that there is a type I error for the fourth hypothesis test H_4, given that there is no type I error for each of the three hypothesis tests H_1, H_2, and H_3. Solving equation (E.2) for the joint probability involving four events reveals

$$P[T_1 = 0 \cap T_2 = 0 \cap T_3 = 0 \cap T_4 = 0]$$
$$= P[T_4 = 0 \mid T_1 = 0 \cap T_2 = 0 \cap T_3 = 0]P[T_1 = 0 \cap T_2 = 0 \cap T_3 = 0] \qquad (E.3)$$

Now we write the dependency measure $D_{4|1,2,3}$ as

$$D_{4|1,2,3} = \sqrt{1 - \frac{\left(1 - P[T_4 = 0 \mid T_1 = 0 \cap T_2 = 0 \cap T_3 = 0]\right)}{\alpha_4}}. \qquad (E.4)$$

$D_{4|1,2,3}$ denotes the measurement of dependency between H_4 given knowledge of H_1, H_2, and H_3. We now solve equation (E.4) for the conditional probability

$$P[T_4 = 0 \mid T_1 = 0 \cap T_2 = 0 \cap T_3 = 0] = (1 - \alpha_4) + D_{4|1,2,3}^2 [1 - (1 - \alpha_4)]$$
$$= 1 - \alpha_4 \left(1 - D_{4|1,2,3}^2\right). \qquad (E.5)$$

We now have an expression for the conditional probability involving the dependence parameter. What remains is to take this expression denoted in (E.5) and substitute it into equation (E.1) using (E.2) to find

$$\xi = 1 - P[T_1 = 0 \cap T_2 = 0 \cap T_3 = 0 \cap T_4 = 0]$$
$$= 1 - P[T_4 = 0 \mid T_1 = 0 \cap T_2 = 0 \cap T_3 = 0]P[T_1 = 0 \cap T_2 = 0 \cap T_3 = 0] \qquad (E.6)$$
$$= 1 - \left[1 - \alpha_4 \left(1 - D_{4|1,2,3}^2\right)\right]P[T_1 = 0 \cap T_2 = 0 \cap T_3 = 0].$$

Finally, recalling that from Section 6.2 that

$$P[T_1 = 0 \cap T_2 = 0 \cap T_3 = 0] = \left[1 - \alpha_3 \left(1 - D_{3|1,2}^2\right)\right]\left[1 - \alpha_2 \left(1 - D_{2|1}^2\right)\right][1 - \alpha_1] \qquad (E.7)$$

we write the familywise error level ξ,

$$\xi = 1 - \left[1 - \alpha_4 \left(1 - D_{4|1,2}^2\right)\right]\left[1 - \alpha_3 \left(1 - D_{3|1,2}^2\right)\right]\left[1 - \alpha_2 \left(1 - D_{2|1}^2\right)\right][1 - \alpha_1] \qquad (E.8)$$

Note that ξ is a function of the four test-specific alpha levels α_1, α_2, α_3, α_4 and the three dependency measures $D_{2|1}$, $D_{3|1,2}$ and $D_{4|1,2,3}$.

    As was the case for three hypothesis tests, it will be useful for us to prospectively compute the test-specific alpha level α_4 for the fourth primary analysis given the levels α_1, α_2, and α_3 for the other three hypothesis tests H_1, H_2, and H_3. Solving (E.8) for α_3 reveals

$$\alpha_4 = \min\left[\alpha_3, \frac{1 - \dfrac{1-\xi}{\left[1-\alpha_1\right]\left[1-\alpha_2\left(1-D_{2|1}^2\right)\right]\left[1-\alpha_3\left(1-D_{3|1,2}^2\right)\right]}}{1-D_{4|1,2,3}^2}\right]. \quad \text{(E.9)}$$

If the value for the dependency measure is the same across the three prospectively planned, primary analyses, then $D_{2|1} = D_{3|1,2} = D_{4|1,2,3} = D$, and equation (E.9) becomes

$$\alpha_4 = \min\left[\alpha_3, \frac{\left[1-\alpha_1\right]\left[1-\alpha_2\left(1-D^2\right)\right]\left[1-\alpha_3\left(1-D^2\right)\right] - \left(1-\xi\right)}{\left[1-\alpha_1\right]\left[1-\alpha_2\left(1-D^2\right)\right]\left[1-\alpha_3\left(1-D^2\right)\right]\left(1-D^2\right)}\right] \quad \text{(E.10)}$$

E.2 Induction Arguments

An induction argument can be used to verify the following formula. Let there be K prospectively declared primary endpoints with the measure $D_{j|1,2,3,...,j-1}$, as the level of dependency for the jth primary analysis given first $j-1$ primary analyses for $j = 1$, 2, 3, ..., K. In this circumstance, the FWER is

$$\xi_K = 1 - \left[\prod_{k=2}^{K}\left[1-\alpha_k\left(1-D_{k|1,2,3,...,k-1}^2\right)\right]\right]\left[1-\alpha_1\right]. \quad \text{(E.11)}$$

This result was proven for $K = 2$, 3, and 4.[1] We must show that the assumption the assumption that equation (E.11) holds for $K - 1$ implies (E.11) is true for K.

Continuing with the notation from chapter five, allow T_j to be a random variable which takes on the value 0 when the jth primary hypothesis test does not produce a type I error and the value 1 when this test does produce a type I error, we can write

$$\xi_K = 1 - P\left[T_1 = 0 \cap T_2 = 0 \cap T_3 = 0 \cap T_4 = 0 \cap ... \cap T_K = 0\right]$$

$$= 1 - P\left[\bigcap_{j=1}^{K} T_j = 0\right]. \quad \text{(E.12)}$$

Using conditional probability, we now write

---

[1] The formulation does not apply for $K = 1$ because the paradigm of dependence requires at least two statistical hypothesis tests.

$$P\left[T_K = 0 \mid \bigcap_{j=1}^{K-1} T_j = 0\right] = \frac{P\left[\bigcap_{j=1}^{K} T_j = 0\right]}{P\left[\bigcap_{j=1}^{K-1} T_j = 0\right]}. \tag{E.13}$$

which can be reformulated as

$$P\left[\bigcap_{j=1}^{K} T_j = 0\right] = P\left[T_K = 0 \mid \bigcap_{j=1}^{K-1} T_j = 0\right] P\left[\bigcap_{j=1}^{K-1} T_j = 0\right]. \tag{E.14}$$

Proceeding as we did for the case of $K = 2, 3,$ and 4, we now define the dependency measure

$$D_{K|1,2,3,4,\ldots,K-1} = \sqrt{1 - \frac{\left(1 - P\left[T_K = 0 \mid \bigcap_{j=1}^{K-1} T_j = 0\right]\right)}{\alpha_K}}. \tag{E.15}$$

letting $D_{K|1,2,3,\ldots,K-1}$ denote the measurement of dependency between hypothesis test H_K given knowledge of $H_1, H_2, H_3\ldots,H_{K-1}$. We now solve equation (E.15) for the conditional probability

$$P\left[T_K = 0 \mid \bigcap_{j=0}^{K-1} T_j = 0\right] = (1 - \alpha_K) + D^2_{K|1,2,3,\ldots,K-1}\left[1 - (1 - \alpha_K)\right]$$
$$= 1 - \alpha_K\left(1 - D^2_{K|1,2,3,4,\ldots,K-1}\right). \tag{E.16}$$

We now have the conditional probability computed in terms of α_K and the dependency parameter. From equation (E.14), we can write

$$P\left[\bigcap_{j=1}^{K} T_j = 0\right] = P\left[T_K = 0 \mid \bigcap_{j=1}^{K-1} T_j = 0\right] P\left[\bigcap_{j=1}^{K-1} T_j = 0\right]$$
$$= \left[1 - \alpha_K\left(1 - D^2_{K|1,2,3,4,\ldots,K-1}\right)\right] P\left[\bigcap_{j=1}^{K-1} T_j = 0\right]. \tag{E.17}$$

and we can write

$$\xi_K = 1 - P\left[\bigcap_{j=1}^{K} T_j = 0\right]$$

$$= 1 - \left[1 - \alpha_K\left(1 - D^2_{K|1,2,3,\dots,K-1}\right)\right]P\left[\bigcap_{j=1}^{K-1} T_j = 0\right]. \tag{E.18}$$

We now use the induction condition,

$$1 - P\left[\bigcap_{j=0}^{K-1} T_j = 0\right] = \xi_{K-1} = 1 - \left[\prod_{k=2}^{K-1}\left[1 - \alpha_k\left(1 - D^2_{k|1,2,3,\dots,k-1}\right)\right]\right]\left[1 - \alpha_1\right]. \tag{E.19}$$

In order to see that

$$P\left[\bigcap_{j=0}^{K-1} T_j = 0\right] = \left[\prod_{k=2}^{K-1}\left[1 - \alpha_k\left(1 - D^2_{k|1,2,3,\dots,k-1}\right)\right]\right]\left[1 - \alpha_1\right], \tag{E.20}$$

we write the familywise error level ξ_K

$$\xi_K = 1 - \left[1 - \alpha_K\left(1 - D^2_{K|1,2,3,\dots,K-1}\right)\right]P\left[\bigcap_{j=1}^{K-1} T_j = 0\right]$$

$$= 1 - \left[1 - \alpha_K\left(1 - D^2_{K|1,2,3,\dots,K-1}\right)\right]\left[\prod_{k=2}^{K-1}\left[1 - \alpha_k\left(1 - D^2_{k|1,2,3,\dots,k-1}\right)\right]\right]\left[1 - \alpha_1\right], \tag{E.21}$$

and the product can be combined from the last line of expression (E.21) to find

$$\xi_K = 1 - \left[\prod_{k=2}^{K}\left[1 - \alpha_k\left(1 - D^2_{k|1,2,3,\dots,k-1}\right)\right]\right]\left[1 - \alpha_1\right]. \tag{E.22}$$

which is the desired result. To verify that

$$\alpha_K = \min\left[\alpha_{K-1}, \frac{1 - \dfrac{1 - \xi}{\left[1 - \alpha_1\right]\prod_{j=2}^{k-1}\left[1 - \alpha_j\left(1 - D^2_{j|1,2,3,\dots,j-1}\right)\right]}}{1 - D^2_{K|1,2,3,\dots,K-1}}\right], \tag{E.23}$$

we need only evaluate (E.22)

$$\xi_K = 1 - \left[\prod_{k=2}^{K}\left[1 - \alpha_k\left(1 - D^2_{k|1,2,3,\dots,k-1}\right)\right]\right]\left[1 - \alpha_1\right]$$

$$= 1 - \left[1 - \alpha_K\left(1 - D^2_{K|1,2,3,\dots,K-1}\right)\right]\left[\prod_{k=2}^{K-1}\left[1 - \alpha_k\left(1 - D^2_{k|1,2,3,\dots,k-1}\right)\right]\right]\left[1 - \alpha_1\right] \qquad \text{(E.24)}$$

and solve for α_K

$$\xi_K = 1 - \left[1 - \alpha_K\left(1 - D^2_{K|1,2,3,\dots,K-1}\right)\right]\left[\prod_{k=2}^{K-1}\left[1 - \alpha_k\left(1 - D^2_{k|1,2,3,\dots,k-1}\right)\right]\right]\left[1 - \alpha_1\right],$$

$$1 - \xi_K = \left[1 - \alpha_K\left(1 - D^2_{K|1,2,3,\dots,K-1}\right)\right]\left[\prod_{k=2}^{K-1}\left[1 - \alpha_k\left(1 - D^2_{k|1,2,3,\dots,k-1}\right)\right]\right]\left[1 - \alpha_1\right], \quad \text{(E.25)}$$

$$1 - \alpha_K\left(1 - D^2_{K|1,2,3,\dots,K-1}\right) = \frac{1 - \xi_K}{\left[\prod_{k=2}^{K-1}\left[1 - \alpha_k\left(1 - D^2_{k|1,2,3,\dots,k-1}\right)\right]\right]\left[1 - \alpha_1\right]}.$$

Continuing,

$$\alpha_K\left(1 - D^2_{K|1,2,3,\dots,K-1}\right) = 1 - \frac{1 - \xi_K}{\left[\prod_{k=2}^{K-1}\left[1 - \alpha_k\left(1 - D^2_{k|1,2,3,\dots,k-1}\right)\right]\right]\left[1 - \alpha_1\right]},$$

$$\qquad \text{(E.26)}$$

$$\alpha_K = \frac{1 - \dfrac{1 - \xi_K}{\left[\prod_{k=2}^{K-1}\left[1 - \alpha_k\left(1 - D^2_{k|1,2,3,\dots,k-1}\right)\right]\right]\left[1 - \alpha_1\right]}}{\left(1 - D^2_{K|1,2,3,\dots,K-1}\right)},$$

and we have the desired result.

E.3 Additional Recursive Relationships

The relationships between α_k, the test-specific alpha level for the kth specific hypothesis test and ξ_k the familywise type I error level after k primary analyses have been carried out can be easily deduced by noting the dependency between the two. We may write in the case of independent hypothesis tests that

$$\xi_{k+1} = 1 - (1 - \xi_k)(1 - \alpha_{k+1}) \tag{E.27}$$

for $k = 1$ to K. This is easily verified. For $k = 1$, (E.27) becomes

$$\begin{aligned}\xi_1 &= 1 - (1 - \xi_0)(1 - \alpha_1) \\ &= 1 - (1 - 0)(1 - \alpha_1) \\ &= \alpha_1\end{aligned} \tag{E.28}$$

since $\xi_0 = 0$.

For $k = 2$, the evaluation becomes

$$\begin{aligned}\xi_2 &= 1 - (1 - \xi_1)(1 - \alpha_2) \\ &= 1 - (1 - \alpha_1)(1 - \alpha_2),\end{aligned} \tag{E.29}$$

the results from equations (E.28) and (E.29) are the anticipated reproductions of the familywise error level for the situation of one and two hypothesis tests, respectively. In the case of dependence, we may write

$$\xi_{k+1} = 1 - [1 - \xi_k]\left[1 - \alpha_{k+1}\left(1 - D_{k+1|1,2,3...k}^2\right)\right], \tag{E.30}$$

See that for $k = 0$

$$\begin{aligned}\xi_1 &= 1 - [1 - \xi_0]\left[1 - \alpha_1\left(1 - D_1^2\right)\right] \\ &= 1 - (1)[1 - \alpha_1(1 - 0)] \\ &= \alpha_1\end{aligned} \tag{E.31}$$

and for $k = 1$

$$\begin{aligned}\xi_2 &= 1 - [1 - \xi_1]\left[1 - \alpha_2\left(1 - D_{2|1}^2\right)\right] \\ &= 1 - [1 - \alpha_1]\left[1 - \alpha_2\left(1 - D_{2|1}^2\right)\right].\end{aligned} \tag{E.32}$$

We can also then easily find that in the case of independence (E.27) reveals that

$$\alpha_{k+1} = 1 - \frac{1 - \xi_{k+1}}{1 - \xi_k}, \tag{E.33}$$

and, in the case of dependent hypothesis testing, working from (E.30) we can write

$$\alpha_{k+1} = \frac{1 - \dfrac{1 - \xi_{k+1}}{1 - \xi_k}}{1 - D^2_{k+1|1,2,3\ldots k}}. \tag{E.34}$$

Of course, considerable simplification is afforded by assuming the test-specific alpha levels are the same and the level of dependence among all of the hypothesis tests is the same. In this circumstance, then (E.30) becomes

$$\xi_{k+1} = 1 - \left[1 - \xi_k\right]\left[1 - \alpha\left(1 - D^2\right)\right]. \tag{E.35}$$

This is a first order, non-homogeneous difference equation which may be solved for ξ_k. Rewrite equation as (E.35) to see that

$$\xi_{k+1} = \alpha\left(1 - D^2\right) + \xi_k\left[1 - \alpha\left(1 - D^2\right)\right] \tag{E.36}$$

To solve this, we will use the generating function argument as presented in [1] and most recently in [2]. Define the generating function $G(s)$ as

$$G(s) = \sum_{k=0}^{\infty} s^k \xi_k, \tag{E.37}$$

where s is a positive real number in $(0,1)$. For this generating function the coefficient of s^k is precisely the value we seek. The goal then is to collapse the infinite number of equations provided in expression (E.36) into one equation that can be written as a function of $G(s)$. We will then consolidate this equation, and solve it for $G(s)$. Once $G(s)$ is identified, it will be inverted to identify the specific values of ξ_k. We begin this process by multiplying side of equation (E.36) by s^k to find

$$s^k \xi_{k+1} = \alpha\left(1 - D^2\right)s^k + \xi_k\left[1 - \alpha\left(1 - D^2\right)\right]s^k \tag{E.38}$$

Since this equation is true for $k = 0$ to infinity[2] we can take the sum over this range from each side of equation (E.38) to find

---

[2] We will just discard the solution for all values of $k > K$ since we are only performing K hypothesis tests.

$$\sum_{k=0}^{\infty} s^k \xi_{k+1} = \sum_{k=0}^{\infty} \left[\alpha\left(1-D^2\right) + \xi_k \left[1-\alpha\left(1-D^2\right)\right] \right] s^k$$

$$= \sum_{k=0}^{\infty} \alpha\left(1-D^2\right) s^k + \sum_{k=0}^{\infty} \xi_k \left[1-\alpha\left(1-D^2\right)\right] s^k \qquad \text{(E.39)}$$

$$= \alpha\left(1-D^2\right) \sum_{k=0}^{\infty} s^k + \left[1-\alpha\left(1-D^2\right)\right] \sum_{k=0}^{\infty} s^k \xi_k$$

We can further simplify the last line of expression (E.39) by recognizing that $\sum_{k=0}^{\infty} s^k \xi_k = G(s)$, and that, for $0 < s < 1$ $\sum_{k=0}^{\infty} s^k = \dfrac{1}{1-s}$. We can now write equation (E.39) as

$$\sum_{k=0}^{\infty} s^k \xi_{k+1} = \frac{\alpha\left(1-D^2\right)}{1-s} + \left[1-\alpha\left(1-D^2\right)\right] G(s). \qquad \text{(E.40)}$$

We now must evaluate $\sum_{k=0}^{\infty} s^k \xi_{k+1}$. Proceeding,

$$\sum_{k=0}^{\infty} s^k \xi_{k+1} = s^{-1} \sum_{k=0}^{\infty} s^{k+1} \xi_{k+1} = s^{-1} \sum_{k=1}^{\infty} s^k \xi_k = s^{-1} \left[\sum_{k=0}^{\infty} s^k \xi_k - s^0 \xi_0 \right]$$

$$= s^{-1} \sum_{k=0}^{\infty} s^k \xi_k = s^{-1} G(s) \qquad \text{(E.41)}$$

since $\xi_0 = 0$. This allows us to write (E.40) as

$$s^{-1} G(s) = \frac{\alpha\left(1-D^2\right)}{1-s} + \left[1-\alpha\left(1-D^2\right)\right] G(s) \qquad \text{(E.42)}$$

Multiplying each side of this equation by s reveals

$$G(s) = \frac{\alpha\left(1-D^2\right)s}{1-s} + \left[1-\alpha\left(1-D^2\right)\right] s G(s). \qquad \text{(E.43)}$$

Simplifying further

$$G(s) - \left[1 - \alpha\left(1 - D^2\right)\right]sG(s) = \frac{\alpha\left(1 - D^2\right)s}{1 - s},$$

$$G(s)\left(1 - \left[1 - \alpha\left(1 - D^2\right)\right]s\right) = \frac{\alpha\left(1 - D^2\right)s}{1 - s},$$ (E.44)

$$G(s) = \frac{\alpha\left(1 - D^2\right)s}{(1 - s)\left(1 - \left[1 - \alpha\left(1 - D^2\right)\right]s\right)},$$

and we are now prepared for the inversion of the generating function G(s). Rewrite $G(s)$ as

$$G(s) = \left[\alpha\left(1 - D^2\right)s\right]\left[\frac{1}{1 - s}\right]\left[\frac{1}{1 - \left[1 - \alpha\left(1 - D^2\right)\right]s}\right].$$ (E.45)

We seek the coefficient of s^k. G(s), as written in equation (E.45) is composed of three expressions. The first expression, $\alpha\left(1 - D^2\right)s$, we can set aside for the moment since its inclusion in the solution will be as a scale factor and adjustment by one for the power of s. The second multiplicative factor in equation (E.45) can be written as

$$\frac{1}{1 - s} = \sum_{k=0}^{\infty} s^k.$$ (E.46)

Analogously

$$\frac{1}{1 - \left[1 - \alpha\left(1 - D^2\right)\right]s} = \sum_{k=0}^{\infty}\left[1 - \alpha\left(1 - D^2\right)\right]^k s^k.$$ (E.47)

Then evaluating the last two expressions of the generating function reveals

$$\left[\frac{1}{1 - s}\right]\left[\frac{1}{1 - \left[1 - \alpha\left(1 - D^2\right)\right]s}\right] = \left[\sum_{k=0}^{\infty} s^k\right]\left[\sum_{k=0}^{\infty}\left[1 - \alpha\left(1 - D^2\right)\right]^k s^k\right].$$ (E.48)

When the right hand side of expression (E.48) is evaluated term by term, the coefficient of s^k is $\sum_{j=0}^{k}\left[1-\alpha\left(1-D^2\right)\right]^j$. It only remains to factor in the first expression ,

$\alpha\left(1-D^2\right)s$, from (E.45). The term $\alpha\left(1-D^2\right)$ does not involve s and is simply a multiplicative constant. Any term involving s denotes that, if we want to find the coefficient of s^k of $G(s)$ we need to identify the coefficient of s^{k-1} from the product of

$$\left[\frac{1}{1-s}\right]\left[\frac{1}{1 - \left[1-\alpha\left(1-D^2\right)\right]s}\right].$$

Thus we find

$$\xi_k =\alpha\left(1-D^2\right)\sum_{j=0}^{k-1}\left[1-\alpha\left(1-D^2\right)\right]^j \qquad (E.49)$$

The following simplification is available,

$$\sum_{j=0}^{k-1}\left[1-\alpha\left(1-D^2\right)\right]^j =\frac{1-\left[1-\alpha\left(1-D^2\right)\right]^k}{1-\left[1-\alpha\left(1-D^2\right)\right]}=\frac{1-\left[1-\alpha\left(1-D^2\right)\right]^k}{\alpha\left(1-D^2\right)}. \qquad (E.50)$$

So

$$\xi_k =\sum_{j=0}^{k-1}\left[1-\alpha\left(1-D^2\right)\right]^j =\alpha\left(1-D^2\right)\frac{1-\left[1-\alpha\left(1-D^2\right)\right]^k}{\alpha\left(1-D^2\right)}, \qquad (E.51)$$

and finally,

$$\xi_k(D) =1-\left[1-\alpha\left(1-D^2\right)\right]^k. \qquad (E.52)$$

If we let $D = 0$, the condition of independence between statistical hypothesis tests, then equation (E.52) simplifies to

$$\xi_k(D = 0) =1-\left[1-\alpha\right]^k \qquad (E.53)$$

the expected result from Chapter 4.

It is useful to note the correspondence between equation (E.52) for $\xi_k(D)$ and $\xi_k(D=0)$ from (E.53). Each of these equations expresses the familywise error level in terms of one minus the product of probabilities. Rewrite these equations as

$$1 - \xi_K(D) = P\left[\bigcap_{j=1}^{K} T_j = 0\right] = \left[1 - \alpha\left(1 - D^2\right)\right]^K.$$

$$(E.54)$$

$$1 - \xi_K(D = 0) = P\left[\bigcap_{j=1}^{K} T_j = 0\right] = \left[1 - \alpha\right]^K.$$

Then in each of the case of dependence and independence, the probability of a type I error is written as the simultaneous occurrence of independent events. In the case of independence between the statistical hypothesis tests, multiplying probabilities is the expected procedure that was first developed in Chapter 3, and we find that the probability for no type I errors among the K hypothesis tests is simply $\left[1 - \alpha\right]^K$.

However, we see that the probability of no type I error among the K primary endpoint analyses when there is dependence among the prospectively planned primary analyses setting can also be written as the product of probabilities, in this case $\left[1 - \alpha\left(1 - D^2\right)\right]^K$. Writing the joint event of $\bigcap_{j=1}^{K} T_j = 0$ as the product of prob-

abilities tells us these events are independent. Thus, using the dependence parameter D as derived in Chapter 5, with the additional assumptions that 1) D is the same for all subgroups of dependent hypothesis testing and 2) the test-specific α is the same for all K primary statistical evaluations, transforms the adjustment in α level for dependence to simply one of multiplying the test-specific alpha by a common factor, that is $1 - D^2$.

This finding produces important formula simplification that will be very useful for us. A simple application of Boole's inequality leads to

$$\xi_K(D) \leq K\alpha\left(1 - D^2\right),$$

$$(E.55)$$

and a Bonferroni style adjustment produces

$$\alpha \leq \frac{\xi_K(D)}{K\left(1 - D^2\right)}.$$

$$(E.56)$$

These simplifications can be generalized. Returning to (E.22).

$$\xi_K = 1 - \left[\prod_{k=2}^{K}\left[1 - \alpha_k\left(1 - D^2_{k|1,2,3,\ldots,k-1}\right)\right]\right]\left[1 - \alpha_1\right],$$

$$(E.22)$$

We now see

$$1-\xi_K = P\left[\bigcap_{k=1}^{K} T_k = 0\right] = \left[\prod_{k=2}^{K}\left[1-\alpha_k\left(1-D_{k|1,2,3,\dots,k-1}^2\right)\right]\right]\left[1-\alpha_1\right].\qquad\text{(E.57)}$$

and the probability of a joint event involving each of the T_j's from $j = 1$ to K can be written as the product of probabilities. We may invoke Boole's inequality to write

$$\xi_K(D) \le \alpha_1 + \sum_{k=2}^{K}\alpha_k\left(1-D_{k|1,2,3,\dots,k-1}^2\right).\qquad\text{(E.58)}$$

If we let $D_{j|1,2,3,\dots,j-1} = D$ for all $j = 2$ to K, then (E.22) becomes

$$\xi_K = 1-\left[\prod_{k=2}^{K}\left[1-\alpha_k\left(1-D^2\right)\right]\right]\left[1-\alpha_1\right].\qquad\text{(E.59)}$$

Under the assumption that $D = 0$ for all of the primary analyses, then equation 17.56 becomes

$$\xi_K = 1-\left[\prod_{k=2}^{K}[1-\alpha_k]\right]\left[1-\alpha_1\right]\qquad\text{(E.60)}$$

a familiar result from Chapter 4. Finally, we may apply Boole's inequality to equation (E.59) to see

$$\xi_K(D) \le \alpha_1 + \sum_{k=2}^{K}\alpha_k\left(1-D^2\right) = \alpha_1 + \left(1-D^2\right)\sum_{k=2}^{K}\alpha_k\qquad\text{(E.61)}$$

and find that when allocating the test-specific alpha levels for the second through the Kth primary analyses, then

$$\sum_{k=2}^{K}\alpha_k = \frac{\xi_K(D)-\alpha_1}{\left(1-D^2\right)}\qquad\text{(E.62)}$$

References

1. Goldberg S. (1958). *Introduction to Difference Equations*. New York. Wiley. p 63-67.
2. Moyé L.A., Kapadia A.S. (2000). *Difference Equations with Public Health Applications*. New York. Marcel Dekker, Inc. Chapter 4.

Index

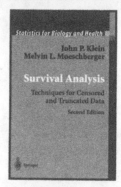
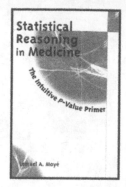
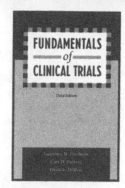
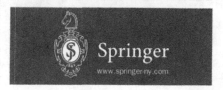